Clinical Skills
for Healthcare
Assistants
and Assistant
Practitioners

Clinical Skills
for Healthcare
Assistants
and Assistant
Practitioners

Clinical Skills for Healthcare Assistants and Assistant Practitioners

Angela Whelan and Elaine Hughes

Faculty of Health and Social Care, Edge Hill University, UK

SECOND EDITION

WILEY Blackwell

Library of Congress Cataloging-in-Publication Data

Names: Whelan, Angela, 1962- , author. | Hughes, Elaine, 1969- , author. |
Ingram, Paula, 1969- Clinical skills for healthcare assistants. Preceded
by (work):
Title: Clinical skills for healthcare assistants and assistant practitioners
/ Angela Whelan and Elaine Hughes.
Description: Second edition. | Chichester, West Sussex ; Hoboken, NJ : John
Wiley & Sons Inc., 2016. | Preceded by Clinical skills for healthcare
assistants / Paula Ingram and Irene Lavery. 2009. | Includes
bibliographical references and index.
Identifiers: LCCN 2015045703 | ISBN 9781118256411 (pbk.)
Subjects: | MESH: Nursing Care–methods | Nurses' Aides | Great Britain |
Handbooks
Classification: LCC RT41 | NLM WY 100 FA1 | DDC 610.73–dc23 LC record available
at http://lccn.loc.gov/2015045703

A catalogue record for this book is available from the British Library.

Wiley also publishes its books in a variety of electronic formats. Some content that appears in print may not be available in electronic books.

Cover image: © Monkey Business Images Ltd/Getty

Set in 9.5/13pt, MeridienLTStd by SPi Global, Chennai, India.

Printed in the UK

Contents

Section II: Core clinical skills

Preface

The Francis Report highlighted the importance of a workforce that was not only caring and compassionate but able to provide care that is underpinned by knowledge. The basis of the broad, generic role that is undertaken by many healthcare workers has alignment with this view of the future nurse and has been included within the Skills for Health and the Skills Certificates.

This book provides background knowledge on the day-to-day care that is provided by those working in caring environments. Clinical skills are fundamental to the role of the care worker, and as the role of the care worker progresses the expansion of the skills that can be undertaken as part of their role continues.

To address this, the book covers both fundamental clinical skills as well as the more complex ones that generally require specific training within the workplace to complete. Therefore this book is aimed at those already engaged in care work and new students in health and social care in a variety of clinical settings and can be used as a resource that will guide the reader through the clinical skill itself through to self-assessment.

Elaine Hughes & Angela Whelan

Acknowledgements

The production of this second edition has been a long and winding road and we would like to acknowledge the work of both Paula Ingram and Irene Lavery in the original book.

The continued support and encouragement form our families, especially Ged and Ruth Whelan, Owen Gallagher and Les McNee has been unwavering, for which we are very grateful.

Enthusiasm from friends and colleagues has been continuous and we would like to offer special thanks to Karen Ellis, Aintree University Hospital Trust, Beth Spencer and Debbie Chadwick, Edge Hill University for their help and support.

Angela Whelan & Elaine Hughes

Introduction

The book has been split into three sections:

1 **Section 1** covers fundamental skills applicable to all staff, and is essential as a prerequisite before performing all clinical skills.
2 **Section 2** contains core clinical skills, which includes most of the clinical skills required for clinical practice that are often taught at a local level.
3 **Section 3** outlines complex clinical skills, which require more in-depth training and may be restricted to specialist areas of practice, and that often require the direct supervision of registered nurses.

Each chapter has the same structure, starting with the aims and objectives of the chapter, followed by the explanation of why the skill is performed, relevant anatomy and physiology, related aspects and terminology, how to perform the skill and common problems. Throughout each chapter case studies and Think about it boxes relating to the topic will be included, encouraging the reader to apply them to their own practice. The final section addresses both self- and formal assessment where required.

The use of checklists, pictures and clear, concise theory is aimed at making the book a comprehensive yet easy to read resource for all.

SECTION I
Fundamental skills

CHAPTER 1

Accountability

LEARNING OBJECTIVES

- Identify the current plans regarding regulation of healthcare assistants and assistant practitioners
- Define accountability
- Relate accountability to the healthcare assistant and assistant practitioner role
- Describe the duty of care and how it relates to negligence
- Discuss consent
- List the key elements of the Mental Capacity Act

Aim of this chapter

The aim of this chapter is to enable healthcare assistants and assistant practitioners to understand the issues and concept of accountability relating both to their role and to others around them.

This chapter covers accountability and issues surrounding accountability in relation to clinical skills. Healthcare assistants, healthcare support workers and assistant practitioners form an integral part of the contemporary flexible 'nursing family' (RCN 2004). A substantial proportion of essential nursing care is now delivered by the unregistered branch of the nursing family with some personnel such as assistant practitioners undertaking work previously performed by registered staff (RCN 2012). Registration and regulation of healthcare assistants, health support workers and assistant practitioners continues to be debated (Vaughan et al. 2014)

Regulation and registration

Registration refers to the process by which professionals such as nurses are registered with a regulatory body. Registered staff are professionally accountable

Clinical Skills for Healthcare Assistants and Assistant Practitioners, Second Edition.
Angela Whelan and Elaine Hughes.
© 2016 John Wiley & Sons, Ltd. Published 2016 by John Wiley & Sons, Ltd.

to their respective regulatory bodies, for example nurses are accountable to the Nursing Midwifery Council (NMC) and allied health professionals to the Health and Care Professions Council (HCPC). Regulation refers to a set of rules that members are required to follow by law (Law Commission et al. 2012: 68): for example, nurses are regulated by the NMC and legally have to follow the rules set out by that specific body; for nurses, therefore, the NMC is the main focus for regulatory accountability (NMC 2015b). The Nursing Midwifery Council regulates nurses and midwives in England, Wales, Scotland and Northern Ireland and exists to protect the public. They set standards of education, training, conduct and performance so that nurses and midwives can deliver high-quality healthcare throughout their careers. The NMC makes sure that nurses and midwives keep their skills and knowledge up to date and uphold a set of professional standards. There is a clear and transparent processes used to investigate nurses and midwives who fall short of those standards. In the event of a serious error, professional misconduct, failure to respect professional boundaries or unethical conduct, a registered nurse is held accountable and can be removed from the register. The NMC hold a register of nurses and midwives allowed to practise in the UK (NMC 2015b).

Healthcare assistants and assistant practitioners

Both assistant practitioners and healthcare assistants remain unregistered and without a regulatory body, unlike registered nurses. They do, however, have codes of conduct and it is imperative practitioners become familiar with them.

In Scotland, since 2011 all new HCAs have been required to meet induction standards and comply with a code of conduct, while employers are required to sign up to a code of practice (Scottish Government 2010). In Wales there is an All Wales Code of Conduct for healthcare support workers (Welsh Assembly Government 2011). In addition, the Hywel Dda Health Board introduced a code of conduct for healthcare support workers, along with an employers' code of practice 'to provide an assurance framework for public protection' (Horner 2012; Hywel Dda Health Board 2015). A voluntary register, but no mandatory regulatory system, exists in Northern Ireland. In England, the Coalition Government rejected the recommendation made in Robert Francis's report into the failings at the Mid Staffordshire Foundation Trust (Francis 2013), that recommended all healthcare support workers should be regulated. Instead Camilla Cavendish (DH 2013b) was asked by the Secretary of State to review and make recommendations on the recruitment, learning and development, management and support of healthcare assistants and social care support workers. The resulting report, published in July 2013, found that the preparation of healthcare assistants and social care support workers for their roles within care settings was inconsistent, and one of the recommendations was the development of the Care Certificate.

In the absence of registration and a regulatory body, all unregistered health and social care workers are recommended to read the chapters of this book and consider them alongside and in addition to the Care Certificate. Local codes have also been developed, please become familiar with your local policy and code(s)

Skills for Health and Skills for Care published the Code of Conduct (2013) for healthcare support workers and adult social care workers. Although this code is voluntary it is seen as best practice. This Code of Conduct sets the standard of conduct expected of healthcare support workers and adult social care workers, outlining the behaviour and attitudes that are expected of those working in health and social care settings to provide safe, compassionate care and support (Skills for Health and Skills for Care 2013).

The role of the assistant practitioner operates at band 4 or above and has emerged since it was first introduced in the Northwest of England in 2002 to cover a number of professions and settings. This role was introduced in the UK to complement the work of registered professionals, working across professional boundaries, and now performs many tasks previously undertaken by registered staff (Vaughan et al. 2014). Skills for Health (2009: 1) defined the role of the Assistant Practitioner as:

> An Assistant Practitioner is a worker who competently delivers health and social care to and for people. They have a required level of knowledge and skill beyond that of the traditional healthcare assistant or support worker. The Assistant Practitioner would be able to deliver elements of health and social care and undertake clinical work in domains that have previously only been within the remit of registered professionals. The Assistant Practitioner may transcend professional boundaries. They are accountable to themselves, their employer, and, more importantly, the people they serve.

THINK ABOUT IT

Identify other professional groups within your clinical area and find out about the professional bodies to which they report. What are your thoughts about registration? What advantages do you think are attached to registration and are there any negatives?

Responsibilities and accountability

Accountability and responsibility are words that are often used interchangeably by health professionals as though they have the same meaning (Griffith 2015). Responsibility means *having control or authority over someone or something* (Griffith and Tenegnah 2010). Carvallo et al. (2012) identify responsibility as accepting a task or duty that you have been given and accepting that task willingly. So it can be seen that responsibilities are linked to your role, which means you require training and assessment of the necessary knowledge, skills, values and ability to undertake a particular task or duty. In order to be responsible, Dimond (2011) asserts it is also necessary to have legal knowledge, as ignorance of the law is no defence. So as an HCA or AP you are responsible for your practice and for ensuring the interventions undertaken are in the best interests of your patients. Responsibility equates to the duty of care in law. Scrivener et al. (2011) explain that the duty of care applies whether the task involves bathing a patient or complex surgery – in each case there is the opportunity for harm to occur. In this context, the question that arises concerns the standard of care expected of practitioners performing these tasks. This is the legal liability the practitioner owes to the patient. By accepting the responsibility to perform a task the practitioner must ensure the task is performed competently, at least to the standard of the ordinarily competent practitioner in that type of task.

Accountability

Accountability is crucial to the protection of the public and individual patients and is a complex concept to understand (Griffith and Tengnah 2010). Nurses are bound by the NMC to be accountable (NMC 2015a). Dimond (2011) reports four arenas of accountability relating to registered nurses:

1 Accountable to the Public via criminal law and criminal courts.
2 Accountable to the Patients via civil law, civil courts.
3 Accountable to the Employer via contract of employment, employment tribunal.
4 Accountable to the Profession via NMC, Conduct and Competence Committee.

   Mullen (2014) points out that HCAs and APs are not accountable to a professional body, but they are accountable to the other arenas. Additionally there are also general responsibilities related to accountability laid out for all staff in the NHS Constitution (see Boxes 1.1 and 1.2 for a summary of responsibilities relating to accountability (Mullen 2014)). Put quite simply, Griffith and Tengnah (2010) define accountability as 'being answerable for your personal acts or omissions to a higher authority with whom you have a legal relationship'.

Box 1.1 Accountability

Code of Conduct for Healthcare Support Workers and Adult Social Care Workers
   (Skills for Health and Skills for Care 2013)

Guidance statements

As a healthcare support worker or adult social care worker in England, you must:
• Be honest with yourself and others about what you can do, recognise your abilities and the limitations of your competence and only carry out or delegate those tasks agreed in your job description.
• Always behave and present yourself in a way that does not call into question your suitability to work in a health and social care environment.

- Be able to justify and be accountable for your actions or your omissions – what you fail to do.
- Always ask your supervisor or employer about any issues that might affect your ability to do your job competently and safety. If you do not feel competent to carry out an activity, you must report this.
- Comply with your employers agreed ways of working.
- Report any actions or omissions by yourself or colleagues that you feel may compromise the safety or care of people who use healthy and care services and. If necessary, use whistle blowing procedures to report any suspected wrongdoing experiences, activities and people across the NHS.

Box 1.2 NHS Constitution staff responsibilities

A summary of the areas related to accountability
- You have a duty to accept professional accountability and maintain the standards of professional practice as set by the appropriate regulatory body applicable to your profession or role.
- You have a duty to act in accordance with the express and implied terms of your contract of employment.
- You have a duty not to discriminate against patients or staff and to adhere to equal opportunities and equality and human rights legislation.
- You have a duty to protect the confidentiality of personal information that you hold.
- You have a duty to be honest and truthful in applying for a job and in carrying out that job.

Remember: you are still 100% accountable for your acts and omissions.

Areas of accountability

Public
Accountability to the public would involve a breach of criminal law and prosecution through the criminal courts (Dimond 2011). An example of this would be if an HCA or AP caused the death of a patient through their practice. The individual would be prosecuted through the criminal courts for that crime.

Patients
Civil law is actionable in the civil courts and may or may not be a crime (Dimond 2011). Individuals can take out legal proceedings against any healthcare professional, including healthcare assistants and assistant practitioners. The organisation will take responsibility for this under a concept known as vicarious liability that will be discussed later, providing the worker has followed policies and procedures. The law imposes a duty of care on a practitioner in circumstances where it is reasonably foreseeable that the practitioner could harm a patient through their action or failure to act (Cox 2010). Healthcare assistants are legally accountable to the patient for any errors that they may make through civil law (RCN 2011).

An example here could be if, during cannulation, a healthcare assistant hit a nerve and caused pain, and the patient wished to take legal proceedings.

Employer

Mullen (2014) points out that HCAs and APs are accountable to their employer and as such are expected to follow their contract of duty, to work within the domain of their job description and to follow the codes of responsibility and behaviour, as laid out in the recent code of conduct for healthcare workers (Skills for Health and Skills for Care 2013) (Box 1.1). It is vital, therefore, that you have an up-to-date copy of your job description and that you are competent and trained to undertake the tasks, behaviours and responsibilities described (Mullen 2014). The need for job/role clarification is essential as employers need to ensure the right processes are in place and staff are trained with the right skills (Vaughan et al. 2014)

Delegation

The Oxford English Dictionary (2012) defines delegation as, 'entrusting a task to another person'. HCAs and APs may be delegated or allocated tasks by another member of staff (usually, but not always from a registered practitioner) or they may delegate a task to somebody else (i.e. they are the delegator) (Mullen 2014). The RCN (2011) states:

> If a practitioner such as a registered nurse should delegate a task, then that practitioner must be sure that the delegation is appropriate. This means that the task must be necessary; and the person performing the delegated task, for example a HCA or nursing student, must understand the task and how it is performed, have the skills and abilities to perform the task competently and accept responsibility for carrying it out.

Delegation must always be appropriate and in the best interest of the patient. Simply put, if you are delegated a task, you must have been trained and assessed as competent to undertake that job. If this is not the case, you must inform the person delegating the task to you. Equally, if you are delegating a task to somebody else you must ensure they are competent to perform that task. It is essential that delegation is appropriate, and the principles of delegation adapted from the RCN document (RCN 2011) are shown in Box 1.3.

THINK ABOUT IT

A registered nurse (RN) delegates the task of taking a patient's temperature using a tympanic thermometer (this measures the temperature in the tympanic membrane in the ear). You have never seen the piece of equipment before. What would your response be? Do you think that this is an appropriate task to delegate?

Box 1.3 Principles of delegation

- Delegation must always be in the best interest of the patient and not performed simply in an effort to save time or money
- The support worker must have been suitably trained to perform the task
- The support worker should always keep full records of training given, including dates
- There should be written evidence of competence assessment, preferably against recognised standards such as National Occupational Standards
- There should be clear guidelines and protocols in place so that the support worker is not required to make a clinical judgement that they are not competent to make
- The role should be within the support worker's job description
- The team and any support staff need to be informed that the task has been delegated (e.g. a receptionist in a GP surgery or ward clerk in a hospital setting)
- The person who delegates the task must ensure that an appropriate level of supervision is available and that the support worker has the opportunity for mentorship. The level of supervision and feedback provided must be appropriate to the task being delegated. This will be based on the recorded knowledge and competence of the support worker, the needs of the patient/client, the service setting and the tasks assigned (RCN et al. 2006)
- Ongoing development to ensure that competency is maintained is essential
- The whole process must be assessed for the degree of risk.

Delegation is the process by which a registered practitioner can allocate work to a healthcare assistant who is deemed competent to undertake that task, and the worker then carries the responsibility for that task. Registered practitioners are accountable for ensuring you have the knowledge and skill level required to perform the delegated task. The healthcare assistant is accountable for accepting the delegated task, as well as being responsible for their actions in carrying it out.

THINK ABOUT IT

In relation to these principles, identify and reflect on the tasks that are delegated to you within your own organisation. Seek out any local policies and procedures that are in place to define the tasks that can be undertaken following competency based training.

Choosing tasks or roles to be undertaken by a healthcare assistant is actually a complex professional activity; it depends on the registered practitioner's professional opinion and, for any particular task, there are no general rules (RCN 2011). The NHS Constitution (Department of Health (DH) 2013), however, applies to registered practitioners who are additionally accountable to their regulatory body for ensuring that the standards of practice, patient care and treatment meet the regulator's standards. The concept of delegation is included within all professional bodies' codes of conduct that the registered practitioner is required to follow (Mullen 2014). For example: Standard 11 of The Code, (NMC 2015a) requires nurses to:

Be accountable for your decisions to delegate tasks and duties to other people

To achieve this, you must;

11.1 only delegate tasks and duties that are within the other person's scope of competence, making sure that they fully understand your instructions

11.2 make sure that everyone you delegate tasks to is adequately supervised and supported so they can provide safe and compassionate care, and

11.3 confirm that the outcome of any tasks you have delegated to someone meets the required standard.

There are a number of aspects to consider in conjunction with the competence of the healthcare assistant and assistant practitioner in relation to the activity to be delegated.

Related aspects and terminology

Competence

Skills for Health develop National Occupational Standards (NOS) to set clear standards for a wide range of activities for healthcare workers. NOS describe the skills, knowledge and understanding needed to undertake a particular task or job to a nationally recognised level of competence. They cover key activities undertaken within the occupation in question under all the circumstances that the job holder is likely to encounter. HCAs and APs must develop the competencies required within their role to a given standard. The introduction of the Care Certificate has already been discussed and is available from SFH's website http://www.skillsforcare.org.uk/Standards/Care-Certificate/Care-Certificate.asp.

Vicarious liability

Vicarious liability means that the employer is accountable for the standard of care delivered and is responsible for employees working within agreed limits of competence appropriate to the abilities of that employee. Therefore, to remain covered by an employer's vicarious liability clause, the HCA or AP must only work within this area of assessed competence and within the responsibilities of their role and job description. This principle operates to make an employer liable, along with the employee, for any negligence caused by the employee provided that they are operating within the organisation's policies and procedures (Samanta and Samanta 2011). For example, you have performed venepuncture (the taking or drawing of blood) from a patient, having completed all the appropriate education and competency required by your employer. Unfortunately, the next day the patient has bruising at the site. As you had followed all policies and procedures, should the patient sue, the organisation would take responsibility for your actions.

Indemnity insurance

Where employers are vicariously liable for the actions of their staff, they need to have insurance to cover the risks of clinical negligence claims arising from employee carelessness. Individual practitioners remain legally accountable for their actions but it is rare for injured patients to sue them rather than their employers (Cox 2010).

The Health Care and Associated Professions (Indemnity Arrangements) Order 2014 No. 1887 (2014) states 'each practising registrant must have in force in relation to that registrant an indemnity arrangement which provides appropriate cover for practising as such'. The NMC Code (2015) standard 12 reflected these new arrangements stating that registered nurses must:

'12.1 make sure that you have an appropriate indemnity arrangement in place relevant to your scope of practice.'

This means, if a patient sues the employing hospital for negligence due to a nurse or healthcare assistant causing injury, the organisation would cover the nurse under vicarious liability (see above). However, the patient can also decide to sue the nurse or healthcare assistant as a separate case and, in this instance, indemnity insurance would pay for the practitioner's legal costs and the compensation paid to the patient. While this currently refers to regulated healthcare professionals, there is discussion as to whether HCAs, APs and other support workers will also require mandatory indemnity insurance. Some union membership includes indemnity insurance; it is advisable that you check whether you are currently covered.

Duty of care and negligence

The term 'duty of care' is used to describe the obligations implicit in the roles of all health or social care workers and is not something that can be opted out of (Mullen 2014). The RCN (2011) guidance highlights the importance of 'duty of care', a term that is described clearly: 'The law imposes a duty of care on practitioners, whether they are HCAs, APs, students, registered nurses, doctors or others, when it is "reasonably foreseeable" that they might cause harm to patients through their actions or their failure to act' (Cox 2010; RCN 2011). Where a patient or relative is dissatisfied with the care received from either an organisation or an individual, they can sue for clinical negligence. So, HCAs and APs have a duty of care and therefore a legal liability with regard to the patient. Mullen (2014) clearly identifies that HCAs and APs are responsible for:

- Always making the care and safety of patients your first concern.
- Ensuring that the task is necessary and in the patient's best interest.
- Ensuring your level of practice is of the standard that is expected of your role and the tasks that you perform.
- Keeping your practice and knowledge up to date.
- Always respecting the public, the patients, the clients, carers, NHS staff and partners in other organisations.

- Demonstrating your commitment to team working by cooperating with your colleagues in the NHS and in the wider community.
- Reporting to the registered professional members of the team any concerns, changes, and developments about the patients/clients.
- If you as an HCA or AP supervise the work of other junior members of the team, you need to be sure that what you ask them to do is within their capability and that you are accessible and supportive.
- If you supervise the work of other junior members of the team, that you report any concerns about their performance to your line manager.

Reasonable care

Reasonable care is the level of care which an ordinary and reasonable person would use under comparable circumstances. In the law, it is used as a standard to assess liability. If it can be demonstrated that someone had a duty of care and failed to exercise reasonable care, that person can be held negligent and may be liable for damages. On the other hand, if someone exhibited reasonable care and something happened anyway, this person would not be considered negligent.

Standards of care

The law imposes a duty of care on practitioners, whether healthcare support workers, registered nurses, doctors or Allied Health Professionals (AHPs), in circumstances where it is 'reasonably foreseeable' that they might cause harm to the patients through their actions or their failure to act (Cox 2010). This applies whether a complex task is being performed or whether the HCA or AP is bathing a patient and injure a patient through a careless act. The law imposes a standard of care in relation to each task and this standard applies no matter where patients receive treatment and is irrespective of the carer's qualifications. The legal standard of care is judged by that of the ordinarily competent practitioner performing the particular task or role. Should practitioners fall below this standard of care, they breach their duty of care.

Consent

In 2009, the Department of Health published the second edition of the *Reference Guide to Consent for Examination or Treatment* (the guide is currently under review, 2015). The Guide describes the process of seeking consent, the importance of establishing whether the person has capacity to give consent, what constitutes valid consent, the form that consent might take and the duration of that consent. It highlights the need to ensure that the consent is given voluntarily and that sufficient information has been imparted to allow valid consent to be made (DH 2009).

The Guide (DH 2009) further identifies that it is a general legal and ethical principle that valid consent must be obtained before starting any treatment, physical investigation, or providing personal care, for a person. This principle reflects the right of patients to determine what happens to their own bodies, and is a fundamental part of good practice. A healthcare professional (or other healthcare staff) who does not respect this principle may be liable both to legal action by the patient and to action by their professional body. Employing bodies may also be liable for the actions of their staff.

Consent is clearly enshrined within the various codes of conduct so that you are working in partnership with patients at all times and that agreement is clearly documented within patient records. For the nursing family, obtaining consent is an opportunity to deliver care, using good communication and interpersonal skills to discuss the procedure fully with the patient, which may involve reassurance and support especially if the procedure is new to the patient, they are anxious or they have had a previous bad experience. Where possible, choose a quiet environment where you will not be interrupted and give the patient plenty of time to be able to ask questions.

Once you are happy that the patient fully understands the procedure and any possible complications, this should be documented. It is important to remember that the patient may refuse to consent: this is their right which must be respected.

There are a number of legal cases that are identified within the Guide (DH 2009) that are worth reading to gain an understanding of the importance and consequences of gaining consent.

Capacity

Capacity means the ability to use and understand information to make a decision, and communicate any decision made. Taylor (2013) points out that it is generally presumed in law that adult patients have the capacity to make decisions, unless there is evidence that they do not (Parliament 2005). A decision made by a patient with capacity must be respected, even if it appears unwise or irrational. A patient may want to sign their own discharge; while not logical to us, this patient may have other priorities such as drug or alcohol misuse or they may want to make some arrangements before being admitted from the Accident and Emergency Department. Although hospitals and other healthcare providers have a legal obligation to provide adequate care for their patients (Cassidy v Ministry of Health, 1951), patients do not generally have to accept any offer of treatment.

It can be very frustrating to respect the patients' rights to autonomy, and healthcare practitioners can feel frustrated by what they see as a foolish or reckless decision. They may also feel uncomfortable knowing that a failure to provide care may lead to liability in civil law (negligence) or a criminal charge of gross negligence manslaughter if the patient dies as a result (R v Adomako, 1994). Ethical awareness and an earnest desire to deliver care in the best interest of the patient can cause healthcare workers to worry about the implications of following a patient's wishes, particularly if the patient has refused potentially life-saving treatment. There is always the worry of what might happen to the patient and of potential legal reprisals.

Capacity must be assessed by the health professional who is seeking consent. The issues to be set decided by any assessment are set out in s. 3(1) Mental Capacity Act 2005. These are whether or not the patient is able to:

(a) understand the information relevant to the decision,

(b) retain that information,

(c) weigh that information as part of the process of making the decision, or

(d) communicate his decision (Gallagher et al. 2012).

Where there is cause to question a patient's decision-making capacity, it can be difficult to decide the best course of action if they refuse treatment. In these situations, cases can be referred for a court declaration on the lawfulness of a proposed course of action (Taylor 2013).

Mental Capacity Act (2005)

The law applies to adults over the age of 16 years in England and Wales and is designed to protect and empower individuals who may lack the mental capacity to make their own decisions about their care and treatment. Examples of people who may lack capacity include those with:

• dementia;

• a severe learning disability;

• a brain injury;

• a mental health condition;

• a stroke;

• unconsciousness caused by an anaesthetic or sudden accident.

If a person has one of the above conditions it does not necessarily mean they lack the capacity to make a specific decision. Someone can lack capacity to make some decisions (for example, to decide on complex financial issues) but still have the capacity to make other decisions (for example, whether they want or need paracetamol for a headache). The person who would normally assess capacity is the person who would implement the decision if the person had capacity and agreed. For example, a surgeon would assess an individual's capacity with regards to surgery.

The HCA and AP need to have an understanding of what mental capacity is and recognise that these are potentially vulnerable people, ensuring they are fully safeguarded and remain at the centre of decision-making. Please check your local policy and if you have any uncertainties discuss this with your manager. The RCN (2013) in their document Making it Work: Shared Decision-making and People with Learning Disabilities discuss shared decision-making, which is a process by which people with learning disabilities, their families, carers and healthcare professionals work in partnership to decide on tests, treatments, management or support packages, based on clinical evidence and the person's

informed choices. This process will very often involve the person's family, supporters and those closest to the person with a learning disability; the aim is to reach an agreement on the best course of action while at the same time acting in the person's best interests. The RCN emphasise the work of Coulter and Ellins (2011: 11)
that:

> The most important reason for practising shared decision-making is that it is the right thing to do. Communication of unbiased and understandable information on treatment or self-management support options, benefits, harms, and uncertainties is an ethical imperative and failure to provide this should be taken as evidence of poor quality care.

Scotland

The Adults with Incapacity (Scotland) Act 2000 permits intervention in the affairs of an adult only if:

> The person responsible for authorising or effecting the intervention is satisfied that the intervention will benefit the adult and that such benefit cannot reasonably be achieved without the intervention. (s.1(2))

> The term adult means a person who has attained the age of 16 years (s.1 (6))

Gallagher et al. (2012) point out the important difference between the Scottish Act and the Act governing England and Wales is the purpose of any intervention – it will 'benefit' the person in Scotland and be in their 'best interests' in England and Wales. Both Acts and relevant Codes of Practice set out similar matters to be taken into account in assessing capacity and in deciding benefit/best interest.

Lack of capacity may occur, with particular reference to mental illness or inability to communicate because of physical disability. It may be the case that you are the first person to notice a loss of capacity in a patient and, in these instances, further advice and help should be sought.

THINK ABOUT IT

Identify patients in your care with possible disabilities that might reduce their capacity. What do you think you can do and what policies should you be aware of?

If the patient is deemed incapable of giving consent then treatment will be strictly undertaken in relation to the Incapacity Act or the Mental Health (Care and Treatment) (Scotland) Act 2003. Part 5 of the Adults with Incapacity Act (relating to medical treatment and research) allows treatment to be given to safeguard or promote the physical and mental health of an adult who is unable to consent.

In England, the Department for Constitutional Affairs published a factsheet in April 2004 that summarises the key principles of the then Mental Incapacity

Bill (now renamed the Mental Capacity Bill). The key principles from this are adapted in Box 1.4.

Box 1.4 Key principles of incapacity (adapted from Department for Constitutional Affairs 2004)

- An assumption of capacity: every adult has the right to make their own decisions and must be assumed to have capacity to do so unless it is proved otherwise.
- Capacity is decision specific: a new assessment must be taken each time that a decision is to be made and no blanket label of incapacity is allowed.
- Participation in decision-making: everyone should be encouraged and enabled to make decisions with help and support given to allow an expression of choice.
- Individuals must retain the right to make what might be seen as eccentric or unwise decisions.
- All decisions must be in the person's best interests, giving consideration to what the person would have wanted.
- Decisions made on behalf of someone else should be those that are least restrictive of their basic rights and freedoms.
www.dca.gov.uk/menincap/mcbfactsheet.htm

Summary

The need for healthcare assistants and assistant practitioners to gain an understanding of accountability and related issues cannot be over-emphasised. It is vital to have an up-to-date copy of a job description, to ensure they have the education and training required to safely and competently deliver care. While healthcare providers have a responsibility to offer the best care possible, it is important to remember that patients have the right to refuse it.

CASE STUDY 1.1

A patient requires a specimen of blood to be taken. You are asked to perform this task. You have had training and done a couple of supervised practices, but have not yet had your final assessment. You take the blood with no injury to the patient. Would this be acceptable, stating your rationale?

CASE STUDY 1.2

Mrs Phillips, a 58 year old, requires an indwelling urinary catheter inserted, but has refused before.

   Discuss how you proceed to try to gain her consent. Are there issues about her capacity that you should consider?

Self-assessment		
Assessment	**Aspects**	
Code of Conduct	*Have you read and understood your Code of Conduct?*	**Achieved ✓**
Accountability	*Have you considered all aspects of this section?* To whom are you accountable? The different areas of accountability The healthcare assistant role and delegation The assistant practitioner role and delegation Vicarious liability	**Achieved ✓**
Patient	*Have you considered all aspects of this section?* Duty of care and negligence Reasonable care Standards of Care Consent Capacity	**Achieved ✓**

References

Carvalho S, Reeves M and Orford J (2012) *Fundamental Aspects of Legal and Ethical and Professional Nursing*, 2nd edn. London: Quay Books.

Coulter A and Ellins J (2011) *Making shared decision-making a reality, no decision about me, without me*, London: The Kings Fund. Available at: www.kingsfund.org.uk (accessed 22 May 2013).

Cox C (2010) Legal responsibility and accountability. *Nursing Management* 17(3): 18–20.

Department for Constitutional Affairs (2004) Mental Incapacity Bill (now renamed the Mental Capacity Bill). Factsheet April 2004. Available at: www.dca.gov.uk/menincap/mcbfactsheet .htm (accessed 10 March 2015).

Department of Health (DH) (2009) *Reference Guide to Consent for Examination or Treatment*, 2nd edn. London: HMSO.

Department of Health (DH) (2013a) *The NHS Constitution – the NHS Belongs To Us All*. London: HMSO.

Department of Health (DH) (2013b) The Cavendish Review. *An Independent Review into Health Care Assistants and Support Workers in the NHS and Social Care Settings*. London: HMSO.

Department of Health (DH) (2014) *The Health Care and Associated Professions (Indemnity Arrangements) Order 2014*. London: HMSO.

Dimond B (2011) *Legal Aspects of Nursing*, 6th edn. London: Prentice Hall.

Francis R (2013) *The Mid Staffordshire NHS Foundation Trust Public Inquiry: Final report*. Mid Staffordshire NHS Trust Public Inquiry. London. http://bit.ly/1bbgTt (accessed 30 March 2015).

Gallagher A, Hodge S and Pansari N (2012) Consent when capacity is compromised. In: Gallagher A and Hodge S (eds) *Ethics, Law and Professional Issues*. London: Palgrave, pp 61–79.

Griffith R (2015) Accountability in direct nursing practice: key concepts. *British Journal of Community Nursing* 20(3): 146–149.

Griffith, R and Tengnah C (2010) *Law and Professional Issues in Nursing*. Padstow: Learning Matters Ltd.

Hywel Dda Health Board (2015) EAGLE Governance Framework for Employer-led Regulation and Registration of HCSW Revised 2015 Available at: http://www.wales.nhs.uk/sitesplus/862/opendoc/215731 (accessed 2 May 2015).

Horner A (2012) A process to ensure public protection. *Nursing Standard* 26(38): 70–71.

Law Commission, Scottish Law Commission, Northern Ireland Law Commission (2012) Regulation Of Health Care Professionals: Regulation Of Social Care Professionals In England, A Joint Consultation Paper. http://tinyurl.com/nqwme34 (accessed 19 February 2015).

Mullen C (2014) Accountability and delegation explained. *British Journal of Healthcare Assistants* 8(9): 450–453.

Nursing and Midwifery Council (NMC) (2015a) *The Code. Professional Standards of Practice and Behaviour for Nurses and Midwives*. London: NMC.

Nursing and Midwifery Council (NMC) (2015b) Our role [online]. Available at: http://www.nmc.org.uk/about-us/our-role/ (accessed 15 April 2015).

Oxford English Dictionary (2012) *Oxford English Dictionary*. Oxford: Oxford University Press.

Parliament (2005) *Mental Capacity Act*. London: Stationery Office. Available at: www.opsi.gov.uk.

Royal College of Nursing (RCN) (2004) *Full Health Care Support Worker*. London: RCN. Available at: https://www.rcn.org.uk/membership/categories/category30 (accessed 3 March 2015).

Royal College of Nursing (RCN) (2006) *Intercollegiate Paper: Supervision, Accountability and Delegation of Activities to Support Workers: A Guide for Registered Practitioners and Support Workers*. London: RCN.

Royal College of Nursing (RCN) (2011). *Accountability and Delegation: What You Need to Know*. London: RCN. Available at http://www.rcn.org.uk/__data/assets/pdf_file/0003/381720/003942.pdf (accessed 30 April 2015).

Royal College of Nursing (RCN) (2012) *The Nursing Team: Common Goals, Different Roles*. London: RCN. Available at: http://www.rcn.org.uk/__data/assets/pdf_file/0010/441919/004213.pdf (accessed 30 April 2015)

Royal College of Nursing (RCN) (2013) *Making it Work: Shared Decision-making and People with Learning Disabilities*. London: RCN.

Samanta A and Samanta J (2011) Patient safety in secondary care. In: Tingle J and Bank P (eds) *Patient Safety, Law Policy and Proceedure*. London: Routledge, pp. 128–136.

Scottish Government (2010) *Healthcare support workers – mandatory standards and codes*. Edinburgh: Scottish Government. Available at: www.healthworkerstandards.scot.nhs.

Scrivener R, Hand T and Hooper R (2011) Accountability and responsibility: Principle of Nursing Practice B. *Nursing Standard* 25(29): 35–36.

Skills for Health (2009) *Core Standards for Assistant Practitioners*. Bristol: Skills for Health.

Skills for Care and Skills for Health (2013) Code of Conduct for Healthcare Support Workers and Adult Social Care Workers in England. Available at: http://www.skillsforcare.org.uk/Document-library/Standards/National-minimum-training-standard-and-code/CodeofConduct.pdf (accessed 30 April 2015).

Taylor H (2013) Determining capacity to consent to treatment. *Nursing Times* 109(43): 12–13.

Vaughan S, Melling K, O'Reilly L and Cooper D (2014) Understanding the debate on regulation of support workers. *British Journal of Healthcare Assistants* 8(4): 185–189.

Welsh Assembly Government (2011) *Code of Conduct for Healthcare Support Workers in Wales*. Cardiff: Welsh Assembly Government. Available at www.wales.nhs.uk (accessed December 2015).

CHAPTER 2
Communication in healthcare

LEARNING OBJECTIVES

- Define effective communication in relation to healthcare settings
- Discuss the importance of communication in effective team working in clinical practice
- Identify appropriate communication methods and their application to practice
- List barriers to communication and identify solutions

Aim of this chapter

The aim of this chapter is to explore communication methods and challenges within the healthcare setting. This will enable the reader to maximise their skills in communicating with patients, families, carers, colleagues and the interprofessional team.

Why good communication is important

The importance of communication is reflected by professional bodies such as the Nursing Midwifery Council (NMC) who recommend that communication is integrated into the education of healthcare practitioners. Communication and interpersonal skills are highlighted as Standards for Competence and are part of the essential skill clusters for registered nurses (NMC 2013). Furthermore, the Code (NMC 2015) clearly states the importance of communication in Statement 7: that to practise effectively you communicate effectively. Similarly, The Code of Conduct for Healthcare Support Workers and Adult Social Care Workers in England, developed by Skills for Health (2013: 7), states that you should 'Communicate in an open and effective way to promote the health, safety and wellbeing of people who use health and care services and their carers'. Patient-centred healthcare revolves around the implementation of effective communication (Hayes and Collins 2013) and healthcare assistants and assistant practitioners, as part

Clinical Skills for Healthcare Assistants and Assistant Practitioners, Second Edition.
Angela Whelan and Elaine Hughes.
© 2016 John Wiley & Sons, Ltd. Published 2016 by John Wiley & Sons, Ltd.

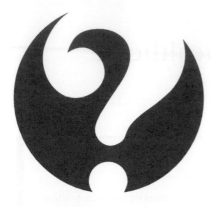

Figure 2.1 Briefly look at Figure 2.1. What can you see? It might depend on your perspective. Refer to the end footnote on this page. Source: www .creativethink.com. 1990. Reproduced with permission of Von Oech.

of the nursing family, are at the heart of the communication process. Casey and Wallis (2011: 35) nicely sum up the importance of communication when they write: 'Communication is central to human interaction. Without it, people cannot relate to those around them, make their needs and concerns known or make sense of what is happening to them.' The Department of Health (2010) clearly identifies that staff should communicate effectively with each other to ensure continuity, safety and quality of healthcare for all (DH 2010).

Communication is possibly the most important skill you can develop, but it is a vast and complex topic and so this chapter focuses on helping healthcare assistants and assistant practitioners improve and develop their communication skills in the context of their roles. Look at Figure 2.1. What can you see? What you see will depend on your perspective.

Figure 2.1 is either a bird, or a question mark, or if you turn it upside down it's a seal juggling a ball on its nose.

Self-knowledge and understanding, that is being self-aware, help us to gain insight into our values and beliefs that mould us as individuals. By becoming self-aware (Iggulden and Sharples 2009) we can develop the understanding we need to have empathy with other people and see things from their perspective; an important facet of communication, especially when we can see why communication is important from somebody else's perspective.

Definition of communication

We tend to take communication for granted; we understand the word, but it is not that easy to define. Oxford Dictionary Language Matters defines communication as 'the imparting or exchanging of information by speaking, writing, or using some other medium', which fails to express its complexity. Schiavo (2013) discusses the difficulty of defining communication, emphasising the importance of behavioural, social, and organisational aspects of communication. Although the focus of this chapter is on work settings, consider the difference with respect to a social, everyday lifestyle communication and a work-related communication. Hayes and Collins (2013) also point out the complexities of communication that relate to how organisational communication feeds directly into the attitudes, relationships and behaviours of staff working within.

Different types of relationships determine the appropriate style of communication, for example how we talk with our family will differ from how we talk with our manager, and so some choices of communication are already made for us by the situation or the context.

THINK ABOUT IT

This is a useful point to stop and consider why we need to communicate.

Communication is essential:
• to give instructions;
• to ask for information;
• to express needs and feelings;
• to exchange ideas and thoughts;
• to entertain;
• to give and seek reassurances;
• to share experiences.

The NMC (2015) states that patients should be informed about their care and that information should be shared appropriately. In order to achieve this, Standard 5 of the Code (NMC 2015) states that you must:

5.1 respect a person's right to privacy in all aspects of their care

5.2 So communication is two way, with sender(s) and receiver(s), with the purpose of passing on a message with information; therefore it needs to be to the right person/people, at the right time and in language that is comprehensible to all.ake sure that people are informed about how and why information is used and shared by those who will be providing care

5.3 respect that a person's right to privacy and confidentiality continues after they have died

5.4 share necessary information with other healthcare professionals and agencies only when the interests of patient safety and public protection override the need for confidentiality, and

5.5 share with people, their families and their carers, as far as the law allows, the information they want or need to know about their health, care and ongoing treatment sensitively and in a way they can understand. (NMC 2015: 6)

Communication is often the main complaint in healthcare, and in 2012 the then newly appointed health service ombudsman, Julie Mellor, reported 'careless', 'insincere' and 'unclear' communication had fuelled a surge in complaints against the NHS in England. These complaints can affect the quality of a patient's care, and this is why this book suggests that communication is a fundamental skill.

Communication methods

Let us now review some key aspects of communication in healthcare.

> **THINK ABOUT IT**
>
> What methods of communication are used in healthcare – make a list of them.

McEwen and Harris (2010) propose that communication is made up of three intricately woven parts: verbal, non-verbal and paralinguistic or paraverbal modes. All three modes are usually used together. Mehrabian's (1981) classic research into body language and non-verbal communication found that:

- only 7% of a message is conveyed by the actual words we speak;
- 38% is by paralinguistic features (e.g. tone and pitch);
- 55% is by other non-verbal factors.

So we can see that attention to non-verbal methods is crucial.

Thus, when communicating, it is important that actions match words because that is what people see; for example, smiling when saying 'Hello, pleased to see you', and not frowning, because the receiver might misunderstand the message. In fact the sender may be frowning because it is a very sunny day and they can't see the other's face clearly, but the receiver will see the frown and may think 'He doesn't really want to talk to me'. The importance of this approach is borne out by the introduction of the '*hello* my name is' campaign, which was started by Dr Kate Granger in 2013 following her experience as a patient.

Non-verbal communication

> **THINK ABOUT IT**
>
> Non-verbal communication is often classified as body language, so name three ways of communicating using body language:
> 1
> 2
> 3

Dickson et al. (1997) in their classical text highlighted the six main functions of non-verbal communication:

1 Replacing speech.
2 Complementing the verbal message: this is considered the main function of non-verbal communication.
3 Regulating and controlling the flow of communication, for example nodding, and eye contact to indicate continue speaking.
4 Providing feedback, as above.

5 Helping define relationships between people, for example a white coat to denote a role such as a doctor.
6 Conveying emotional states.

Components of non-verbal communication include: touch, proximity, orientation, posture, body movements, facial expressions, eye contact and appearance.

Touch

Healthcare professionals are increasingly wary of touching patients, other than when undertaking a task such as dressing a wound. In healthcare, however, touch is therapeutic and one of the most powerful ways that we have of communicating non-verbally (McEwen and Harris 2010). Here culture and gender issues may arise, and so the healthcare assistant should observe the patient for cues as to comfort and acceptance. Kitching (2012) highlights the importance of touch in caring for vulnerable patients. However, if you read and consider the scenario in Box 2.1, Sara could have sat down with Annie and held her hand while they had the same conversation, and certainly then Annie would have felt really listened to and cared for.

Box 2.1 Scenario

It is 07:15 on a busy Saturday shift in an acute hospital ward, when Mrs Annie Wilson, a 54-year-old patient with acute asthma, rings her bedside buzzer.
  Healthcare assistant Sara Smith goes into the single room in response to the buzzer.

Annie: 'Thank goodness, you've come.'
  Sara: 'Hello Annie, what's the problem?'
Annie: 'I can't breathe.'
  Sara: 'Can't breathe? Oh dear, let me check your oxygen.'
Annie: 'I'm so frightened, I haven't slept a wink.'
  Sara: 'Why are you frightened, Annie?'
Annie: 'Because of my asthma, I feel I can't breathe, like I'm choking.'
  Sara: 'Now, Annie, you know you are on treatment for your asthma and you are safe in hospital as we are around all the time.'
Annie: 'I still feel like I'm choking, it's terrible ....'
  Sara: 'I'm sure it must be. What can I do to help make you feel better? Would it help if I put on your fan as it's a bit stuffy in here?'
Annie: 'I was cold and it made too much noise.'
  Sara: 'Let's try it, and I'll get you a blanket. How would that be?'
Annie: 'OK, if you think that'll help. Don't leave me please.'
  Sara: 'I am only going to get you a blanket.'

Proximity

Proximity is about space, and Dickson et al. (1997) suggest that in Western cultures we have four zones:
1 Intimate zone of 0–50 cm.
2 Personal zone of 50 cm–1.2 m.

3 Social/consultative zone 1.2–3.5 m.

4 Public zone 3.5 m and above.

They further noted, interestingly, that in healthcare, patients' personal space and even intimate space is regularly invaded by staff, often without seeking the patient's permission, and they say that this can increase the vulnerability and loss of control that a patient feels in healthcare. Thus always consider when approaching the patient, particularly if about to undertake a clinical skill, that they should be allowed to give permission; for example ask, 'Is it alright if I take your blood pressure?' Then the healthcare assistant can proceed and the patient feels in control of the situation.

Orientation

Orientation is about where and how the communication takes place. Thus, when talking to a patient in a wheelchair, consider the level and where possible make sure that you communicate at eye level and so sit down too. Often in healthcare we talk over objects, for example the patient is on one side of a desk or bed and the healthcare assistant is on the other; this artificial barrier can affect the quality of communication too, so consider how to minimise this.

Posture

Posture includes how one stands or sits, looking relaxed and interested, for example leaning forward to listen. This links to orientation and, again, if a patient is in bed and we approach them to talk, remember that we are towering above them and this can look very dominating or controlling, and so sit down.

Body movements

Body movements are a powerful means of conveying non-verbal communication; imagine if Sara (see Box 2.1) had stood with her arms folded during the conversation, what message would Annie have picked up? Probably that Sara does not care or is not interested. However, body language can be misunderstood, as Sara may have had her arms crossed because she was tired and cold after a long night shift.

Be aware also that cultural variances might play a part, for example hand gestures in some cultures might offend; Sobiechowska (2010) states that cultural or ethnic experience and heritage may imbue us with strong beliefs about a number of matters, for example the role of women or the capacity of gender. Similarly, Hindle (2003) uses the example of a gesture that we commonly use in the UK for OK, which is a circle made with our index finger and thumb; with the other fingers pointing up, this means to a Tunisian 'I am going to kill you'. The NMC (2015: 7) states that to communicate effectively one must use 'a range of verbal and non verbal communication methods and consider cultural sensitivities, to better understand and respond to people's personal health needs'.

Facial expressions

Think of facial expressions: one example has already been used with frowning, but our faces are often said to tell a story, as we roll our eyes we may not even realise that we are doing so. So, when someone says, 'I see you're unhappy about my idea', it is because of the cue that they have observed; but cues can be misread, so, for communication to be effective, it is about all aspects of communication working together, delivering the same message.

Eye contact

Many suggest that the eyes are a powerful means of communicating non-verbal messages, for example the child misbehaving becomes aware of a glare from a parent and swiftly knows that she is in trouble! Eye contact can include or exclude. Toocaram (2010) also points out that some people with severe learning disabilities may be able to point to symbols or pictures to explain how they are feeling (e.g. the Wong Baker visual analogue pain chart that uses faces) and what they want or need. Good eye contact and 'eye pointing' can become meaningful and communicative and can speak volumes.

Appearance

Finally, appearance is a means of communicating non-verbally, for example how we dress may reflect our mood or task. In a hospital setting we often ask the patient to get undressed and take away that form of expression (communication). Think of dressing for a night out with friends versus a first date; I bet that your wardrobe choice is very different!

So non-verbal cues can be important for the observant healthcare assistant; for example while taking a venous sample of blood, the healthcare assistant notices that the patient is looking away and is restless – this body language may tell the healthcare assistant that the patient is nervous or frightened and so they can give reassurance and explanations.

Tone in communication

Now let us briefly think about tone and its importance in effective communication; again vigilance and self-awareness are necessary. How do we sound to others? If we speak loudly because a person is hard of hearing, will they hear the tone as angry? In healthcare a conversation might be carried out over the phone with a patient's family member so consider how much of the message is lost if they can hear only the tone and words.

Email is another form of communication. Kraszewski (2010) highlights the advantages of communication via email as being cheaper, faster, more convenient and less obtrusive than a phone call. Email also allows the recipient time to consider and think about their response while providing a written record of communication, enhancing record keeping. However Kraszewski (2010) does advise caution: the use of humour may cause offense and lead to misunderstanding, plus there is the possibility of sending the email to an incorrect recipient. Although email lacks the subtlety of tone, there are a series of symbols to denote expressions such as a smiley face ☺ or :) which may not be appropriate in a formal email. The NMC (2015: 16) requests to 'use all forms of spoken, written and digital communication (including social media and networking sites) responsibly, respecting the right to privacy at all times'. More guidance on the use of social media and networking sites can be found at: www.nmc-uk.org/guidance.

In terms of healthcare, Crow (2010) reports that professionals often use jargon, abbreviations and acronyms that are meaningless to patients, carers and even their colleagues in other departments. This jargon can help us to be specific in our work, but the choice of words can create confusion to others. Imagine that you have been sent a clinic appointment and are a young teenager, so, on arrival at the reception, you ask for Nurse Led, because printed at the top of your appointment card is Nurse Led Clinic. This is an example of jargon and, if the receptionist finds it funny and laughs while explaining, the tone may cause the young teenager to become embarrassed or even angry, resulting in a total breakdown in communication and creating a humiliated and possibly angry patient.

Verbal communication

The written word is still classed as verbal communication. There are many advantages to written language as it allows distribution and uniformity of instruction and information, and so can be re-read and thought over or reflected upon and is also a permanent record.

THINK ABOUT IT

Consider restrictions on the effectiveness of the written word. Write down what these might be.

People's reading skills need to be considered: can they read – have they lost their spectacles or is the font size too small, are they literate (able to read), do they have dyslexia (disorder in reading or writing), is the information too technical, or is English not their first language? All these factors will affect the quality of the written word as a means of communication, which the NMC (2015) emphasises in statement 7.2: 'take reasonable steps to meet people's language and communication needs, providing, wherever possible, assistance to those who need help to communicate their own or other people's needs'.

No matter whether care plans are computer held or paper copies, the writing needs to be legible, clear, concise and understandable. There are a number of tools available to help you to improve the readability of any piece of work including the Gunning FOG Index and the SMOG Readability Formula. Both tools are similar and relate to the use and length of words and simple sentence structure. Writing is explored in more detail in Chapter 4 in relation to record-keeping purposes.

Strategies to improve communication

This section reviews some of the challenges facing effective communication in healthcare.

THINK ABOUT IT

What might be barriers to effective communication in healthcare?

Let us consider the three aspects related to communication (each of these aspects is reviewed in the scenario in Box 2.1):

- the sender;
- the receiver(s);
- the situation: includes environmental factors.

THINK ABOUT IT

What recommendations might you suggest to enhance the conversation in Box 2.1?

Let us pause here and think over the short conversation:

- Is there evidence of active listening?
- Is there evidence of open questions?
- Is there evidence of any leading questions?
- Is this conversation effective?

Related aspects and terminology

Active listening

Active listening is a process and the most important aspect is to *accept* what is heard, so that the conversation is heard from the sender's (e.g. in Box 2.1, the patient Annie's) point of view (McEwen and Harris 2010). The receiver is listening for clues – words or phrases – that say what the sender is feeling and expressing. Listening is therefore crucial for effective communication.

Table 2.1 figures SOLER, a theory that was developed by Gerard Egan who describes techniques for active listening. In the form of non-verbal communication, SOLER theory can be valuable when helping another person and can make that person feel cared for, involved in what is going on, feel respected and understood. SOLER theory can also be learned by anyone who wishes to become a better listener.

Table 2.1 Checklist for effective communication

SOLER	Achieved ✓
Sit **S**quarely in relation to the patient	
Maintain an **O**pen posture	
Lean slightly towards the patient	
Maintain reasonable **E**ye contact with the patient	
Relax (sit comfortably and supported)	

Source: Egan 1990. Reproduced with permission of Cengage Learning.

In Annie's case she says, 'I'm frightened' and the receiver (Sara) shows that she has heard by acknowledging this; one way is to repeat the word or phrase, so Sara replies, 'Why are you frightened?' Here Sara has used Annie's word and asked her a question to allow her to expand on this initial statement; this is defined as an 'open' question.

An open question

An open question is phrased in a way that invites the other person to open up and say more, and usually starts with what, why, how, when or where. The framing of questions is crucial; Harris and McEwan (2010) maintain that if people are asked open-ended questions and are rushed, they may respond more freely. Using a non-judgemental approach coupled with active listening is important. Closed questions, which usually require a yes or no answer or confirmation of details, such as 'Tell me your name', are useful for confirming what is known or for being specific. In this situation it is more helpful to allow Annie 'space' to tell you why she is frightened. 'How' is a useful way of starting a question, but take care because this can sometimes lead to one-word answers, for example 'How are you feeling?' 'Tired!' Harris and McEwan (2010) also remind us it is important to know when to refer an issue on to others, especially when dealing with sensitive issues.

Leading questions

This links to leading questions; the risk with these is getting the answer that was wanted and maybe not what was needed, for example 'You do want to get up now, don't you?' There was an example in Box 2.1 with the fan suggestion and, although it may be helpful, Sara has possibly missed the cue about Annie's fear of choking. So care must be taken to use questions that allow the person to expand and go beyond a simple statement.

In one author's experience, a real conversation led to the identification that the patient thought that if she fell asleep her breathing would become poorer and so her oxygen levels would drop, and she would then fall into a coma and die. Only through open questions did we arrive at this fear and so were able to discuss and allay it.

Common problems or communication barriers

There are a numerous barriers to effective communication; Toocaram (2010) highlights the challenges faced in caring for disadvantaged and vulnerable groups of people, including those with learning difficulties, physical difficulties, sensory deprivation and cross-cultural issues. Furthermore we have to consider prejudice and stereotyping that may affect communication – and that includes our own. Consider a normal shift: think of how much time you could spend with one patient, compared to how much time you actually have. Are there any resource issues, are you feeling stressed by targets to meet or staff shortages? What kind of mood are you in; perhaps you had an argument before you came into work? And can you really fit all that you need to do into one day? Are there any organisational or professional barriers? Hayes and Collins (2013) recognise the necessity for cultivating the ability to professionally disagree with colleagues without personally offending them, which can impact on the organisation, the team, the individual as well as, perhaps most importantly, the patient. Good communication is an ongoing process particularly in stressful situations where it can be difficult to see the non-verbal messages of the patients with whom we mostly communicate (Kourlouta and Papathanasiou 2014).

When nursing, communication requires:
1 Being self-aware – what are we doing, why and how.
2 Developing the knowledge that informs our behaviour and our skills. There are formal courses or you can access resources and undertake some self-directed study. Have a chat with your manager and/or your clinical educator.
3 Be clear – if you are not certain and muddled, you are not going to communicate anything other than your own lack of ability. If you are clear, you will have more confidence and present yourself in a positive manner.

Physical barriers
Other barriers to effective communication might relate to a patient's condition, for example Annie may find talking difficult due to her asthma and acute breathlessness. Other factors that may affect the patient's ability to communicate or understand communication range from poorly fitting dentures, poor hearing, to poor sight or maybe not wearing hearing aids or glasses.

Conditions such as cerebral vascular accidents (stroke) may affect a patient's speech (dysphasia) and also a patient may be less able to process a conversation, or the words that they choose may not be appropriate or 'fit' the conversation. A stutter or other form of speech impediment may cause poor communication. A patient who suffers from dementia or acute confusion may be unable to process a message and so responds less appropriately, as could a patient with a brain or head injury or illness, and the patient in an intensive setting on a ventilator will also have a communication challenge. A learning disability may impede or hinder the ability to understand and process a message. You must communicate any concerns you have if you believe a patient is vulnerable or at risk and needs extra support and this is clearly identified in Statement 17 of the Code (NMC 2015).

We also need to consider environmental barriers. These will depend on the environment; however, broadly we might consider noise as a barrier, for example machines bleeping, other people talking, trolleys clattering.

Allied to this might be the lack of privacy, especially in a hospital setting. Lighting and room space are other factors and, in the community setting, environmental factors may include other family members or pets!

If it is too cold or hot people can become distracted, blocking effective communication. Talking to someone while you stand in front of a window can create a shadow over your face and poor-sighted or hearing-impaired or deaf people will lose the ability to see your face and your mouth, and so limit their ability to 'see' the conversation.

Case study 2.1 will help in consideration of some environmental aspects.

CASE STUDY 2.1

Mr Wang, a Chinese man in his 60s, is being admitted to his bed in the ward. Part of the admission requires asking about his bowel habits; he appears not to understand the question and answers with a 'yes'.

What action might the healthcare assistant admitting him need to consider?

Possible factors might be that the patient is embarrassed in a public place, is hard of hearing or does not understand English. Never assume anything.

The options available to the healthcare assistant would again depend on the setting, but there might be a private room where he could be admitted. If hearing were identified as a problem, writing the question down could possibly help. If English were not his first language, a professional (trained) translator could help. It is recommended not to use family members or friends even when their English is good, because this may breach confidentiality and also cause embarrassment between the family or friends and the patient. Harris and McEwen (2010) note that translators maybe required when communicating with people for whom English is not their first language. In this case, it is important to clarify the role of the interpreter or translator and to address the patient, not the translator.

Some situations might be aided with the use of pre-prepared cards with symbols and words; however, these would have limited application. A drawing instead of words may also assist, but take care not to patronise or use inappropriate pictures.

So, environmental barriers need careful attention, including:

- layout;
- lighting;
- ventilation;
- distractions in the area.

All these are known to affect communication, for example if the lighting is poor a patient with a sight problem might not be able to see and so communication may break down.

Skills for the Health Care Certificate

In the wake of the Francis Inquiry into the Mid Staffordshire NHS Foundation Trust, Camilla Cavendish was appointed to undertake an independent review of healthcare assistants and support workers across health and social care. Consequently a partnership was formed led by Health Education England, working closely with Skills for Care and Skills for Health. The partnership developed the standards and framework for the delivery of the Care Certificate, with guidance from the Department of Health and its Cavendish Governance Assurance Board. Standard 6 of the Care Certificate (Skills for Health 2015) is about Communication, which incorporates themes discussed within this chapter. Further information about the Care Certificate can be found at www.skillsforhealth/qualifications@skillsforhealth.org.uk.

Summary

All of the points below are embedded within the Code of Professional standards of practice and behaviour for nurses and midwives (NMC 2015: 1) which 'set the standards that patients and members of the public tell us they expect from healthcare professionals'. A healthcare professional:

- is respectful of the person being talked to;
- is clear;
- does not use jargon, technical words or abbreviations;
- is empathic and sensitive to the receiver's (patient) needs;
- takes account of the receiver's abilities/disabilities.

Self-assessment

Table 2.1 is a simple checklist that would aid any communication and ensure it is effective.

References

Casey A and Wallis A (2011) Effective communication: Principle of Nursing Practice E. *Nursing Standard* 25(32): 35–37.

Crow J (2010) Communication: the essence of care. In: Kraszewski S and McEwen A (eds) *Communication Skills for Adult Nurses*. London: McGraw Open University Press, pp. 37–54.

Department of Health (2010) Essence of Care 2010: Benchmarks for Communication https://www.gov.uk/government/uploads/system/uploads/attachment_data/file/216695/dh_119973.pdf (last accessed 15 March 2015).

Dickson D, Hargie O and Morrow N (1997) *Communication Skills Training for Health Professionals*. London: Chapman & Hall.

Egan G (ed.) (1990) *The Skilled Helper: A Systematic Approach to Effective Helping*, 4th edn. Pacific Grove, CA: Brooks Cole.

Hayes C and Collins M (2013) Organisational contexts of communication in health care. *British Journal of Health Care Assistants* 7(11): 553–555.

Hindle S A (2003) Psychological factors affecting communication. In: Ellis R B, Gates B and Kenworthy N (eds) *Interpersonal Communication in Nursing*, 2nd edn. Edinburgh: Churchill Livingstone, pp. 53–72.

Iggulden H and Sharples N (2009) Communication. In: Iggulden H, MacDonald C and Staniland K (eds) *Clinical Skills The Essence of Caring*. London: McGraw Hill Open University Press.

Kitching A (2012) Good communication enhanced: a vulnerable patient's hospital stay. *Nursing Standard* 26(33): 28.

Kourkouta L and Papathanasiou I (2014) Communication in nursing practice. *Mater Sociomed* 26(1): 65–67.

Kraszewski S (2010) Using technology to communicate. In: Kraszewski S and McEwen A (eds) *Communication Skills for Adult Nurses*. London: McGraw Open University Press, pp. 54–71.

McEwen A and Harris G (2010) Communication: fundamental skills. In: Kraszewski S and McEwen A (eds) *Communication Skills for Adult Nurses*. London: McGraw Open University Press, pp. 1–22.

Mehrabian A (1981). *Silent Messages: Implicit Communication of Emotions and Attitudes*, 2nd edn. Wadsworth, Belmont, California. Available at: http://www.kaaj.com/psych/smorder.html (accessed 6 February 2015).

Nursing Midwifery Council (2013) Standards for Competence for Registered Nurses. Available at: http://www.nmc.org.uk/globalassets/siteDocuments/Standards/Standards-for-competence.pdf (accessed 10 February 2015).

Nursing & Midwifery Council (NMC) (2015) The Code. *Professional Standards of Practice and Behaviour for Nurses and Midwives*. London: NMC.

Oxford Dictionary Language Matters (online) Available at: http://www.oxforddictionaries.com/definition/english/communication (accessed 30 March 2015).

Schiavo R (2013) *Health Communication: From Theory to Practice*, 2nd edn. London: John Wiley & Sons.

Skills for Care & Skills for Health (2013) Code of Conduct for Healthcare Support Workers and Adult Social Care Workers in England www.skillsforcare.org.uk & www.skillsforhealth.org.uk (accessed March 2015).

Skills for Health (2015) The Care Certificate Framework (Assessor) Health Education England, Skills for Care and Skills for Health.

Sobiechowska P (2010) Communication in learning and teaching. In: Kraszewski S and McEwen A (eds) *Communication Skills for Adult Nurses*. London: McGraw Open University Press, pp. 123–142.

Toocaram J (2010) Communication in learning and teaching. In: Kraszewski S and McEwen A (eds) *Communication Skills for Adult Nurses*. London: McGraw Open University Press, pp. 90–106.

Von Oech R (1990) *A Whack on the Side of the Head*. London: HarperCollins Publishers.

Addendum

Gunning FOG Index (Gunning 1952)

Gunning FOG Index: from http://en.wikipedia.org/wiki/Gunning-Fog_Index, accessed 27/02/08 and permission obtained from wikipedia. Also available at: www.tasc.ac.uk/sdev1/drobis/profcom/fog.htm (accessed 11 January 2006).

Step 1	Count out a 100-word passage. Make sure that the passage ends with a full stop, even if you go slightly above or below exactly 100 words
Step 2	Find the average sentence length by dividing 100 by the number of sentences in the selected passage, e.g. 8 sentences = $100 \div 8 = 12.5$
Step 3	Count the number of words with three or more syllables (e.g. syllables). This number gives you the percentage of 'hard words' in the passage, e.g. 9
Don't count	Proper nouns, e.g. Irene, Paris
	Combinations of easy words such as typewriter or newsletter
	Verb forms with ends: es, ing or ed, e.g. transmitted
	Jargon familiar to your reader
Step 4	Add the average sentence length (Step 2) to the number of 'hard words' (step 3), e.g. $12.5 + 9 = 21.5$
Step 5	Multiply the total in Step 4 by 0.4 to get the reading level for the passage, e.g. $21.5 \times 0.4 = 8.6$
Note	Easy reading range is 6–10. The average person reads at level 9. Step 5 score was based on a sample from this chapter

Remember, when writing, that the aim is to be understood, so keep to the KIS principle = keep it simple. Aim for a reasonable FOG score, because the last thing we need is the lack of clarity and confusion that we often get with fog!

CHAPTER 3

Psychological well-being

Aim of this chapter

The aim of this chapter is to explore the importance of the psychological health and well-being of the people in our care. This will allow the healthcare assistant to consider the patient in a holistic and compassionate manner when supporting people and undertaking clinical skills in the workplace.

What is meant by psychological care?

Consideration of the patient's psychological health and well-being is essential in delivering holistic, person-centered care. Maslow discussed the concept of human motivation in 1943 and this has often been used as the foundation for discussion of holism in nursing. Maslow's Hierarchy of Needs clearly identifies how all the elements of the person's life need to be fulfilled to achieve what he defines as 'self actualisation' or to feel as a whole person. Maslow's (1943) theory provided the basis for the Activities of Living Model (Roper et al. 1985) which is often used in Adult and Child settings to assess patients' needs. The underpinning concept of this model was to provide care that was holistic in nature, focusing on the biopsychosocial elements of the individual's needs across the lifespan. Frequently the biological aspects of nursing are focused on, for example, the performance of a task such as undertaking venepuncture. However it is essential that the psychological elements of care are not forgotten when providing high-quality,

Clinical Skills for Healthcare Assistants and Assistant Practitioners, Second Edition.
Angela Whelan and Elaine Hughes.
© 2016 John Wiley & Sons, Ltd. Published 2016 by John Wiley & Sons, Ltd.

compassionate nursing care as this allows nurses to add the human dimension to care in understanding their patients' behaviour in response to health and illness.

Walker et al. (2012) describe psychology as the study of human behaviour, thought processes and emotions. However, when psychological care is discussed it can have many dimensions all rooted within the individual's 'behaviour'. Psychological care can range from caring for people with mental health disorders (psychiatry and psychology) to health psychology, which looks at behaviour responses in health and illness (Taylor 2009; French et al. 2010) and holism. Therefore this chapter will review how a fundamental psychological assessment can be undertaken and how this can aid the healthcare assistant to ensure that the patient receives a holistic package of care, enhancing the patient experience.

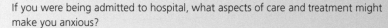

THINK ABOUT IT

If you were being admitted to hospital, what aspects of care and treatment might make you anxious?

Individuals are unique, so assessment is critical to identify their concerns or fears. When patients are admitted to hospital or attend a GP surgery, they may be experiencing stress, which could result from their illness, fear of the unknown, fear about painful treatments or concerns over the impact that a potential illness may have on their life, family, work and social community. The skill for the healthcare assistant is to identify and support a patient through this stressful period, and to do that they must first ensure that they have a clear understanding of patient's holistic needs and their concerns.

Psychological assessment in the healthcare setting

Consider, as Mitchell (2007) describes, patients entering a strange and often sterile environment such as a hospital, where they will probably be partially undressed, for example for 12-lead ECG, and unsure about what is happening or about to happen. They will be waiting for instructions and procedures (often unpleasant) from a variety of healthcare staff (many strangers to them), all the while trying to retain information and ask questions. It is known that anxiety can prevent people from retaining information and for this reason it is important to check the patient's understanding of any nursing procedure before it is undertaken.

Mitchell (2007) identifies that the belief in one's own ability to cope with a stressful situation or challenging demand is often based on past experiences. Therefore, when assessing the patient pre-procedure, the healthcare assistant should identify this and the ways in which the patient may cope or maintain control over their own health, particularly if they have a long-term condition; for example through the use of music or reading for relaxation before investigations or surgery, or patients could continue to manage their own blood sugar tests. *Please check that this is acceptable policy locally.*

Mitchell (2007) also suggests considering environmental factors, noting that the friendliness of staff is crucial, especially in busy, sterile clinical areas because they often feel impersonal and unfriendly. These thoughts have been fundamental to care since the publication of the Francis Report (Francis 2013) and have been central to the adoption of the 6 Cs in nursing (DH 2012) as well as in NHS core values (DH 2013) and quality strategies such as the 15 Steps Challenge (Williams 2013), which was born from a mother stating that she could tell what kind of care her daughter would receive within 15 steps of walking onto a ward. The principles contained within the 6 Cs, the NHS core values and the 15 Steps Challenge can all help to ensure that care and compassion is at the heart of care delivery in any health and social care settling and reduce feelings of anxiety that many patients will have.

Noise can often increase stress and distract patients (and staff), and although distraction can be a strategy to help patients cope, here it may be a problem, for example when the healthcare assistant explains the preparation for a 12-lead ECG and the patient misses important information because of distraction or background noise making it difficult for them to hear or concentrate.

Preparation of children and their families is essential in healthcare. The psychological care of the child is paramount and reduces stress and anxiety before procedures and helps to prevent further distress when clinical skills are undertaken. Part of the preparation may be undertaken by a play specialist. The role of the play specialist is to work with children and families to prepare them for procedures and help develop mechanisms to cope with anxiety, as structured play is known to improve recovery times (Howard 2013; Stonehouse 2014). However, the point of preparation is equally important, and those working in children's settings should be aware of the developmental stage of the child. For some children, preparation too far in advance can cause greater anxiety and this should be discussed with the child's parents or guardians (Trigg and Mohammed, 2010)

Parents' knowledge of how their children react to stressful situations will help the healthcare assistant determine the appropriate timing of the preparation, as well as which coping strategies would be most useful. Crowley (2014) suggests that having a knowledge of child development is important in preparing children for tests and clinical interventions. This can be used during the preparatory period and communication with the child and parents adjusted accordingly. Before any procedure such aspects must be considered because they will help the healthcare assistant identify and plan or offer strategies to help the patient cope.

The importance of psychological care in the healthcare setting

Psychological factors
Some factors have already been mentioned, for example fear and stress; however, there is a range of factors that the healthcare assistant should consider.

Stress
The symptoms of stress are based on the body's autonomic nervous system response (fight or flight) of arousal. Table 3.1 shows the body's autonomic responses.

Clancy and McVicar (2009) state that a person's response to stress is individual to them and therefore subjective. However, what is clear is that the individual responds in a cognitive, behavioural and physiological way to their stressor (Walker 2012). In the healthcare environment, stress can affect many patients. The role of the healthcare worker is important in helping patients develop coping strategies. It has long been recognised that the more information a patient is given, the more anxiety levels are reduced. This is particularly relevant in pre-operative patients where direct care is often provided by healthcare assistants. Spending extra time listening to patients and recognising their fears can reduce stress and anxiety levels (Renouf et al. 2014: Mendes da Mata 2014). Stress is also known to have direct effects on the immune system, which may delay recovery for some patients, and the importance of health promotion around lifestyle can have a positive impact on recuperation (Walker 2012). Walker et al. (2012) identified a range of symptoms from the stress response, which is discussed in Table 3.2.

Often patients can be unaware of the effects of stress until careful questioning, commonly at admission but also before some procedures, when the healthcare assistant checks that the patient understands the procedure.

Table 3.1 Body's autonomic responses.

Body organ/system	Effect
Heart and cardiac system	Heart rate and blood pressure increases
Lungs	Respiratory rate and depth of breathing increases
Liver	Glucose is released for muscular activity
Brain	Blood re-routed here to aid decision making
Eyes	Pupils dilate to aid visualisation of threat
Stomach and digestive system	Blood diverted to the major organs
Skin	Blood diverted – leads to pallor and sweating

Adapted from Walker et al. (2012) and Clancy and McVicar (2009).

Table 3.2 Stress response symptoms.

Aspects	Symptoms
Physiological	Altered sleep pattern, e.g. insomnia, waking early or not getting to sleep
	Indigestion, nausea, diarrhoea, constipation
	Headaches, muscle tension
	Panic attacks
	Increased heart rate
	Weight loss or gain
Cognitive	Feeling a failure, low self-esteem or confidence
	Worrying a lot, perhaps about things that didn't normally matter
	Not wanting to be bothered, apathetic about issues
	Difficulty in making decisions, forgetfulness
Emotional	Feeling upset, crying more than normal
	Feeling irritable or short tempered
	Unreasonable behaviour or negative attitude
	Fears that are not rational
	Tiredness
	Loss of being able to see life in a fun way or loss of sense of humour
Behavioural	Irregular eating habits, e.g. comfort eating, not eating at all or overindulging
	Taking time off for minor illnesses (which would not normally result in absence)
	Using stimulants, e.g. drugs, alcohol, tobacco
	Withdrawing from usual activities, e.g. not seeing friends or going out as much
	Being accident prone

Adapted from Walker et al. (2012) and Clancy and McVicar (2009).

THINK ABOUT IT

Look through the clinical skills in the other chapters and list the ways that stress and anxiety might affect the tests or results, the patient's response to the test itself or your ability to undertake the test with an anxious patient

---

Pain

Walker et al. (2012) describe pain as not only a physical experience but an emotional one too. From childhood, pain is associated with injury and acts as a warning that something has gone awry with the body (Brooker and Waugh 2013). With children, pain can be very difficult to assess as they may not have the verbal ability to communicate, yet pain can be associated with stress, fear and anxiety (Trigg and Mohammed 2010).

Walker et al. (2012) suggest that pain-related fear is often more disabling than the pain itself. Both adults and children may experience anticipatory pain before a procedure and become stressed and anxious. This can have an effect on the procedure, for example inserting a cannula in a patient who is tense is likely to be more painful and can lead to avoidance behaviour (Solowiej 2010) unless this is recognised and managed.

Chronic pain is associated with a range of psychological problems, for example depression and social isolation (Brooker and Waugh 2013). Chronic pain can have effects on both adults and children. The child with chronic pain can become isolated from their peer groups and pain can potentially delay their development, while pain in an adult can have a wide-ranging impact on their holistic well-being and affect many aspects of their lives (Brooker and Waugh 2013; Trigg and Mohammed 2010). It is not within the scope of this book to explore this area in depth, but some aspects are worth reviewing relating to the patient's response to healthcare.

Phobias
Walker et al. (2012) describe phobias as irrational fears that lead to avoidance. Brooker and Waugh (2013) state that both adults and children can develop a phobia towards needles which is influenced by prior experiences. For this reason, when undertaking any clinical skill it is essential to assess each patient and provide as much information as the patient requires to prevent the development of healthcare-associated phobias. It should also be noted that the healthcare assistant should ensure that each patient is given enough time to discuss any fears they may have around a procedure.

Panic or anxiety
This is described as a consequence of uncertainty and unpredictability. It is often the result of a new situation, for example emergency admission to hospital, where the person lacks the appropriate information, or the ability to make sense of what's happening, for example a patient with dementia (Walker et al. 2012).

Confusion
Confusion can occur for several reasons within the healthcare setting and having an understanding of the reason for confusion will assist the healthcare assistant in helping patients to make a recovery or undertake a clinical skills. Patients may be confused because of their clinical condition, for example because of diabetes, epilepsy, dehydration, medication or dementia. For those who have any form of dementia, taking them from familiar surroundings can make confusion worse and good communication skills are essential when caring for any patient who is confused. It should also be noted that it may be necessary to change the method of communication to meet the patient's needs (Nazarko 2014).

Culture
Culture can be interpreted in different ways and can be linked to religion. However, countries also have their own cultures with associated beliefs and norms of behaviour and this can influence how a patient may react to healthcare

Table 3.3 Stages of grief and possible outcomes.

Stage	Possible outcome examples
Denial and isolation	'I can't possibly have bowel cancer, I feel well'
Anger	'It's all your fault, you should have sent me for tests sooner'
Bargaining	'If I could turn the clock back I would eat better food and stop smoking and this cancer would never have happened'
Depression	'I can't cope with this, what if I need surgery, how will my family manage without me if I die?'
Acceptance	'Now that the operation is scheduled I feel less uncertain as I know this cancer will be gone soon and I can focus on getting better again'

(Brooker and Waugh 2013). Therefore healthcare assistants need to be respectful of their patient's cultural values, especially where privacy and dignity is concerned, without making assumptions (Trigg and Mohammed 2010; Brooker and Waugh 2013). Brooker and Waugh (2013) point out that the acceptance of healthcare can be based on cultural beliefs, for example around blood transfusions, certain medications that are animal derivatives or the preference of traditional therapeutic interventions such as herbalism or acupuncture.

However, in terms of pain and pain expression, there is evidence to suggest that culture plays a role in the patient's experience of pain. Yet Brooker and Waugh (2013) point out that when an individual is away from their original culture their response to pain changes. Although the relevance of culture in the experience of pain is useful for the healthcare assistant to acknowledge, it should also be pointed out that this can lead to stereotyping of specific cultures and therefore care should be taken to prevent this from occurring (Trigg and Mohammed 2010).

Grieving process

In 1969, Elisabeth Kubler-Ross identified five stages of grief that could encompass different types of behaviour: denial and isolation, anger, bargaining, depression, and acceptance (Kubler-Ross 1989). Table 3.3 outlines this process.

Throughout the stages the person who experiences loss will attempt to find meaning, enabling adaptation to the new status quo (Neimeyer et al. 2011).The final stage is often described as acceptance, as the person comes to terms with loss, but timeframes vary considerably and may not necessarily follow any logical progression. A patient may react to bad news, such as being told that they have a heart condition after tests such as a 12-lead ECG and blood tests, in different ways, so it may be helpful to be aware of these stages. This can help the healthcare assistant to respond in a supportive and caring manner, and to suggest or offer coping strategies.

Conflict

This may occur as part of grieving or anxiety about the loss of family member or because of a diagnosis. Showing compassion and empathy to patients can help avoid conflict and where this does occur the use of good communication skills can help deescalate the situation.

Strategies to optimise psychological well-being

Many patients, particularly those with long-term conditions, can be affected psychologically by their health. It is important for healthcare assistants to ensure effective communication with their patients at all times and this can act as a signpost to help patients cope with their condition. Some patients may benefit from adopting mindfulness techniques to help them cope with their illnesses, and these techniques can then be utilised by the patients when in stressful situations such as in a healthcare environment (Coffey et al. 2010).

Communication

Effective and compassionate communication is an essential skill for all healthcare assistants. Part of this is active listening skills that will enable the patient to be clearly understood by those caring for them and can help build a therapeutic relationship (Boyd and Dare 2014). Healthcare assistants need to be able to communicate with patients in a language they understand without technical jargon as this will help reduce anxiety. Working in a multicultural and inclusive society will inevitably bring healthcare assistants into contact with patients who either do not speak English or communicate via sign language. As all patients have a right to information about their condition, and a lack of information can cause anxiety, in instances such as this the local policy should be followed regarding the use of interpreters (Boyd and Dare 2014).

Information

When providing children with information it is essential that this is done in a truthful way. If a clinical skill you are undertaking is likely to hurt then telling the child this will help to form a trusting relationship (Trigg and Mohammed 2010). Information provides a greater understanding of the procedure for children and their families and helps eliminate fear (Dawson et al. 2012). As Trigg and Mohammed (2010) point out, age friendly and accurate information is particularly important with children as their active imaginations and lack of knowledge can actually cause a greater level of fear. It should also be noted that stress can prevent retention of information in both children and adults and therefore it can be useful to repeat information to ensure it is understood and retained (Mohammed and Trigg 2010).

In addition, the person's cognitive ability will also determine how information is provided, and for those patients with learning disabilities information may need to be given in manageable chunks with the support of the key worker (Brooker and Waugh 2013). Pre-information can be helpful, to prepare the patient in advance of the procedure, for example for catheterisation. Information can allow a patient more control, choice and understanding of what is happening, which is why many of the chapters identify patient education aspects, for example peripheral cannulation. A review of Chapter 2 may also be of value.

Thus, the intent of effective communication and appropriate information is to have a patient who is aware and reassured about what is happening or going to happen.

Assessment

Careful assessment includes both communication and information; this is not just to inform, educate and gain consent, but also to ensure that all factors have been assessed, both physically and psychologically.

Trigg and Mohammed (2010) and Dawson (2012) suggest that assessing the readiness of both the parents and child to undergo any clinical skill can help the healthcare assistant to prepare them more effectively. Methods that can be used to assess readiness and prepare families could include photographs, play with actual equipment, videos of clinical areas and pre-admission clubs where available.

These methods may help identify the child's, as well as the parents', understanding and acceptance of the procedure, and allow healthcare staff to assess what strategies might be most suited to the child, for example if a child shows fear of a catheter, discuss the use of local anaesthetic gel and clinical holding (see Chapter 11).

In adults Dougherty and Lister (2011) noted the use of open questions (discussed in Chapter 2) to assess psychological care needs such, as:

- How have you been feeling since your treatment?
- What concerns you most about your health?
- What do you find helps you to relax the most?

Patient involvement

It is now embedded in healthcare that all patients have a fundamental human right to make their own decisions and participate within their own healthcare (McKinnon 2013). The exceptions to this would be those who are not deemed to have mental capacity or are of a young age (McKinnon 2014). This is particularly important in terms of gaining consent when undertaking clinical skills. Here the patient can make choices that are appropriate to their own needs, such as when a test will be undertaken or even whether to have it at all. This is very closely linked to the provision of information and all patients have the right to be fully informed in their care as well as a participant in their choices (McPeake et al. 2014).

THINK ABOUT IT

You are preparing a 13-year-old boy for a peak flow test. How could you check out his understanding of the procedure?

Timing/pacing

As mentioned earlier, ensuring that the patient has the right information and communication at the right time are important. Mitchell (2007) highlights this and points out that the healthcare assistant must ensure that the patient is not too sleepy, for example under post-procedure sedation or following an epileptic seizure, as they may not be able to fully absorb the information that is given.

This is particularly important when dealing with children, as different age ranges will be able to process information at varied rates. The healthcare assistant needs to be aware of their level of development and adjust the timing and pacing accordingly (Crowley 2014).

Pharmacological (drug-related) options

Medicines that may be used might be limited to registered nurses or doctors only; please check your local policies.

Hands et al. (2010) state that children undergoing venepuncture, can suffer from both physical and psychological stress and suggest that local anaesthetics, such as creams/gels, should be used in venepuncture and cannulation in children – which must be prescribed and administered by an authorised healthcare professional. Zempsky (2008) also discusses non-invasive needle-free local anaesthesia called iontophoresis, which uses a mild electric current to numb the area before cannulation or venepuncture. Please check your local policy about this equipment and its use.

Sedation is another pharmacological option. However it does have the side effects of patients becoming too drowsy to respond, and in research from intensive care settings it has been found that sedation can have negative long-term effects on a person's psychological health (Croxall et al. 2014).

One final option may be the use of general anaesthesia; however, this is unlikely to be used for any of the clinical skills listed and discussed within this book.

It should be noted that pharmacological options are unlikely to be within the scope of a healthcare assistant.

Table 3.4 Non-pharmacological options.

Option	Action
Massage	Can be helpful for all ages, but only if patient wishes and is not contraindicated by their condition; can reduce pain and anxiety, and increases relaxation
Guided imagery	Most effective with adults and children 8 years and over. The patient imagines a positive place or setting, e.g. playing on a beach, sitting by a gently flowing river
Relaxation	Works well with adults and older children because they can be taught to breathe slowly and relax different muscle groups; younger children can be asked to slowly blow out imaginary birthday candles; relaxation can work well with soothing music that is chosen by the patient. However, recordings that provide the sound of birds chirping, waves rolling or soft heartbeat can be very soothing to small infants
Distraction	Can be provided through reading, music, conversation or through play – specifically with children
Visualisation	Positive thoughts can dispel false or unfounded fears, and similar to guided imagery, patient thinks of a personal positive situation
Hypnosis	Helps to reduce pain perception and aids relaxation. Should only be attempted by a trained hypnotherapist

Adapted from Brooker and Waugh (2013) and Trigg and Mohammed (2010).

Non-pharmacological options

There are several options for patients to utilise before, during and after any treatment or tests. Trigg and Mohammed (2010) suggest the use of distraction, guided imagery and visualisation, and relaxation techniques. Brooker and Waugh (2013) suggest that similar strategies can be employed by adults, which may include relaxation, distraction, hypnosis, imagery and massage where appropriate for the patient's condition. Table 3.4 lists the options.

Therapeutic sense of self

Mitchell (2007) describes this as the beneficial effects that the presence of a healthcare worker, such as an assistant, can have on a patient, especially in the acute care setting. This is due to the support and reassurance that a healthcare assistant can provide, offering supportive, positive communications and providing some coping strategies; for example, a patient with a fear of needles before sampling (venepuncture) is supported by the healthcare assistant using a breathing technique and topical local anaesthetic gel. Having a partner or friend present while waiting can help ease anxiety and, in some cases, such as children or a patient with a learning disability, being present (if willing and it is suitable) during a procedure may also help. With children, a parent can hold the child while the procedure is carried out, for example insertion of a peripheral cannula or blood being sampled from a finger for blood sugar testing. The presence of a friend, parent or family member can often reassure, and make the person, especially a child, feel safe. Walker et al. (2012) noted the importance of social support, which offers a sense of belonging gained from family and friends.

This aspect should not be overlooked, and it is often the presence of a health-care assistant, or any other healthcare staff, that is of great benefit to the patient's psychological well-being. It is also good practice with many invasive procedures; acting as a chaperone and being able to answer questions, or just *being there*, can be a huge relief to an anxious patient.

Instrumental support

Walker et al. (2012) suggest that this is about offering practical and tangible support. This could include signposting them to self-help groups where patients can receive support to take control of their own health. The healthcare assistant should also be wary about offering advice as it is essential that patients make their own decisions around healthcare or patients can become passive in managing their own conditions.

Common problems

As noted earlier by Mitchell (2007), when the patient's physical needs are met, but their emotional and psychological ones are not, holistic care is not being provided. The patient may not respond to treatment or communications in the manner expected (Walker et al. 2012). The patient's feeling of loss or anxiety may lead to unexpected behaviours, which could cause disruption in a healthcare setting, for example coping with anger can be threatening to the healthcare assistant and others because this behaviour, if not handled effectively, may escalate into verbal or physical aggression where knowledge of conflict resolution would be advantageous. Likewise, the patient who withdraws due to confusion or fear will also pose a challenge to all healthcare staff, and effectively care, compassion and communication are essential.

Staff may lack confidence in assessing psychological needs, but by use of open questions, as suggested by Dougherty and Lister (2011), the healthcare assistant can invite patients to discuss any fears or concerns that they have. From this initial dialogue, the patient, together with the healthcare assistant, can identify what strategies are available and suitable. An associated aspect is recording this information, because many staff may not recognise documentation as an essential part of practice (Skills for Care & Skills for Health 2013). This is an area where the healthcare assistant must ensure good practice and record any communications promptly and clearly. These should be factual reports and not contain subjective statements.

Summary

This chapter has a narrow focus of just clinical skills; we acknowledge this and suggest that the reader explores wider aspects of psychological care. It is not within the scope of this book to explore mental health issues, but further reading around this area may be beneficial to your practise as a healthcare assistant and ultimately patient care.

   If you do not know the patient, some mental health symptoms may be 'masked' or hidden by the process of admission and undergoing procedures, particularly invasive ones such as peripheral cannulation (inserting a cannula). If you have any concerns about your patient's psychological well-being, always seek advice from a registered practitioner.

CASE STUDY 3.1

Mr Helmut Jung has been admitted as an emergency with chest pain, while on holiday from Germany. He is 66 years old and seems to speak reasonable English. His wife is back at the hotel, calling his family in Hamburg and gathering his medicines and nightclothes. He is in pain and very anxious.

   You have been asked to prepare him for a standard 12-lead ECG procedure. What aspects would you need to consider to help prepare him psychologically?

You do not need to understand the actual procedure of recording a standard 12-lead ECG for this task. This asks you to consider the situation and the psychological preparation required.

Self-assessment		
Assessment	**Aspects**	**Achieved ✓**
Psychological care	*Have you considered all aspects of this section?*	
	Patient assessment	
	Psychological factors	
	Coping strategies	
	Problems and reporting concerns	

References

Boyd C and Dare J (2014) *Communication Skills for Nurses*. Chichester: John Wiley & Sons.

Brooker C and Waugh A (2013) *Foundations of Nursing Practice: Fundamentals of Holistic Care*. Oxford: Mosby.

Clancy J and McVicar A (2009) *Physiology and Anatomy for Nurses and Healthcare Practitioners: A Homeostatic Approach*. London: Hodder Arnold.

Coffey K, Hartman M and Fredrickson B (2010) Deconstructing mindfulness and constructing mental health: understanding mindfulness and its mechanisms of action. *Mindfulness* 1: 235.

Crowley, K (2014) *Child Development: A Practical Introduction*. Los Angeles: Sage.

Croxall C, Tyas, M. and Garside J (2014) Sedation and its psychological effects following intensive care. *British Journal of Nursing* 23(14): 800–804.

Dawson P (2012) *Oxford Handbook of Clinical Skills for Children's and Young People's Nursing*. Oxford: Oxford University Press.

Department of Health (DH) (2012) Compassion in Practice: Nursing, Midwifery and Care Staff. Our Vision and Strategy. Available at: www.commissioningboard.nhs.uk (accessed December 2015).

Department of Health (DH) (2013) *The NHS Constitution*. London: Department of Health.

Dougherty L and Lister S (eds) (2011) *The Royal Marsden Hospital Manual of Clinical Nursing*. Oxford: Wiley-Blackwell.

Francis R (2013) *Report of the Mid Staffordshire NHS Foundation Trust Public Inquiry*. London: The Stationary Office.

French D, Vedhara K, Kaptein A and Weinman J.(2010) *Health Psychology*, 2nd edn. Chichester: Blackwell.

Hands C, Rounds J and Thomas J (2010) Evaluating venepuncture practice on a general children's ward. *Paediatric Nursing* 22(2): 32–35.

Howard J (2013) *The Essence of Play. A Practice Companion for Professionals Working with Children and Young People*. London: Routledge.

Kubler-Ross E (1989) *On Death and Dying*. London: Routledge.

Maslow A (1943) A theory of human motivation. *Psychological Review* 50: 370–396.

McKinnon J (2013) The case for concordance: value and application in nursing practice. *British Journal of Nursing* 22(13): 776–771.

McKinnon J (2014) Pursuing concordance: moving away from paternalism. *British Journal of Nursing* 23(12): 677–684.

McPeake J, Quasim T and Daniel M (2014) User involvement: beyond the tick-box. *British Journal of Nursing* 23(14): 810.

Mendes da Mata A. (2014) Psychology in nursing: an inherent part of practice and care. *British Journal of Nursing* 23(17): 951.

Mitchell M (2007) Psychological care of patients undergoing elective surgery. *Nursing Standard* 21(30): 48–55.

Nazarko L (2014) Dementia series 2: how dementia affects the ability to communicate. *British Journal of Healthcare Assistants* 8(12): 614–619.

Neimeyer R, Harris D, Thornton G and Winokeur, H (2011) *Grief and Bereavement in Contemporary Society: Bridging Research and Practice*. London: Routledge.

Renouf T, Leary A and Wiseman T (2014) Do psychological interventions reduce preoperative anxiety? *British Journal of Nursing* 23(22): 1208–1212.

Roper N, Logan W and Tierney A. (1985) *The Elements of Nursing*, 2nd edn. Edinburgh: Churchill Livingstone.

Skills for Care & Skills for Health (2013) Code of Conduct for Healthcare Support Workers and Adult Social Care Workers in England. Available at: www.skillsforhealth.org.uk (accessed December 2015).

Solowiej K (2010) Pain induced stress in wound care- part 1. *British Journal of Healthcare Assistants* 4(8): 384–386.

Stonehouse D (2014) Support workers have a vital role to play in play. *British Journal of Healthcare Assistants* 8(3): 137–139.

Taylor S (2009) *Introduction to Health Psychology*. New York: McGraw-Hill.

Trigg E and Mohammed T (2010) *Practices in Children's Nursing: Guidelines for Hospital and Community*. Edinburgh: Churchill Livingstone.

Walker J, Payne S, Jarrett N and Lay, T (2012) *Psychology for Nurses and the Caring Professions*, 4th edn. Maidenhead: Open University Press.

Williams A (2013) A toolkit to assess first impressions of healthcare. *Nursing Times* 109 online issue: 1–2.

Zempsky W (2008) Pharmacological approaches for reducing venous access pain in children. *Paediatrics* 122 supplement 3: S.140–153.

CHAPTER 4

Documentation and record keeping

LEARNING OBJECTIVES

- Identify why accurate and prompt records are essential
- Outline the standards for good record keeping
- Discuss the types of documentation in relation to clinical skills
- Describe legal requirements in relation to record keeping

Aim of this chapter

The aim of this chapter is to explore the standards required for patient documentation and record keeping, focusing on records and documentation relating to clinical skills, such as recording observations on the T, P, R (temperature, pulse and respiration) chart. The importance of recording and maintaining accurate and prompt records along with legal aspects are also discussed.

The importance and purpose of documentation in relation to clinical skills

Beach and Oates (2104) describe health records as documented evidence about the care and treatment patients receive, including care plans. They are not only written communications between colleagues about patients and evidence of care, but are also clinical tools, enabling continuity of care and the setting of goals and plans to deliver care. From a governance and commissioning perspective, health records also provide evidence that care is meeting quality and safety standards set and monitored by regulators in addition to the contractual requirements set by commissioners (Unite the Union 2014).

As a member of the wider healthcare team, the healthcare assistant (HCA) and assistant practitioner (AP) or student nurse is personally accountable for good record keeping so that they can document their care. The HCA or AP should only be delegated a task if they fully understand what is being asked of them,

---

Clinical Skills for Healthcare Assistants and Assistant Practitioners, Second Edition.
Angela Whelan and Elaine Hughes.
© 2016 John Wiley & Sons, Ltd. Published 2016 by John Wiley & Sons, Ltd.

Table 4.1 Examples of records.

Poor example	Good example
Upset today	Patient states: 'feeling upset'
Appears depressed	Patient says: 'I am concerned about my treatment and how it will affect me'

Source: Adapted from Dougherty 2011. Reproduced with permission of Wiley Blackwell.

they have had relevant training, are competent and the task is within their scope of practice. The Code (NMC 2015) emphasises the responsibility of registered nurses when delegating tasks. Furthermore, in relation to record keeping and documentation, the Code (NMC 2015: 9) states that to keep clear and accurate records you must:

10.1 complete all records at the time or as soon as possible after an event, recording if the notes are written some time after the event
10.2 identify any risks or problems that have arisen and the steps taken to deal with them, so that colleagues who use the records have all the information they need
10.3 complete all records accurately and without any falsification, taking immediate and appropriate action if you become aware that someone has not kept to these requirements
10.4 attribute any entries you make in any paper or electronic records to yourself, making sure they are clearly written, dated and timed, and do not include unnecessary abbreviations, jargon or speculation
10.5 take all steps to make sure that all records are kept securely, and
10.6 collect, treat and store all data and research findings appropriately.

In relation to clinical skills, records are maintained in order that a patient's condition can be observed and monitored, for example the record of a patient with diabetes would contain information about blood sugar levels in the urine or blood. These ongoing records, at defined times such as before meals, will allow the patient to receive the correct treatment. In a person with diabetes, this might be to adjust the dose of insulin that the patient receives. Hutson and Millar (2009) and NMC (2015) emphasise that record keeping should not be viewed as something that is done if time allows and that they should be written as soon as possible after the procedure. Recording vital signs such as temperature, pulse and blood pressure can determine future actions. The HCA or AP must understand why these particular signs have to be checked and recorded. A blood pressure record may be 'routine' as part of a general observation of the patient's condition; which is different from a patient returning from major surgery, where a change in blood pressure may indicate an internal bleed.

As noted above, records ensure that members of the healthcare team are aware of what is happening to that patient, of any treatment(s) that they are receiving, and the effects – both positive and negative – for example, whether analgesia (pain medication) has reduced pain or not. The NMC (2015: 9) states you must keep clear and accurate records relevant to your practice and you must attribute any entries you make in paper or electronic records to yourself, making sure they are clearly written, dated and timed, and do not include unnecessary abbreviations, jargon or speculation. Hutson and Millar (2009) point out that individual Trusts and organisations may have their own local policy about which abbreviations can be used. Care should be taken, however, as any mistakes in their meaning may have serious repercussions. Beach and Oates (2014) suggest writing should be clear and succinct, in short sentences using simple words and sticking to the facts.

Effective records allow staff to monitor patients over 24-hour periods for every day that they receive healthcare (NMC 2015). If a patient was suffering from chest pain and part of the care was to have the patient's vital signs observed (e.g. temperature, pulse and respiratory rate), and they received an analgesic, monitoring can help develop a picture of the patient's response to the treatment. Thus, if the pain were not responding to the analgesic, the pulse and respiratory rate could remain elevated, showing the potential need for more analgesia. Only through keeping accurate records and reviewing them on an ongoing basis can healthcare staff provide the most effective and responsive care possible. Dougherty and Lister (2011) emphasise that documents help in assessing patients and can hold a baseline (a reading that acts as a reference for future readings) of data, for example BP, and allow ongoing monitoring of a patient's condition and needs. This is crucial as a patient's condition can be unpredictable and complex.

Dougherty and Lister (2011) identified examples of subjective statements in records (Table 4.1).

One of the challenges in healthcare is the variety of staff involved in any one patient's care and the fact that the information each person needs to carry out their role varies; this means confidentiality must be considered. The Data Protection Act 1998 and the Freedom of Information Act (FOIA) 2005 are important, and healthcare assistants must be aware of the impact that these acts have on their role. It is important to remember that the Data Protection Act 1998 gives patients the right to access personal information held about them. Hutson and Millar (2009) point out that confidentiality, security and access to records are governed by legislation not only from the UK but also from the European Convention on Human Rights. The various legislation is incorporated within local policies, therefore it is important to read these and be aware of when and to whom information is made available or withheld.

Information sharing is vital to safeguarding and promoting the welfare of children and young people. A key factor identified in many serious case reviews (SCRs) has been a failure by practitioners to record information, to share it, to understand its significance and then take appropriate action. In March 2015, HM Government produced non-statutory advice – Information Sharing Advice for Practitioners Providing Safeguarding Services to Children, Young People,

Parents and Carers to support practitioners in the decisions they take when sharing information to reduce the risk of harm to children and young people. Please check your local policies relating to safeguarding, documentation and information sharing.

Confidentiality in records and documentation

Healthcare assistants must always be aware that information might be accessed by the patient and in some cases friends or visitors – for example via the TPR chart as it is often hanging on a patient's bed or wall. When patients are being admitted, they should be informed that data (their personal details) is shared with other members of the healthcare team where relevant to ensure that they receive the best care possible.

The patient should be reassured that these confidential notes are kept safe and, with the development of computerisation, given added reassurance that these are password protected, so only staff who have authorisation can access their records. Always consider the security of this information: do not leave a patient's records (e.g. nursing or case notes) lying around or walk away from a computer if it is on and still open at a patient record. Check what documents can be left safely at a patient's bedside, such as a urine chart or peak flow chart. *Please check your local policy.*

Improper use of social media, especially Facebook, is leading to disciplinary action against staff at a number of English trusts. Figures released to Guardian Healthcare show that 72 separate actions were taken by 16 trusts against staff that inappropriately used social media between 2008–09 and October 2011. The data, released in response to freedom of information (FoI) requests, reveals Facebook to be the main medium for misdemeanors. The largest number of incidents took place in 2010–11, indicating the growing use of social media and the difficulties it presents to the NHS.

THINK ABOUT IT

Consider who needs the patient records and why they are necessary.

Types of documentation

The key aspect with regard to documentation is to *check your local practice area* and identify what is deemed acceptable and has been approved. In relation to clinical skills, focus would be on charts for recording TPR, urinalysis, peak flow, blood glucose levels, faecal occult blood (FOB) tests and patient care plan/case notes for recording, for example, peripheral intravenous cannulation: date, time, site, cannula gauge, reason for insertion, any issues and signature. The standard 12-lead ECG record is often noted on the recording itself and stored securely within the patient's record – local variations may apply. *Always check your local policy.*

Another type of documentation that may be used is a care pathway or integrated care pathway (ICP). The development of clinical protocols, care pathways, patient-held records or shared documentation emerged to help improve the patient's experience of care and service delivery. Dougherty and Lister (2011) noted that these offer a consistent method of assessment, which enables communication among the various healthcare staff. Beach and Oates (2014) identify that the aim of a care plan is to enable the team providing care, as well as the author of the plan, to meet the assessed needs or goals of the person receiving care. The care plan needs to be current, accurate and evidence based, with SMART (specific, measurable, achievable, realistic and timed) objectives (refer to Figure 4.1 for an example).

The chapters in Section 2 of this book explore a range of clinical skills; within each there is a review of the knowledge and skills necessary to perform the procedure(s) (clinical skill(s)) safely and competently. All require competent record keeping.

THINK ABOUT IT

What clinical skills will you be required to undertake? Consider what types of records or documentation you will need to maintain in your practice area.

Legal aspects relating to documentation

The underpinning principle in record keeping is that *if it has not been recorded, it has not been done*. Documentation and records are therefore essential legal documents that should record and support individual actions, while maintaining a conversation between the multidisciplinary team about the patient. The Department of Health (DH 2006) stipulates that all individuals who work for NHS organisations are responsible for any records they create or use in the performance of their duties. Furthermore, any record an individual creates is a public record. Dimond (2011) states a legal document is 'any document requested by the court', which includes patient records. Therefore it is essential to follow local policy and ensure documentation is accurate and of the highest standard possible. Local policies about record keeping and documentation should reflect relevant legislation and regulations as well as national and regional/organisational policy. Local policy should also reflect the national policies on information governance, confidentiality, information security, records management and the NHS constitution (DH 2003, 2006, 2007, 2013a, 2013b).

Integrated Care Pathway for the Management of Diabetes in the Perioperative Period	UHD, NHS Lothian Addressograph or Name Dob Address
Site : RIE □ WGH □ St Johns □	Unit number CHI

INSTRUCTIONS *Insert information into appropriate spaces as required & complete 'Initial Key'*
Do not initial until actually done!

This ICP is an action checklist & a clinical record & requires a Kardex & SEWS chart

---

Date initiated: ___/___/___   **PRE-ASSESSMENT CLINIC**

PROPOSED DATE OF SURGERY   ...../......./.......

Type of Diabetes Type 1   □ Type 2 □   Usual treatment: Insulin □   Tablet(s) □   Diet □

HbA1c □   result..................: if HbA1c > 9%, discuss with Diabetes Specialist Nurse

Anaesthetist aware that patient has Diabetes Mellitus   □

Ensure patient is first on the list when possible   □
                             To be **Nil By Mouth** from:.......... on............

Patient on Metformin Yes   □, No □   To be stopped on ..../........./.......

To be commenced on:
    SHORT Fast: when immediate post-operative resumption of oral intake is likely   □
    LONG Fast: when immediate resumption of oral intake after surgery not planned   □

Information leaflets provided   □

DATE OF SURGERY   ...../......./....... **Peri-operative SHORT Fast**

When immediate post-operative resumption of oral intake is likely following protocol may be used

	initial
Omit breakfast & morning dose of insulin (and oral hypoglycaemic agents, if taking these) □	
Check blood glucose hourly from 8am □	
If blood glucose remains between 5–12 mmol/l, no action □	
If blood glucose is above 12 mmol/l, consider intravenous insulin □	
See Intravenous Insulin protocol sheet.	

DATE OF SURGERY   ...../......./....... **Peri-operative LONG Fast**
        The following protocol should be used for major surgery, when immediate resumption of oral
                               intake after surgery is not planned:

	initial
The patient should be first on the operation list (preferably am) □	
Omit breakfast & morning dose of insulin (and oral hypoglycaemic agents if taking these) □ [**Note**: oral hypoglycaemic agents = OHA]	
Intravenous Insulin regime □	
Time of commencement of Intravenous insulin: 8am □, or, on arrival in theatre □	

              Note any Variances from Pathway with 'VAR' & explain fully

Name *sign*		*print*	initial
Profession	designation	date	

Figure 4.1 The diabetic care pathway. Source: Reproduced with kind permission of Suzanne Delaney, Diabetic Nurse Specialist, NHS Lothian.

Those working in regulated care settings, such as care homes, should adhere to the standards set by the relevant regulator. In England, care is regulated by the Care Quality Commission under the Health and Social Care Act 2008 (Regulated Activities) Regulations 2010, and in Scotland care is regulated by Health Care Improvement Scotland. Regulation 20 of the Health and Social Care Act 2008 (Regulated Activities) Regulations 2010 stipulates, 'that service users are protected against the risks of unsafe or inappropriate care and treatment arising from a lack of proper information about them by means of the maintenance of an accurate record in respect of each service user, which shall include appropriate information and documents in relation to the care and treatment provided to each service user'. Effectively this means that whether you work within or outwith the NHS, record keeping and documentation must be of a high standard.

Caldicott Guardians was set up within the NHS to oversee access to patient identifiable information and should be seen as the gatekeeper for patient information held within a healthcare setting (Hutson and Millar 2009). In England, Wales and Northern Ireland this role is mandatory and is usually undertaken by a senior clinician, but it is only advisory in Scotland. This person is also responsible for the protection of and uses of patient identifiable information by staff, and for the developing and monitoring policies of interagency disclosure. The Caldicott principles (Department of Health 2013a) are

1 Justify the purposes.
2 Don't use personal confidential data unless it is absolutely necessary.
3 Use the minimum necessary personal confidential data.
4 Access to personal confidential data should be on a strict need-to-know basis.
5 Everyone with access to personal confidential data should be aware of their responsibilities.
6 Comply with the law.
7 The duty to share information can be as important as the duty to protect patient confidentiality.

THINK ABOUT IT

Who is designated to release patient records in your organisation? If a patient asks to see their documents, what is your local policy and what would you do?

Beach and Oates (2014) also highlight that clinical records have been discussed in several recent serious case reviews and public inquiries, including the reviews of NHS complaints (Clywd and Hart 2013); the Liverpool Care Pathway (Neuberger 2013); the reviews of care at the University Hospitals of Morecambe Bay NHS Foundation Trust (Care Quality Commission (CQC) 2012) and Mid Staffordshire NHS Foundation Trust (Mid Staffordshire NHS Foundation Trust Inquiry 2010; Francis 2013) – all of which related poor practice to poor record keeping, including incomplete and inconsistent records, inaccurate recording of patient information and discussions with patients and families, and poor recording of transfer information.

Common problems

The quality of nursing documentation has consistently been found to be failing to meet recommended standards (Prideaux 2011). Bridget Dimond (2011) has noted the following common errors in record keeping:

- Date, time and signature omitted.
- Inaccuracies/lack of name, date of birth, address, NHS number.
- Lack of evidence of discussions/agreement with patient.
- Illegible handwriting.
- Lack of entry in the record when an abortive call/visit has been made.
- Ambiguous abbreviations.
- Record of phone calls (e.g. to social services) that omitted the name and designation of the recipient (e.g. social worker).
- Covering up errors.
- Absence of relevant information.
- Inaccuracies, especially of date.
- Delay in completing the record, sometimes more than 24 hours have elapsed before the records are completed.
- Record completed by someone who did not deliver the care.
- Unprofessional terminology, for example 'dull as a doorstep'.
- Meaningless phrases, such as 'lovely child', 'appears', 'slept well', 'encouraged'.
- Opinion mixed with facts.
- Reliance on information from others without identifying the source.
- Subjective not objective comments, for example 'normal development'.
- Main dataset fields on the Patient Administration System (PAS) incomplete.

Related aspects and terminology

The main areas of concern in relation to information governance are consent, information sharing and confidentiality (Beach and Oates 2014). Therefore it might be useful at this point to revisit Chapter 4 and then consider this terminology in relation to your record keeping and documentation.

Strategies to improve standards of record keeping

Electronic records and standardised approach

Both unitary (single) patient records and electronic formats are becoming the 'norm', which has the potential to standardise format, minimising confusion, giving uniformity and allowing staff to record information in a recognisable way that is easy to locate and act upon (Dougherty and Lister 2011; Beach and Oates 2014). This approach allows information to be shared, reducing duplication and repetition, which is better for the patient who does not have to repeat name, address, DOB, and so on over and over. Another advantage of electronic records is that they can be shared promptly across healthcare teams, for example a GP can send a patient's records when they are being admitted to hospital. This can allow data to be compared, for example the peak flow record of a patient with asthma will allow staff to monitor and observe changes (e.g. deterioration from home/baseline) and response to treatment (Dougherty and Lister 2011). Beach and Oates (2014), however, emphasise the importance of not sharing passwords and logging out of computers following use.

Good time-management skills

Time constraints and workload are often cited as reasons for poor documentation; as previously stated, the recording of care is an integral part of care, not an add on, using and developing good time-management skills will help to allocate time for documentation.

Cultural change

The UK Government's health information strategy (DH 2012), arising from the 'no decision about me without me' approach (DH 2010), reflects the move away from healthcare providers being in sole control towards a more involved approach including patients and service users in decisions about their health and care. As of 2015, GP practices offer patients access to online services, communication with the practice and personal records (Royal College of General Practitioners (RCGP) 2013).

Audit and education/training

Regularly auditing documentation acts as an incentive for staff to maintain a good standard of record keeping and also provides evidence of areas of poor practice so that measures can be taken to improve performance. Education and training are important, organisations need to ensure that staff know what to do and are giving adequate training to enable them to do the job

---

THINK ABOUT IT

How could you audit your records? What formal audit process and tools does your organisation use relating to record keeping?

Summary

Record keeping is not something separate from clinical care but is the documented reflection of the care provided, and together they co-exist and are

Table 4.2 Competency framework: record keeping.

Competency	First assessment/reassessment					Date/competent signature
Steps	**Demonstration/supervised practice**					
Record keeping	Date/signed 1	Date/signed 2	Date/signed 3	Date/signed 4	Date/signed 5	
Information was						
1 Held securely and confidentially						
2 Obtained fairly and efficiently						
3 Recorded accurately and reliably						
4 Used effectively and ethically						
5 Shared appropriately and lawfully						
Supervisors/Assessor(s):						

Source: Hutchinson 2006. Reproduced with permission of RCN Publishing Company.

integral to holistic practice (Prideaux 2011). Healthcare assistants and assistant practitioners must recognise the importance of good documentation and record keeping. Very simply, to conclude and sum up this chapter: health records should demonstrate and be a part of high-quality patient care.

Hutchinson and Sharples (2006) described a model called HORUS, indicated within the NHS's Connecting for Health, which is used as the basis for a competency checklist (Table 4.2).

CASE STUDY 4.1

John Simms is a healthcare assistant in your team. He reports to you that he was recording Mr Jung's urinalysis results in his records when he realised that he had written this information in the wrong record. He has been working in your clinical area for only six weeks and is unsure what he should do. What would you advise?

Self-assessment

Assessment	Aspects	Achieved ✓
Records	Have you considered all aspects of this section? Purpose and importance of accurate records Access to and completion of appropriate records Types of documentation in practice area Ensuring security and safety of information	
Patient	Have you considered all aspects of this section? Consent aspects Confidentiality Patient education, e.g. access to health records	**Achieved ✓**

References

Beach J and Oates J (2014) Maintaining best practice in record-keeping and documentation. *Nursing Standard* 28(36): 45–50.

Care Quality Commission (2012) *Investigation Report. University Hospitals of Morecambe Bay NHS Foundation Trust*. London: CQC.

Clwyd A and Hart T (2013) *A Review of the NHS Hospitals Complaints System: Putting Patients Back in the Picture*. London: The Stationery Office.

Department of Health (DH) (2003) *Confidentiality: NHS Code of Practice*. London: The Stationery Office.

Department of Health (DH) (2006) *Records Management: NHS Code of Practice, Parts 1–2*. London: The Stationary Office.

Department of Health (DH) (2007) *NHS Information Governance: Guidance on Legal and Professional Obligations*. London: The Stationery Office.

Department of Health (DH) (2010) *Equity and Excellence: Liberating the NHS*. London: The Stationery Office.

Department of Health (DH) (2012) *The Power of Information: Putting All of Us in Control of the Health and Care Information We Need*. London: The Stationery Office.

Department of Health (DH) (2013a) *Information: To Share or Not to Share. The Information Governance Review*. London: The Stationery Office.

Department of Health (DH) (2013b) *The NHS Constitution for England*. London: The Stationery Office.

Dimond B (2011) *Legal Aspects of Nursing*, 6th edn. Harlow: Pearson Education Limited.

Dougherty L and Lister S (eds) (2011) *The Royal Marsden Hospital Manual of Clinical Nursing Procedures*, student edn. Oxford: Blackwell Publishing.

Francis R (2013) *Report of the Mid Staffordshire NHS Foundation Trust Public Inquiry: Executive Summary*. London: The Stationery Office.

Hand T and Casey A (2012) Delegating Record Keeping and Countersigning. Royal College of Nursing Records. Available at http://www.rcn.org.uk/__data/assets/pdf_file/0003/472719/Delegating_and_countersigning_records 2012.pdf (accessed 26 March 2015).

The Health and Social Care Act 2008 (Regulated Activities) Regulations (2010) Available at: www.legislation.gov.uk/search?title=The+Health+and+Social+Care+Act+2008+%28Regulated+Activities%29+Regulations+2010&year=&number=&type=uksi (accessed April 2015).

HM Government (2015) *Information Sharing Advice for Practitioners Providing Safeguarding Services to Children, Young People, Parents and Carers*. Crown copyright, London.

Hutson M and Millar N (2009) Recording keeping. In: Iggulden H, MacDonald C and Staniland K (eds) *Clinical Skills. The Essence of Caring*. London: McGraw Hill, pp. 27–54.

Hutchinson C and Sharples C (2006) Information governance: practical implications for record-keeping. *Nursing Standard* 20(36): 59–64.

Mid Staffordshire NHS Foundation Trust Inquiry (2010) *Independent Inquiry into Care Provided by Mid Staffordshire NHS Foundation Trust*. January 2005 – March 2009. Volume I. London: The Stationery Office.

Neuberger J (2013) *More Care, Less Pathway: A Review of the Liverpool Care Pathway*. London: The Stationery Office.

Nursing and Midwifery Council (NMC) (2009) *Record Keeping – Guidance for Nurses and Midwives*. London: NMC.

Nursing and Midwifery Council (NMC) (2015) *The Code Professional Standards of Practice and Behaviour for Nurses and Midwives*. London: NMC.

Prideaux A (2011) Issues in documentation and record-keeping. *British Journal of Nursing* 20(22): 1450–1454.

Royal College of Nurses (RCN) (2012) Record Keeping (online) Available at: http://www.rcn.org.uk/development/health_care_support_workers/professional_issues/record_keeping (accessed April 2015).

Royal College of General Practitioners (2013) *Patient Online: The Road Map*. London: RCGP.

Unite the Union (2014) *Record Keeping and Documentation: A Guide for Health Professionals*. London: Unite the Union.

SECTION II
Core clinical skills

CHAPTER 5

Pulse

LEARNING OBJECTIVES

- Define what a pulse is
- Explain how a pulse is initiated by the heart
- List the different locations where a pulse can be felt
- Identify common factors that can affect the pulse rate

Aim of this chapter

The aim of this chapter is to understand how a pulse is generated and felt within the body, the common sites and factors influencing its rate, rhythm and amplitude (strength).

What is a pulse?

A pulse can be felt where an artery is near the surface of the body and lies over a bone or another firm background. A pulse is the rhythmic expansion of the artery wall as it is stretched by a wave of blood that is pumped through the vessels with each heartbeat (Waugh and Grant 2010; Thibodeau and Patton 2007; Rawlings-Anderson and Hunter 2008). The heartbeat occurs when the ventricle of the heart (see 'Relevant anatomy and physiology') pumps blood into the aorta, which is already full with blood, and then into the arterial system (Maddex 2009). In normal cardiovascular health, one heartbeat corresponds to one pulse beat (Maddex 2009).

Reasons for performing a pulse reading

A pulse rate is often requested as part of 'routine' observations. It can be taken as a baseline (a reading taken that acts as a reference for future readings), to monitor changes in a patient's condition (e.g. after surgical intervention) or to check that medication is working correctly (e.g. after administration of a medication to correct an abnormal heartbeat (Marieb and Hoehn 2007).

Clinical Skills for Healthcare Assistants and Assistant Practitioners, Second Edition.
Angela Whelan and Elaine Hughes.
© 2016 John Wiley & Sons, Ltd. Published 2016 by John Wiley & Sons, Ltd.

Relevant anatomy and physiology

The pulse is strongest in the arteries closest to the heart, becoming weaker in the arterioles and then disappearing altogether in the capillaries (Tortora and Derrickson 2011). The most common location for taking a pulse reading is the radial site (located inside of the wrist and underneath the thumb). It is often the first choice because many patients are familiar with this site and it is easily accessible and non-invasive. However the choice of site will often vary with the patient and the presenting clinical situation. If the patient was acutely unwell, perhaps with a condition that reduces blood volume – such as shock, haemorrhage or a collapse with unknown cause – a pulse may not be easy to palpate at sites away from the heart because blood will be directed to the major organs. In such instances the radial pulse may be weak or difficult to find and the carotid or femoral site would be more appropriate (Figure 5.1). In children under the age of 2 the heartbeat is usually auscultated (listened to) via a stethoscope at the apex of the heart. In adulthood the apex can be located on patients' left-sided chest wall in the space between the fifth and sixth ribs (fifth intercostal space) on a line with the midpoint of the left clavicle (collar bone) (Herbert and Sheppard 2005) (Figure 5.1). In children up to the age of 7 the location of the apex beat can be found at the fourth intercostal space (Kyle 2008). Listening to the apex is deemed more appropriate because the vessel walls in neonates and infants are not fully developed, making palpation difficult. However, it is good practice in children's nursing to check for the presence of the brachial pulse (Ball and Bindler 2008). Pulses in the lower legs are usually palpated only when assessing the circulation (flow of blood) to the limbs, which may be affected by vascular problems or after surgery or trauma to the limbs (Maddex 2009).

In some patients locating a pulse may prove challenging, despite them being clinically well. This can be due to slightly unusual anatomy or the presence of cardiovascular disease. It is also a skill that can prove difficult initially and practise is recommended, especially when accessing the carotid pulse, because locating this may be necessary in an emergency situation.

THINK ABOUT IT

Ask your friends and family if you can practise taking their pulse at various sites. Note the difference in the pulses, including the rate, rhythm and strength (amplitude). Is there anything that might be causing these differences?

The heart generates an electrical impulse that causes it to contract (the muscles within the heart structure shorten and pulls inwards, compressing the chambers). Figure 5.2 shows the important structures involved in generating this impulse. The sinoatrial (SA) node is often described as the natural 'pacemaker' of the heart because it initiates impulses of contraction (Waugh and Grant

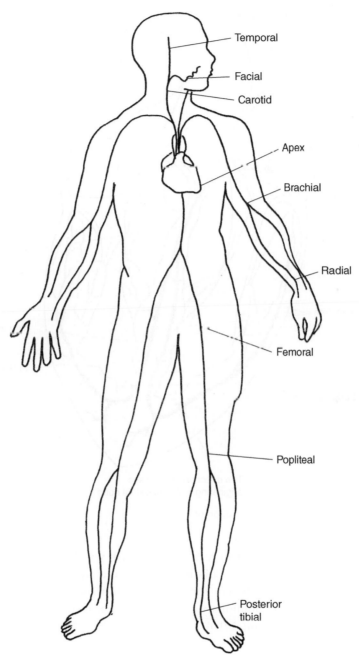

Figure 5.1 Sites for taking a pulse.

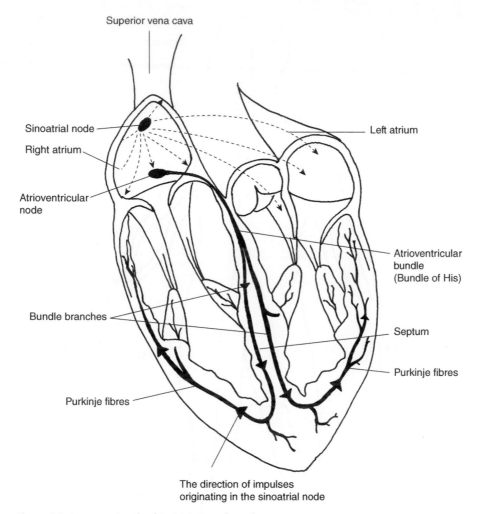

Superior vena cava

Sinoatrial node

Right atrium

Left atrium

Atrioventricular node

Atrioventricular bundle (Bundle of His)

Bundle branches

Septum

Purkinje fibres

Purkinje fibres

The direction of impulses originating in the sinoatrial node

Figure 5.2 Structure involved in initiation of a pulse.

2010). This causes the atria (Figure 5.2) to contract, which then stimulates the atrioventricular (AV) node. The Purkinje fibres then convey this impulse to the apex of the myocardium, where the wave of ventricular contraction begins pumping blood into the pulmonary artery and aorta, resulting in a heartbeat and pulse (Waugh and Grant 2010).

Related aspects and terminology

Maddex (2009) suggests that the following be considered when obtaining a pulse.

The rate of the pulse

This indicates the frequency of contraction of the left ventricle and is affected by age, exercise, stress, injury and disease. In acute practice patients may have hypovolaemic shock, which is a circulatory disturbance where there is usually a reduction in blood volume. This leads to a rapid, thready pulse which is a characteristic sign of shock (Scales and Pilsworth 2008; Boulanger and Toghill 2009).

The amplitude

This indicates the strength of the ventricular contractions. A weak contraction may not generate a pulse at the limbs (peripheral) or, if present, it may be weak. It can also occur when there is a lack of blood volume, for example if the patient is bleeding heavily or dehydrated. Where a full and bounding pulse is felt, this may be indicative of complications such as anaemia, heart failure or the early stages of septic shock (Jevon and Ewens 2007).

The rhythm

The rhythm of the pulse is determined by assessing the regularity of the pressure waves from the heart and can assist in establishing whether the heart is beating regularly (Rawlings-Anderson and Hunter 2008). In health, the heartbeats with regular coordinated contractions, which is referred to as sinus rhythm (Marieb and Hoehn 2007). An irregular pulse can be caused by problems in the heart's conduction system, such as atrial fibrillation where the chambers of heart fails to contract together (Marieb and Hoehn 2007).

When listened to through a stethoscope, the sound of the heartbeat comes primarily from blood turbulence caused by closing of the heart valves, although only the first two are loud enough to be heard through a stethoscope (Tortora and Derrickson 2010). The sounds are heard as 'lubb dupp', followed by a pause, with the pause interval reducing when the pulse increases (Tortora and Derrickson 20101).

POINT FOR PRACTICE

As anxiety can increase the pulse rate, before taking a pulse try to ensure that the patient is as relaxed as possible. Ensure that the patient is fully informed as to why the pulse is being taken and give reassurance if necessary. If the patient is unduly anxious, consider a delay to provide them with time to settle into the surroundings and relax before the pulse is recorded

---

Factors affecting the pulse rate

Pulse rates can alter due to many factors, both physical and psychological, and may indicate conditions that are life threatening, for example cardiac arrest, or long-term cardiac conditions such as angina. Factors that increase and decrease pulse rates are the following:

- Exercise: this increases the heart rate (Marieb and Hoehn 2007).
- Anxiety: a patient's heart rate can increase due to anxiety.
- Medication: some medication can both increase and decrease heart rates.
- Trauma: the loss of blood and fluid volume causes the heart to beat faster to circulate the fluid around the body.
- Pain: this can cause an increase in heart rate.
- Infection.
- Cardiac abnormalities; for example, if atherosclerosis (build-up of plaque) is present in the arteries, this can influence the pulse rate (Maddex 2009).
- Circulation problems.
- Temperature: increased body temperature (pyrexia) will increase the pulse rate (Jevon and Ewens 2007), whereas decreased body temperature (hypothermia) will decrease it (Waugh and Grant 2010).
- Reduced consciousness: coma will decrease the pulse rate.
- Fitness: if a person is very fit, the heart becomes very efficient and a lower pulse rate can deliver the required blood to the body.
- Metabolic diseases: these affect the body's metabolic rate, for example over/underactive thyroid.
- Breathing pattern: in some patients inspiration (breathing in) can increase the pulse rate due to changes in intrathoracic pressure (Rawlings-Anderson and Hunter 2008).
- Smoking can increase the heart rate as this can cause a narrowing of the arteries.
- Age: see Table 5.3.

THINK ABOUT IT

Take your resting pulse rate. Now run on the spot for 2 minutes and take your pulse again.

What implications do you think this may have for patients attending the GP surgery or hospital?

How would you ensure that you are measuring an accurate pulse rate for your patient?

Terminology

- *Irregular pulse*: this is a pulse that does not have a clear pattern and may have 'gaps' as if beats were being omitted. Because this cannot be detected on standard automated machines, it is important that pulse readings should be taken manually as relevant clinical information can otherwise be missed (Boulanger and Toghill 2009).

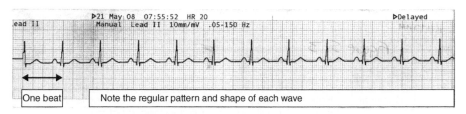

Figure 5.3 Rhythm strip for normal heartbeat – 'sinus rhythm': note the regular pattern and shape of each wave. Source: NHS Lothian (2008). Reproduced with permission from NHS Lothian.

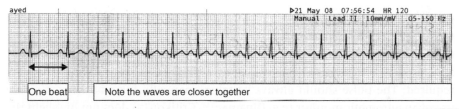

Figure 5.4 An increased heart rate – tachycardia: note that the waves are closer together. Source: NHS Lothian (2008). Reproduced with permission from NHS Lothian.

- *'Normal' pulse*: the normal adult heart rate is between 60 and 100 beats/min, but at rest is usually between 60 and 80 beats/min depending upon the individual (Waugh and Grant 2010). When assessing a patient's pulse, it is important to look at what is considered 'normal' for every individual, bearing in mind the many factors discussed previously. Figure 5.3 shows the normal pattern of a pulse on an electrocardiograph (ECG) reading (see also Chapter 17).
- *Tachycardia*: this is an increased pulse rate of over 100 beats/min (Maddex 2009; Rawlings-Anderson and Hunter 2008). Atrial tachycardia relates to an increased rate in the upper chamber of the heart. On an ECG this would be seen as having an increased number of contractions on the strip (Figure 5.4).
- *Bradycardia*: a reduced heartbeat of less than 60 beats/min (Maddex 2009; Rawlings-Anderson and Hunter 2008). This will result in a decreased number of contractions shown on the ECG (Figure 5.5).
- *Weak pulse*: this is when the pulse is not strong on palpation with two fingers placed over the site.
- *Thready pulse*: this is when the palpated pulse is weak and can be irregular.
- *Fibrillation*: a condition of rapid and irregular contractions (Dougherty and Lister 2011).
- *Respiratory sinus arrhythmia*: a harmless increase in the pulse rate due to inspiration (breathing in) can be seen in patients with good cardiovascular health (Woods et al. 2005).

The contraction of the heart, which gives rise to a pulse, can be shown on ECG readings (see Chapter 17). The strips in Figures 5.3–5.5 show how normal,

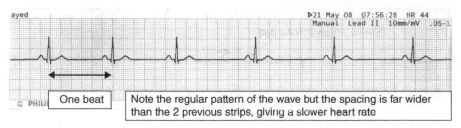

Figure 5.5 Bradycardia – slow heartbeat: note the regular pattern of the wave, but the spacing is far wider than the strips in Figures 5.3 and 5.4, giving a slower heart rate. Source: NHS Lothian (2008). Reproduced with permission from NHS Lothian.

fast and slow pulses affect the ECG. It is not the intention that individuals read ECGs (see also Chapter 17); these are merely to show how the pulse rate presents with different pulse values.

If a pulse is being taken manually, a watch or clock with a second hand is required. The pulse should always be taken manually for a baseline, because use of an automatic monitor (e.g. Dinamap™, Critikon™) does not highlight the amplitude (depth), volume or whether it is regular (Boulanger and Toghill 2009). Always seek advice as to which method of recording the pulse is being requested if not for a baseline recording. The procedure for taking a manual pulse is shown in Table 5.1 (note that for apex and radial pulse, this is shown in Table 5.5).

Automated devices

Pulse recording is a feature on many machines including automated blood pressure machines (see Chapter 6) and pulse oximetry machines (see Chapter 8). The machine takes the reading automatically without the user needing to palpate (feel) the pulse. To ensure accurate readings the following points should be considered:

- The machine should be clean, appear undamaged and have been serviced regularly (usually annually, but check local policy). When the machine is switched on it may do a self-test, and if any error codes are displayed the machine should not be used.
- The machine must be used in accordance with the manufacturer's instructions and appropriate accessories used where applicable; for example, a blood pressure cuff or the finger probe of the pulse oximeter.
- Competency based training should be completed before unsupervised use of the device on a patient to ensure correct placement of the accessories and competent use of the device.
- Some machines will have a timespan in which they make an assessment before showing the pulse rate. This means that, in some instances, the pulse rate given by the machine will be the pulse rate 5–10 seconds before the reading is shown.

Table 5.1 Procedure for taking a manual pulse reading.

Action	Rationale
Wash hands with soap and water or cleanse with alcohol gel	To prevent the spread of infection
Inform the patient and gain verbal consent (for children parent or guardian consent is required)	The patient is fully informed and has given consent voluntarily
Ensure access to a watch or clock with a second hand	To ensure accurate timing
Choose the site (usually radial) and, if necessary, explain the reasoning to the patient	Choose an appropriate site dependent on clinical presentation Children aged under 2 will require the apex site to be used (see Table 5.3)
For the radial pulse: place the first, second or third fingers along the appropriate artery and press gently (Figure 5.6)	The fingertips are sensitive enough to feel the pulse accurately
To record a manual pulse rate, count the number of beats for 60 seconds. The number counted will be the actual pulse rate, e.g. if 84 beats are counted in 60 seconds the pulse rate would be 84	This is more accurate than counting for 15 seconds and multiplying by 4 because it allows enough time for irregularities or other defects to be detected (Dougherty and Lister 2011)
Document the reading as per local policy and any other details, e.g. missed beats, irregular or thready pulse (Figure 5.7)	To ensure accurate record keeping and for good communication
Help patient to redress, if necessary	To maximise patient comfort and dignity
Reassure patient if necessary	Patient comfort
Report to nurse in charge	Patient may require further management

- If the pulse is very fast or irregular, the pulse rate or abnormality may not be detected.
- Where patients have poor circulation to their arms or legs, for example peripheral vascular disease, an inaccurate reading may be obtained due to poor blood flow.
- If the patient moves while the reading is being taken, this may interfere with the signal, and movement may be wrongly interpreted as a heartbeat.
- A pulse should always be checked manually to ensure that it relates to the wave/pulse generated by the machine.

The procedure for taking a pulse rate using a machine is described in Table 5.2.

When taking a pulse reading, either manually or with a machine, it should also be remembered that the value of the pulse measurement should be assessed together with other observations of the patient, including the following:

Table 5.2 Procedure for taking a pulse reading using an automated machine.

Action	Rationale
Wash hands with soap and water or cleanse with alcohol gel	To prevent the spread of infection
Inform the patient and gain verbal consent	The patient is fully informed and has given consent voluntarily
Collect the appropriate machine and, where applicable, accessories. Ensure that the machine is clean and in good working order, and has been serviced as per local policy	To ensure machine is in good working order before use
Ensure that user has had competency training with the machine being used	Correct accessories are essential for the machine to function accurately To ensure that the machine is operated as the manufacturer intended
Apply the machine to the appropriate site, e.g. BP machine to arm, pulse oximeter probe to finger	To allow reading to be taken
Note the value of the recording, taking the patient's physical well-being and other observations into consideration, e.g. temperature, BP, pallor (colour) of patient	To assist in identification of incorrect recordings
Document the reading as per local policy (Figure 5.7)	To ensure accurate record keeping and for good communication
Help patient to redress, where necessary	To maximise patient comfort and dignity
Reassure patient if necessary	Patient comfort
Report to nurse in charge if abnormal	Patient may require further management

- Assess the patient's circulation; if the patient's hands are cold this could indicate poor circulation and if competent to do so a capillary refill time (CRT) test can be done to establish this.
- Is the patient alert? Assessment of the patients AVPU score (alert, responds to voice, responds to pain only, unconsciousness) can be performed if one is competent to do so.
- What are the values of other observations that have been performed, for example BP and temperature recordings? A correlation between these may indicate a more serious clinical condition such as shock or haemorrhage.
- In Acute Hospital Trusts these measurements are the basis of the Early Warning Score (EWS), which is a track and trigger score recommended for use by National Institute for Health and Clinical Excellence (NICE 2007).

Table 5.3 Pulse rates in relation to age.

Age	Average heart rate (beats/min)
Fetus	160
Newborn	140
1–12 months	120
12 months–2 years	110
2–6 years	100
6–12 years	95
Young person	80
Adult	80

Adapted from Trimby (1989).

The role of the healthcare assistant will be to report findings, not to diagnose conditions, and therefore any reading that is unexpected or outside the expected range should be reported to a registered nurse to allow further investigation and/or management.

Fetal heartbeat

In both infants and children, the normal heartbeat range is higher than that of adults (Rawlings-Anderson and Hunter 2008). Before being born, a baby's heartbeat can be heard by using a stethoscope or an electronic machine. The value is around 150 beats/min, which is significantly higher than in adults (see Table 5.3).

Neonates and young children

Once born, babies continue to have an increased heartbeat up until adolescence, with the pulse rate gradually decreasing until a more constant reading is reached in adulthood (see Table 5.3). As mentioned earlier, a stethoscope is used to hear the apex heartbeat of a child under the age of 2 because, if taken manually, the rapid pulse rate and small area for palpation result in inaccurate data (Dougherty and Lister 2011). The procedure for taking an apex beat is detailed in Table 5.4.

Apex and radial pulse measurement

Where patients have a pulse deficit, that is an atrial fibrillation (AF) where the heartbeat does not match the heart rate at the radial pulse, apex (heart) and radial (wrist) pulses may be taken together to assess the number of beats that are not transmitted. This will require two people, with a watch that both individuals

Table 5.4 Procedure for taking an apex pulse recording.

Action	Rationale
Wash hands with soap and water or cleanse with alcohol gel	To prevent the spread of infection
Inform the patient and gain verbal consent (for children parent or guardian consent will be required)	The patient is fully informed and has given consent voluntarily
For very young children involving a play specialist may be helpful	Practising the procedure on, for example, a soft toy may reduce anxiety in the child and increase compliance
Collect equipment: watch/clock, and stethoscope; the stethoscope must be in good condition with clean, well-fitting earpieces. clean the stethoscope as per local policy	So procedure can be performed without delay If the stethoscope is contaminated this presents an infection risk. If the stethoscope is broken it will not perform the function adequately
Draw the screens Check that the stethoscope is positioned correctly	To protect patient privacy and dignity Smooth and accurate facilitation of the procedure
Count the number of apex beats heard in 1 minute. The number counted will be the pulse rate, e.g. if 120 beats are counted in 60 seconds the pulse rate would be 120	This is more accurate than counting for 15 seconds and multiplying by 4 because it allows enough time for irregularities or other defects to be detected (Dougherty and Lister 2011)
Document the reading and any other details as per local policy, e.g. missed beats or irregular (Figure 5.7). Note that it may not be necessary to write apex or abbreviate to 'A' on individual readings as this may be documented at the top of the chart	To ensure accurate record keeping Patient may require further management
Help patient to redress, where necessary	To maximise patient comfort and dignity
Reassure patient if necessary	Patient comfort
Report to nurse in charge if abnormal	To ensure correct clinical management of the patient

can see, and a stethoscope for the person assessing the apex beats. The procedure is shown in Table 5.5.

This is a skill that may require practise, especially when assessing the apex heartbeat, and competency should be achieved in this skill before performing it on a patient. In patients with AF the apex reading will always be higher than the radial pulse because some contractions may not be strong enough to transmit the pulse wave to the radial pulse (Figure 5.6). It is because of this that beats

Table 5.5 Recording apex and radial heartbeats.

Action	Rationale
Wash hands with soap and water or cleanse with alcohol gel	To prevent the spread of infection
Inform the patient and gain verbal consent	The patient is fully informed and has given consent voluntarily
Collect equipment: watch/clock, stethoscope – the stethoscope must be in good condition with clean, well fitting earpieces, clean as per local policy as per local policy	Allow the procedure to be performed without delay If the stethoscope is contaminated this presents an infection risk. If the stethoscope is broken it will not perform the function adequately
Draw the screens	Patient privacy and dignity
Both individuals should be able to see the watch and agree when they will start counting beats	To ensure that the same time period is used to count the heartbeats.
Check that the stethoscope is positioned correctly and that a radial pulse is felt	Smooth facilitation of the procedure
Procedure commences with staff agreeing when counting will start, e.g. when the second hand gets to 12 we will count for a minute, or one person can also control the procedure by saying 'start' and 'stop'	To ensure that the same time period is used to count the heartbeats
Document the reading; this will involve using either different colours, e.g. blue/red, or different letters, e.g. A (for apex) or R (for radial) as per local policy (see Figure 5.8)	To clearly identify which reading relates to apex and radial recording
Help patient to redress, where necessary	To maximise patient comfort
Reassure patient if necessary	Patient comfort
Report to nurse in charge if abnormal	To ensure correct management of the patient

can become lost, resulting in a deficit between pulse and apex measurements (Jevon 2007).

Documentation

The pulse may be recorded in the patient's notes (these may be held by the patient if they are in the community). In a hospital setting, the recordings will be noted on either a temperature, pulse and respiratory chart (TPR) or a EWS chart; the readings often take the form of a graph (see Figure 5.7), where the A (atrial) and R (radial) are clearly marked (Figure 5.8). Many Trusts' record keeping policies

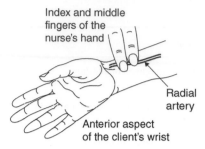

Index and middle
fingers of the
nurse's hand

Radial
artery

Anterior aspect
of the client's wrist

Figure 5.6 Taking a radial pulse.

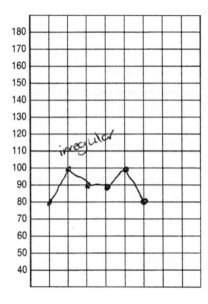

Figure 5.7 Observation chart with 'normal' and
'irregular' pulse charted. Source: NHS Lothian
(2008). Reproduced with permission from NHS
Lothian.

state that records should be made in black ink so they can easily be photocopied
should the need arise. Therefore advice should be sought from the registered
nurse regarding the approved workplace method of documentation.

Common problems

Problems of ensuring an accurate pulse rate can be divided into those concerning
technique, patient and equipment.

Technique

The technique is one that will require practise, especially when accessing sites
other than the radial pulse. Both the thumb and forefinger have pulses of their
own and are very sensitive, therefore practitioners must be aware that this can
be confused for the patient's pulse (Dougherty and Lister 2011). Recognising and

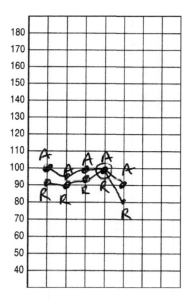

Figure 5.8 TPR (temperature, pulse and respiratory) chart with apex (Λ) and radial (R) pulse charted. Source: NHS Lothian (2008). Reproduced with permission from NHS Lothian.

having the confidence to report an irregular pulse rate will also require practise and the healthcare assistant should work to their code of practice and seek help when unsure (WUTH 2011). Competency based training should be completed before performing this task independently to ensure that the correct technique is performed.

Patients

Where patients have an underlying condition, such as poor circulation, the pulse may be more difficult to find at the radial site and other sites may prove more successful. If the patient is acutely unwell as a result of, for example, a major haemorrhage (blood loss), this will reduce the circulating blood volume and may make the radial site difficult to palpate. In preparation for a pulse rate being taken the patient should not have exercised or smoked before the procedure; if they have done so the reading may not be accurate (Rawlings-Anderson and Hunter 2008).

Equipment

Equipment being used should have been serviced, should be clean and when switched on should not display any error codes. Local policy will dictate when a machine can be used but it is not recommended if performing the reading for the first time on a patient because irregularity, depth and amplitude cannot be identified, as mentioned earlier. If the reading obtained does not appear correct, the pulse rate should be taken manually to check. When taking a pulse manually it is essential that a watch with a second hand is used to enable the pulse to be taken for a full 60 seconds. Universal precautions should always be taken before

Table 5.6 Competency: recording a pulse rate.

Pulse	First assessment/reassessment					
Steps	**Demonstration**					**Date/competent/ signature**
	Date/sign 1	Date/sign 2	Date/sign 3	Date/sign 4	Date/sign 5	
Pulse – manual						
1 Describe what a pulse is and how the heart initiates this						
2 List the sites for taking a pulse with rationale						
3 Describe activities that affect the pulse rate						
4 State the difference in pulse rate for different age groups						
5 Collect equipment for manual or automated device						
6 Correctly identify the patient and explain procedure, and give an effective explanation about the procedure						
Recording pulse	**Demonstration**					**Date/competent/ signature**
	1	2	3	4	5	
7 Demonstrate accurate recording for manual and/or automated machine						
8 Demonstrate tidying away of equipment if applicable						
9 Complete appropriate documentation applicable to the clinical area						

and after contact with a patient and hands should be washed with soap and water or cleaned with alcohol gel using the Ayliffe technique.

Summary

A pulse should always be taken manually for the first time to feel its depth and ensure that it is regular. Subsequent readings can be taken using automated equipment if the pulse is regular and stable according to your workplace policy. As with all other clinical skills, users must be competent in a pulse measurement and understand the factors that influence its value before practising this skill independently on patients. Table 5.6 is an example of a competency framework for recording pulse.

CASE STUDY 5.1

Mr Gary Johnstone has been admitted for planned investigations to his knee. He is 28 years old and enjoys playing sport competitively. He is fairly relaxed about his admission. His pulse rate is taken and it is 48. What factors do you think are influencing his pulse rate?

CASE STUDY 5.2

Mrs Celia Jones is 45 years old, married with two children, and has come into hospital for investigations into suspected stomach cancer. She explains that she has had to rush here after dropping her children at school. Her pulse rate is 104. What factors do you think are influencing her pulse rate and what further actions would you take?

Self-assessment

Assessment	Aspects	Achieved ✓
Patient	*Have you considered all aspects of this section?*	
	What initiates a heartbeat?	
	The possible sites to take a pulse	
	The normal pattern of a pulse on an ECG and	
	how a slow/fast heartbeat alters the pattern	
Procedure	*Have you considered all aspects of this section?*	**Achieved ✓**
	Factors that can affect the pulse reading	
	The factors that should be taken into	
	consideration if using an automated device to	
	take a pulse reading	
	Recording and reporting concerns	

References

Ball J and Bindler R (2008) *Pediatric Nursing. Caring for Children*, 4th edn. London: Pearson.

Boulanger C and Toghill M. (2009) How to measure and record vital signs to ensure detection of deteriorating patients. *Nursing Times* 105(47): 10–12.

Dougherty L and Lister S (eds) (2011) *The Royal Marsden Hospital Manual of Clinical Nursing Procedures*, 8th edn. Oxford: Blackwell Publishing.

Herbert R A and Sheppard M. (2005) Cardiovascular function. In: Montague SE, Watson R and Herbert RA (eds) *Physiology for Nursing Practice*, 3rd edn. London: Baillière Tindall, pp. 383–463.

Maddex S (2009) Measuring vital signs In: Baillie L (ed.) *Developing Practical Adult Nursing Skills*, 3rd edn. London: Hodder Education, pp. 116–157.

Jevon P (2007) Cardiac monitoring part 4: Monitoring the apex beat. *Nursing Times* 103(4): 28–29.

Jevon P and Ewens B (2007) *Monitoring the Critically Ill Patient: Essential clinical skills for nurses*, 2nd edn. London: Blackwell.

Marieb E M and Hoehn K. (2007) *Human Anatomy and Physiology*. San Francisco: Benjamin Cummings.

Kyle T (2008) *Essentials of Pediatric Nursing*. Philadelphia: Lippincott Williams and Wilkins.

NHS Lothian (2008) *Observations Chart*. Edinburgh: NHS Lothian.

National Institute for Health and Clinical Excellence (NICE) (2007) *CG50 Acutely Ill Patients in Hospital*. London: NICE.

Rawlings-Anderson K and Hunter J (2008) Monitoring pulse rate. *Nursing Standard* 22(31): 41–43.

Scales K and Pilsworth J (2008) The importance of fluid balance in clinical practice. *Nursing Standard* 22(47): 50–57.

Thibodeau G A and Patton K T (2007) *Anatomy and Physiology*, 6th edn. St Louis, MO: Mosby Elsevier.

Tortora G J and Derrickson B (2011) *Principles of Anatomy and Physiology*, 13th edn. Hoboken, NJ: Wiley & Sons.

Trimby B (1989) *Clinical Nursing Procedure*. Philadelphia, PA: JB Lippincott.

Waugh A and Grant A (2010) *Ross and Wilson Anatomy and Physiology in Health and Illness*, 11th edn. Edinburgh: Churchill Livingstone.

Woods S L, Sivarajan Foelicher E, Underhill Motzer S and Bridges E (2005) *Cardiac Nursing*, 5th edn. Philadelphia, PA: Lippincott, Williams & Wilkins.

WUTH (2011) *Code of Conduct for Assistant Practitioners*. Wirral England.

CHAPTER 6

Blood pressure monitoring

LEARNING OBJECTIVES

- Discuss the anatomy and physiology of the heart and its major vessels, relating this to blood pressure measurement
- List the factors that affect blood pressure readings
- Identify why lying and standing blood pressure readings are taken
- Identify the correct method for taking blood pressure
- Identify how to document blood pressure readings correctly

Aim of this chapter

The aim of this chapter is to review the principles for undertaking blood pressure (BP) monitoring, the related anatomy and physiology, and the skills required to measure, record and report findings.

What is blood pressure?

Blood pressure can be defined as the force or pressure that the blood exerts on the walls of the blood vessels (Waugh and Grant 2010; Tortora and Derrickson 2011).

Reasons for monitoring blood pressure

Blood pressure is taken to obtain a baseline (a reading that acts as a reference for future readings) or as an ongoing measure of cardiovascular (heart) function in order to make comparisons, aid diagnosis and evaluate the management of medical conditions. It is also used to screen patients for underlying disease or complications, or as a precaution for side-effects to certain medications (e.g. the contraceptive pill).

Who requests the test?

A BP reading can be requested in the community setting by a GP, practice nurse or community nurse. This may be part of patients' care when they are discharged

Clinical Skills for Healthcare Assistants and Assistant Practitioners, Second Edition.
Angela Whelan and Elaine Hughes.
© 2016 John Wiley & Sons, Ltd. Published 2016 by John Wiley & Sons, Ltd.

from hospital, or to assess their health in relation to a long-term condition, for example hypertension (high blood pressure) as a result of heart disease. In an acute setting, such as a hospital, doctors or nursing staff may request blood pressure to be taken due to the patient's clinical presentation, or it may be part of a specific routine, such as admission procedure or after surgical intervention. Other professionals may also take a reading as part of an assessment, for example an occupational therapist or physiotherapist taking a reading to assess a patient after a history of frequent falls.

Who can take a BP reading?

Any healthcare professional can undertake BP measurement, the most important criteria being that they are competent in the skill. Incorrect recordings or poor technique in blood pressure measurement can result in inappropriate treatment or undiagnosed conditions that may have a severe effect on the patient's health. Accurate blood pressure readings, on the other hand, can give important clues about health and well-being, and NICE (2011) recommends that patients with suspected or confirmed hypertension who are appropriately trained use home blood pressure monitoring devices to accurately record their blood pressure, which may influence treatment more appropriately.

What is done with the readings/information?

'Routine' BP recordings will be written in different documents, depending on the purpose of the recording and whether in hospital, the GP surgery, the community or the patient's own home. The documentation may take the format of patient records (can be held by the patient, e.g. antenatal notes during pregnancy), admission documentation, care plans, care pathways or as a specific chart for observations – commonly referred to as a TPR (temperature, pulse and respiratory rate) chart or in acute settings an EWS chart (early warning system). (The recording on the TPR chart is shown in Figure 6.4.) If the result is outside 'normal' parameters for the patient (see notes later) the reading must be verbally reported to the nurse in charge immediately.

Relevant anatomy and physiology

Structure of the heart
The heart is best described as a pump and to assist this function it is made almost entirely of muscle (Figure 6.1). This muscle works automatically, thus it does not need the brain to tell it to work but does so under what is known as 'involuntary

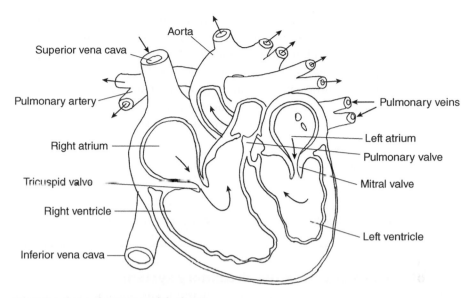

Figure 6.1 Internal structure of the heart.

action'. The heart is situated in the thorax (chest cavity) between and in front of the lungs (Waugh and Grant 2010). It is centrally placed but tilted, which is why the heartbeat is heard to the left, and is roughly the size of a fist (Tortora and Derrickson 2011; Thibodeau and Patton 2007).

Within the heart, there are two top chambers known as the right and left atria and below two further chambers known as the right and left ventricles (Thibodeau and Patton 2007) (Figure 6.1). The right atrium receives blood that does not contain oxygen (deoxygenated) from throughout the body. The deoxygenated blood enters the right atrium from the superior vena cava, which brings blood from the top half of the body, the inferior vena cava, which carries blood from the bottom half of the body and the coronary sinus, which is a collection of vessels that drains blood from the heart into the right atrium. The blood then passes into the right ventricle under pressure through the tricuspid valve. After the blood leaves the right ventricle it is then taken to the lungs via the pulmonary arteries where the lungs add oxygen to the blood. Once the blood has combined with oxygen (oxygenated blood) it is returned to the heart via the pulmonary veins to the left atrium. Again, under pressure it enters the left ventricle through the mitral valve. The oxygenated blood is then expelled from the left ventricle through the aortic valve into the aorta to supply oxygen and blood to the tissues. This results in the left side of the heart having oxygenated blood and the right side deoxygenated blood. The two sides are completely separated by the septum so the blood cannot meet, resulting in the heart functioning as two pumps (Tortora and Derrickson 2011). An independent blood supply delivers blood to the heart muscle itself.

The amount of blood ejected from the ventricle in one contraction is called the 'stroke volume', and this volume is estimated to average 70 millilitres (ml) per beat in the average adult (Tortora and Derrickson 2011). To estimate the cardiac output, this is multiplied by the heart rate, giving the amount of blood ejected from the left ventricle in one minute (Box 6.1) (Jevon and Ewens 2007). Non-invasive blood pressure (involves a machine being applied externally) gives an early sign of a fall in cardiac output (Jevon and Ewens 2007).

Box 6.1 Cardiac output formula

Example
A man has a heartbeat of 72 and a stroke volume of 70 ml (millilitres) Cardiac output = Heart rate × Stroke volume 72 × 70 = 5040 ml/min or 5.04 litres per minute (l/min)

The role of valves within the circulatory system

There are four sets of heart valves, two sets guarding the openings between the atria and ventricles (the tricuspid and mitral valves), and two located inside the pulmonary artery and aorta (called the aortic and pulmonary valves or semilunar valves collectively). Thibodeau and Patton (2007) describe heart valves as mechanical devices that permit the flow of blood in one direction only.

Defective heart valves can cause heart murmurs and this leads to regurgitation (blood leaking backward through the valve when it should be closed). Diagnosis can result after unusual sounds are first heard through a stethoscope before, between or after normal heart sounds, or they may mask the normal heart sounds (Tortora and Derrickson 2011). These sounds are commonly known as 'innocent heart murmurs', because they do not present any health problems at all and the sounds are made by the blood circulating through the heart's chambers and valves, or through blood vessels near the heart. Heart murmurs can be common in children, often disappearing later in life (Tortora and Derrickson 2011).

However some people can develop problems with their valves. Valves that narrow and reduce blood flow have valve stenosis, while valves that fail to close properly have valve incompetence. Valve incompetence allows blood to flow backwards, these are often called 'leaky valves'. The degree of valve incompetence varies with the individual and can have different effects on the body. Because of this some valve problems will not require treatment and for others valve replacement will be necessary.

The cardiac cycle

The heart maintains constant circulation by a series of events known as the cardiac cycle (Waugh and Grant 2010). The cycle consists of atrial systole, which is when the atrium contracts lasting around 0.1 second, followed by ventricular systole, contraction of the ventricles that lasts around 0.3 s. Finally complete relaxation of both atria and ventricles occurs, lasting 0.4 s. It is this sequence of contraction and relaxation of the heart muscle that allows blood to flow around the body.

When the left ventricle contracts and pushes blood into the aorta, the resulting pressure is called the systolic blood pressure. This is the maximum pressure of the blood against the wall of the artery (Waugh and Grant 2010). It is expressed as the top figure when quoting blood pressure (think of a fraction: this is the first number above the line). When complete cardiac diastole occurs and the heart is resting following the ejection of blood, the pressure within the arteries is called diastolic blood pressure (the bottom number below the 'fraction' line). This is the minimum amount of pressure exerted against the wall of the artery, after closure of the aortic valve (Marieb and Hoehn 2010). An example of a blood pressure reading is shown in Box 6.2.

Box 6.2 Example of how a blood pressure is written

$\dfrac{132}{80}$ Systolic
Diastolic

Arterial blood pressure is what is commonly referred to as blood pressure and is measured in millimetres of mercury (mmHg) using a sphygmomanometer or electronic device (Marieb and Hoehn 2010). When measuring blood pressure for the first time it is good practice to take a reading from both arms. It can then be determined if there is a discrepancy in the reading and when this occurs the arm with the highest reading should be used for measurement (British Hypertension Society 2006). It should also be noted that NICE (2011) recommends that readings with a discrepancy greater than 20 mmHg systolic require further investigation. Any discrepancies should be reported to the nurse in charge as this may indicate that the patient has an undiagnosed medical condition. This should also be documented in the patient's records.

Normal blood pressure

Blood pressure can fluctuate within a wide range and still be considered within normal limits. Normal systolic pressure should be between 100 and 140 mmHg and diastolic between 60 and 90 mmHg (Waugh and Grant 2010). Often there can be variance in the definition of normal BP with individual BP fluctuating (Wallymahmed 2008). Systolic readings of around 120 mmHg and diastolic of about 80 mmHg are considered 'normal'. However people with a reading at the high end of the normal range – with a systolic blood pressure between 135–139 mmHg systolic and a diastolic reading between 85–89 mmHg – are likely to benefit from lifestyle advice, with 'at risk' patients requiring medication to control their blood pressure further (Joint British Societies 2005).

Related aspects and terminology

Maintenance of normal blood pressure

Blood pressure is maintained within normal limits through fine adjustments by the body with a number of factors affecting the value recorded; this is detailed in Box 6.3.

Box 6.3 Factors affecting blood pressure readings

- **Blood volume**: this relates to the amount of blood that is circulating around the body. Where the blood volume is reduced dramatically, such as haemorrhage (rapid blood loss), this causes a drop in BP. Tortora and Derrickson (2011) state that even losses of 10 per cent or more, for example in instances of trauma, haemorrhage or severe dehydration, can result in a fall in BP.
- **Peripheral resistance**: this relates to the pressure that is presented against the flow of blood and can reduce the efficiency of blood returning to the heart.
- **Elasticity of the artery walls**: this is how much 'give' the blood vessels have; and in cases of stenosis (narrowing of the artery) of the vessels elasticity is lost (Waugh and Grant 2010). Atherosclerosis, commonly called 'hardening of the arteries', is a build-up of fat and cholesterol deposits within the vessels. This directly affects the elasticity of the arteries and it is caused by lifestyle factors that are related to diet and smoking and may be influenced by a previous family history (Clancy and McVicar 2009).
- **Respiratory centre**: when this centre is stimulated in the brain, particularly during inspiration, the blood pressure will rise (Jevon and Ewens 2007).
- **Nicotine**: as nicotine is a vasoconstrictor (reduces the diameter of the blood vessel), the BP increases (Jevon and Ewens 2007).
- **Age**: Clancy and McVicar (2009) reports that BP increases throughout the lifespan thus affecting the 'normal reading' for any specific patient. In addition, arteries harden with age and therefore an increase in BP is also expected.
- **Gender**: men generally have higher BP than women (Clancy and McVicar 2009).
- **Weight**: obesity is a risk factor in the development of hypertension.
- **Emotional factors**: stress, fear, anxiety and excitement can all increase a person's blood pressure (Maddex 2009). This is due to the body's 'fight or flight' response caused by release of adrenaline from the adrenal glands (Tortora and Derrickson 2011). Although relaxation has been shown to be beneficial for patients' emotional well-being, Dickinson (2008) has identified that relaxation therapy does not reduce blood pressure to a level that is statistically significant.
- **Diet/medications**: high salt intake has been shown to increase blood pressure (ERPHO 2008) while diuretics can also reduce BP by decreasing sodium content in the blood through filtration in the kidneys and by decreasing circulatory volume (Tortora and Derrickson 2011).
- **Time of day**: BP is known to be lowest in the morning, rising throughout the day, reaching its peak in the afternoon, and then falling in the evening. This is linked to the body's own circadian rhythm and research suggests that taking antihypertensive medication at bed time may improve patient's blood pressure levels during the day (Hermida et al. 2011).
- **White coat hypertension**: this is when the individual's BP is consistently higher when measured in a hospital or community practice setting rather than the individual's home, due to anxiety or fear of the medical environment. NICE (2011) acknowledges this importance in its guidelines in suggesting how to determine accuracy of blood pressure readings

- **Gravity**: with postural hypotension the systolic BP can fall more than 20 mmHg within three minutes of standing (Sathyapalan et al. 2011). This is also known as 'orthostatic hypotension'. Baroreceptors, which are situated throughout the body and monitor changes in BP, raise the BP with increased stimulation (Valler-Jones and Wedgbury 2005). However, if this mechanism is lost, for example after prolonged bed rest, the patient may faint on standing (Jevon and Ewens 2007). (See 'Lying and standing BP measurement.')
- **Hormones**: there are also various hormones that affect BP and aid its regulation by altering cardiac output, changing systemic vascular resistance or adjusting the total blood volume, for example the hormones renin and aldosterone from the kidneys (Tortora and Derrickson 2011).
- **Family history**: this can be related to coronary heart disease, which can cause resistance to blood flow and increased peripheral resistance as mentioned earlier (Loscalzo et al. 2008).
- **Sleep**: this is when systolic BP is at its lowest (Hermida 2011).

Terminology

Hypertension

Hypertension is an elevation in the blood pressure and may be acute or chronic. It is based not on one reading but on readings that are taken over several days, and where the value exceeds the upper limits of what is considered normal for the patient (NICE 2011). Hypertension increases the risk of having a stroke or heart attack and can be a result of lifestyle choices, stress, anxiety or recent strenuous activity. The National Institute for Health and Clinical Excellence (NICE) defines hypertension as elevated BP above 140/90 mmHg (NICE 2011) (see also Joint British Societies 2005). If the BP reading is higher than 140/90, NICE (2011) guidelines suggest that further readings should be taken through home ambulatory blood pressure monitoring (ABPM), where two measurements per hour while the patient is awake should be taken. This can also be determined through home blood pressure monitoring (HBPM), where the community team visit patients twice a day for a period between four and seven days to establish trends in blood pressure to enable an accurate diagnosis to be made.

Hypotension

This refers to when the systolic BP is below 100 mmHg and can be the first indicator of shock in an acutely ill patient (where vital body processes shut down in response to a reduction in blood volume), the result of good physical health, caused by medications such as beta blockers, severe congestive cardiac failure or a heart attack affecting a large part of the myocardium (Dougherty and Lister 2011). It can also indicate that there is not sufficient pressure to pump blood around the body. As the blood carries the oxygen with it, organs can become under-perfused and this can cause the individual to faint (see 'Postural hypotension').

Table 6.1 Blood pressure classification.

Category	Systolic BP (mmHg)	Diastolic BP (mmHg)
Optimal blood pressure	<120	<80
Normal blood pressure	<130	<85
High normal blood pressure	130–139	85–89
Grade 1 hypertension (mild)	140–159	90–99
Grade 2 hypertension (moderate)	160–179	100–109
Grade 3 hypertension (severe)	>180	>110
Isolated systolic hypertension (grade 1)	140–159	<90
Isolated systolic hypertension (grade 2)	>160	<90

Postural or 'orthostatic' hypotension

The symptoms of postural hypotension may be dizziness and in some instances fainting. When this occurs BP is measured when the patient is both standing (erect) and lying (supine), to detect a deficit when the patient stands up. Postural hypotension is defined as a reduction in blood pressure measurement of at least 20 mmHg systolic when the patient stands compared to their blood pressure when lying down (Sathyapalan et al. 2011). The procedure for measuring lying and standing blood pressure is shown later in Table 6.4.

The British Hypertension Society (2004), supported by the World Health Organization, classify blood pressure in Table 6.1.

Twenty-four-hour monitoring

Monitoring a patient's blood pressure over a 24-hour period can be done for various reasons that include where patients:

- have suspected white coat hypertension (where blood pressure is normal away from healthcare practitioners but increases in their presence);
- have fluctuating BP readings (Hypertension Influence Team 2007);
- have a BP that is poorly controlled despite medication (Hypertension Influence Team 2007);
- require an initial diagnosis of hypertension (NICE 2011).

The device used is called an ambulatory monitor, which means that the patient is fully mobile while the device is recording the BP at regular intervals. This has the advantage of monitoring the patient's BP while they are participating in normal daily activities.

Korotkoff's sounds

When taking a BP reading manually, sounds known as Korotkoff's sounds are listened for to establish a reading. These can only be heard through a stethoscope during deflation of the inflated cuff. The five phases are in Table 6.2.

Table 6.2 Korotkoff's sounds.

Phase	Description
1	This is the systolic blood pressure. It is heard as repetitive, faint yet clear tapping sounds, which gradually increase in intensity
2	This is the softening of sounds, which may sound like blowing or swishing
3	This is the return of sharper and perhaps crisper sounds that do not regain the intensity of phase 1
4	This is where a distinct muffled sound is heard, which may become soft and blowing
5	No sounds are heard. This is the diastolic blood pressure

Adapted from O'Brien et al. (2003).

In most instances all phases will be heard; however, Williams et al. (2004) state that if, during phase 5, the reading reduces to zero, phase 4 should be used. The British Hypertension Society (BHS 2006) and Dieterle (2012) state that this can occur in pregnancy; if so phase 4 sounds should be used for the systolic reading. It is essential that the skill of taking BP is both practised and assessed to ensure that the technique is correct and that the phases are heard correctly as this is an essential aspect of practice in obtaining an accurate reading.

Care must be exercised when taking patients' BP to ensure that efforts are taken to reduce anxiety, and that a period of time has elapsed after activity and smoking as they both influence the BP value.

Equipment

Blood pressure is taken with a manual mercury sphygmomanometer, an aneroid sphygmomanometer or a fully automatic device (see Table 6.3 for the procedure). When using any equipment, it is necessary before use to check that the machine has been serviced as per local policy and appears in good working order. It is also essential that the correct size of cuff be used to ensure accuracy of the BP readings. Table 6.5 shows correct sizing of cuffs.

If the cuff is too small, the reading could be falsely high and if too large a cuff is selected the reading could be too low (SCENIHR 2009).

Mercury sphygmomanometers

Standard mercury sphygmomanometers are becoming less common as mercury presents a health and safety hazard – and since 2009 they have been removed from the market for purchase – but those already available in the clinical setting can continue to be used if they are in a good state of repair (MHRA 2009). Because of the risk associated with mercury leakage the procedure for dealing

Table 6.3 Procedure to measure blood pressure with mercury, aneroid or electronic machines.

Action	Rationale
1. The patient	
Explain the procedure to patients, paying particular attention to informing them of the tightness of the cuff and the need to stop eating, talking and moving during measurement (Dougherty and Lister 2011; Wallymahmed 2008)	To fully inform the patient, gain verbal consent and cooperation
The patient should not have been participating in strenuous activity for 30 minutes before taking the reading (Jevon and Ewens 2007)	This would give an inaccurate reading
Let the patient rest for 5 minutes before the procedure (Wallymahmed 2008)	Anxiety will give an inaccurate reading
Wash and dry hands (Jevon and Ewens 2007)	Prevent the spread of infection
2. Equipment/accessories	
Ensure that the machine is in good working order, has been serviced as per local policy and is clean	To ensure accuracy of the machine
Choose an appropriate cuff (for both the type and model of the machine and the patient)	BP cuff should be appropriate for the patient (see Table 6.5) to ensure accuracy. The equipment should be in good condition
A stethoscope will be required for a manual reading and must be in good condition with clean, well-fitting earpieces	To ensure that it is fit for purpose and to prevent infection
Bladder length should be 80% of the arm's circumference but no more than 100% (Wallymahmed 2008)	To ensure accurate readings
For mercury position the manometer within 1 metre of the patient with the level of the mercury clearly visible and resting at the zero level (Wallymahmed 2008)	To ensure that the scale is easily visible (Wallymahmed 2008)
For aneroid, ensure that the dial can be seen when operating the machine	
3. Patient	
Expose the arm to the shoulder, removing tight or restrictive clothing (British Hypertension Society 2006; Jevon and Holmes 2007)	Restrictive clothing may produce inaccurate readings
The arm should be supported at the level of the heart; a pillow is ideal (Jevon and Holmes 2007; Wallymahmed 2008)	To ensure accuracy of the reading (see Box 6.1)
The same arm should be used each time to allow comparison	To ensure consistency if there is a variance between arms. The arm with the highest reading should be used (NICE 2011)
The bladder cuff should encircle the arm just above the antecubital fossa (crook of the elbow) 2.5 cm above the brachial artery (Dougherty and Lister 2011). The centre of the bladder cuff should be positioned over the brachial artery at the point of maximum pulsation (Dougherty and Lister 2011). It is recommended that a space of two fingers should be evident between the cuff and where the stethoscope is placed	To ensure correct placement

Table 6.3 (*continued*)

Action	Rationale
Connect the cuff tubing to the manometer tubing and loosen the valve of the inflation ball	To ensure smooth facilitation of the procedure
4. Procedure	
For mercury/aneroid: to estimate systolic blood pressure – palpate the brachial artery which can be located in the middle of the arm at the inner elbow, slightly inwards towards the body. By placing two or three fingers at this site the pulse can be found, as it is the site of maximum pulsation (Dougherty and Lister 2011). Inflate the cuff until pulsation disappears. Inflate a further 10 mmHg and release the valve slowly, taking a note of the reading on the mercury column when the brachial pulse returns	Provides an estimate of the systolic pressure
Deflate the cuff completely allowing all the air to escape	Residual air in the cuff many give an inaccurate reading
Palpate the brachial artery and place the diaphragm of the stethoscope lightly over the site. Inflate the cuff to 30 mmHg above previous estimated systolic pressure	Excessive pressure can distort sounds or make them persist for longer
Listen through the stethoscope releasing the valve on the cuff by approximately 2–3 mmHg/s (Wallymahmed 2008)	At faster rates of deflation if using mercury it may fall too quickly, resulting in an inaccurate reading
When the first sound is heard the level should be noted; this is the systolic pressure. Continue to deflate the cuff and, at the point that the sounds disappear altogether, this is the diastolic pressure	Ensure knowledge of Korotkoff's sounds (see Table 6.2)
BP should be measured to the nearest 2 mmHg (Wallymahmed 2008)	Provides a more accurate reading
Electronic device:	
Switch on the device and press start	To obtain the reading
Read the systolic and diastolic blood pressure as displayed on the machine but ensure the reading is consistent with patient's overall general condition	To ensure that the reading is accurate and the machine functioning correctly
5. Documentation	
Document the systolic and diastolic BP on the appropriate chart (Figure 6.4)	To ensure record of BP reading is available
Report any abnormal readings to nurse in charge or medical staff	To allow further intervention where necessary
6. Remove equipment	
Remove the cuff and make the patient comfortable	Patient comfort
Return the equipment to appropriate store, cleaning as per local policy if required. Plug in electronic device	To allow equipment to be in good working order for next patient

with this should be detailed in local policies and procedures within organisations that use mercury sphygmomanometers. To ensure accurate readings using a mercury sphygmomanometer, it is important that the following points should be noted:

- Ensure that the gauge of the manometer which contains mercury is kept in a vertical position as this will result in an overestimation of the blood pressure reading (SCENIHR 2009; Dougherty and Lister 2011).
- The control valve must tighten and loosen easily and not leak because this would cause an underestimation of the systolic pressure and overestimation of the diastolic pressure (Jevon and Holmes 2007).
- The rubber tubing and bladder centre should be intact and not perished (Dougherty and Lister 2011).
- Deflation of the cuff should be slow at a rate of 2–3 mmHg per second (Jevon and Holmes 2007).

Aneroid sphygmomanometer

This device is commonly used in the community and sometimes patients may have these in their own homes. It works by measuring the cuff pressure using bellows connected to a cuff via rubber tubing, and the pressure is transferred to a dial to give the reading (Dougherty and Lister 2011). Like any other sphygmomanometer, these machines must be calibrated correctly as they can result in inaccurate readings due to damage that is not visible to the user. Therefore, the patient's clinical presentation should also be considered, and readings rechecked using another machine if they do not correlate with the BP reading obtained. To promote accurate readings in these machines it is recommended that:

- the indicators sit at the '0' correctly before use (Dougherty and Lister 2011);
- the faceplate is not damaged; commonly it can be cracked, which will affect readings (Dougherty and Lister 2011);
- the rubber tubing is not defective or leaking (Dougherty and Lister 2011).

Automated devices

An alternative to the manual sphygmomanometer is the use of automated devices, which can be fixed or portable. An example of one model is given in Figure 6.2. They are sometimes referred to as monitors, with some models capable of taking ECG (electrocardiograph), pulse and pulse oximetry readings. The machines can operate by battery, mains power or both. Some machines have functions allowing BP readings to be measured at regular intervals, for example every 15 minutes, and may have a facility to store the readings. It is essential that the machine is used in the way that the manufacturer intended, so individuals must ensure that they are taught how to use it correctly and refer to the manufacturer's instructions. The machine displays the systolic and diastolic values, and in some instances the mean value that is referred to as the 'mean arterial

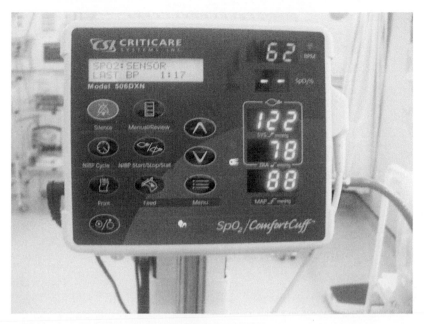

Figure 6.2 An automated blood pressure measuring machine.

pressure'. The machine measures the blood pressure by detecting pressure oscillations (waves) in the cuff, which are generated by arterial wall movement, with each arterial pulsation beneath an occluding cuff. The amplitude (depth) of the oscillation depends on the relationship between the cuff pressure and the arterial BP, reaching a maximum when the cuff pressure equals the mean arterial pressure. Therefore, if the pulse is weak, thready or irregular the reading may not be accurate, and NICE (2011) recommends that the reading should be checked with a manual sphygmomanometer. Validated automated devices can also be used by patients for home blood pressure monitoring where patients are known to have hypertension and for ABPM (NICE 2011).

Sites for recording blood pressure

- Either arm, situating the cuff on the upper arm using the brachial artery (most common) to hear the Korotkoff sounds.
- At the wrist where the radial and ulnar arteries are situated, placing the cuff on the forearm; this would not be expected from a healthcare assistant.
- The foot, placing the cuff above the ankle where the dorsalis pedis artery is situated; this would not be expected from a healthcare assistant.
- On the thigh where the cuff is placed in the centre of the thigh and the Korotkoff sounds are listened for at the popliteal artery. However this would not be expected from a healthcare assistant.

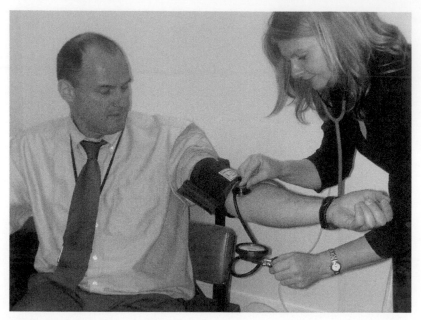

Figure 6.3 Inappropriate positioning for a blood pressure recording. The arm should be supported on a pillow and below heart level.

Taking blood pressure

The cuff is usually placed on the upper arm at the heart level for both adults and children, with the thigh used only when the upper arm cannot be used, and this would not be expected of a healthcare assistant without further training. When using all BP measuring machines the arm should be supported for optimum readings to be obtained (Jevon and Ewens 2007). Figure 6.3 shows inappropriate positioning for taking a BP reading.

> **THINK ABOUT IT**
>
> Get someone who has completed competency based training for blood pressure to take your blood pressure. How did it feel? Did the cuff become uncomfortable? Imagine how this could feel for your patient group. Is there any way you can help to improve their experience here?

As mentioned earlier, where a patient has a variance in lying and standing BP a reading should be obtained for both lying and standing. Where the patient has a history of fainting or collapse when standing it is recommended that another person be available to ensure patient safety. Table 6.4 details the procedure for lying and standing BP measurement.

Table 6.4 Procedure for lying (supine) and standing (erect) blood pressure recordings First ensure that you follow the procedures detailed in Table 6.2 for the specific machine that you are using.

Action	Rationale
1. Explain the procedure and rationale to the patient	To fully inform the patient, gain verbal consent and cooperation
2. For lying (supine) blood pressure: Lie the patient down for 5 minutes (Jevon and Holmes 2007)	To prepare the patient for the procedure and ensure an accurate reading. It may also relax the patient
3. Complete the procedure as per Table 6.3 dependent on the device being used	To ensure that an accurate reading is obtained
4. Document the reading ensuring that you are recording it for lying (supine) reading (Figure 6.4) Leave the cuff in place	Accurate record of the BP reading Preparation for the next part of the procedure
5. Allow the patient to stand for 1 min, supporting the patient where necessary (Jevon and Holmes 2007)	To ensure that an accurate reading is obtained. Supporting the patient will ensure patient safety should they fall
6. Complete the procedure as per Table 6.3 Document the reading ensuring that you are recording it for standing (erect) reading (Figure 6.5)	To ensure that an accurate reading is obtained. Either a code of E (erect) and S (supine) should be recorded on the chart or in some workplaces it is common to record (L) lying and S (standing) (Figure 6.5)
7. Explain the readings to the patients if they want this information	To ensure that the patient is fully informed and allow further information to be given, where necessary

---

THINK ABOUT IT

What factors would you consider when taking a blood pressure reading on a patient who is agitated and who has an intravenous infusion (drip) in place? What other groups of patients might you need to adapt your practice for?

The Joint British Societies (2005) summarise the main points regarding BP measurement using a standard mercury sphygmomanometer or semiautomated device as follows:

- Use a properly maintained, calibrated and validated device.
- Measure sitting BP routinely: standing BP should be recorded at the initial estimation in patients who are older or have diabetes.
- Remove tight clothing, support the arm at heart level, ensure that the patient's hand is relaxed and avoid talking during the measurement procedure.

Table 6.5 Sizes of cuff.

Indication	Bladder width × length (cm)	Arm circumference (cm)
Small adult/child	12 × 18	<23
Standard adult	12 × 26	<33
Large adult	12 × 40	<50
Adult thigh cuff	20 × 42	<53

Source: Hypertension Influence Team 2007. Reproduced with permission of British Hypertension Society.

- Use a cuff of appropriate size (see Table 6.5).
- Read BP to the nearest 2 mmHg.
- Measure diastolic BP during disappearance of Korotkoff sounds (phase 5).
- Take the mean of at least two readings; more readings are needed if marked differences between initial measurements are found.
- Do not treat on the basis of an isolated reading.

Documentation

Charting blood pressure readings

Once the systolic and diastolic BP values have been obtained they should be recorded promptly. If they need to be charted on an observation chart, this takes the format of a graph. Despite variations of the chart being available, the principles are the same. The systolic pressure is marked by an arrow at the top and the diastolic value by an arrow at the bottom. The space between the readings is drawn in a dotted line. After several readings have been charted this method allows trends to be seen clearly. Figures 6.4 and 6.5 show examples of charts with BP readings recorded.

THINK ABOUT IT

A blood pressure reading is taken with a cuff that is too large for the patient. How do you think this will affect the readings obtained? What implications might this have for the patient's treatment?

Common problems

Common complications can occur when using non-invasive blood pressure devices and it is important to identify these promptly and then reporting them to the nurse in charge to ensure patient safety. Box 6.4 shows the common complications.

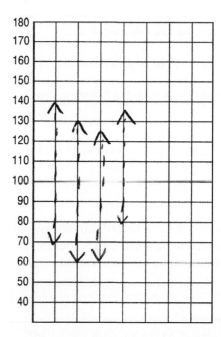

Figure 6.4 A TPR (temperature, pulse, respiratory rate) chart with blood pressure readings charted. Source: NHS Lothian 2008. Reproduced with permission of NHS Lothian.

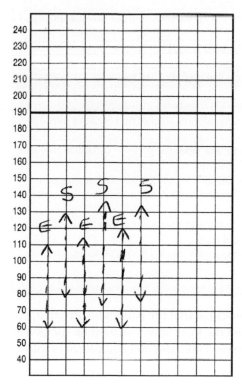

Figure 6.5 TPR (temperature, pulse, respiratory rate) chart with erect (standing: E) and supine (lying: S) blood pressure readings charted. Source: NHS Lothian 2008. Reproduced with permission of NHS Lothian.

Box 6.4 Common complications of non-invasive blood pressure measuring devices

- Swelling at the site where the cuff is placed, known as limb oedema, can occur (Jevon and Ewens 2007).
- Friction blisters can occur if the blood pressure machine is used very frequently causing irritation at the site (Jevon and Ewens 2007).
- Nerve damage can occur to the nerves within the arm, known as ulnar nerve palsy (Jevon and Ewens 2007).
- Excessive bruising and even wounds can result due the frequent overinflation of the cuff where the patient is receiving anticoagulant therapy that 'thins' the blood (e.g. heparin or warfarin) or due to peripheral neuropathy in diabetes (Uzun 2012).

Many patients who are having a BP recorded have underlying diseases or are receiving medical intervention that will need to be taken into account when considering a suitable site. Box 6.5 summarises some of the main considerations.

Box 6.5 Inappropriate sites and rationale

- **Intravenous infusion running:** taking blood pressure on this arm could interfere with fluid delivery.
- **Pulse oximetry machine being used**: taking BP on the same arm will alter the readings, because blood flow will be occluded.
- **Fistula/shunt**: shunts are used for renal dialysis and taking BP at this site may cause damage to the shunt.
- **Trauma**: where there has been injury to a site that could be used for BP measurement the cuff could cause further injury.
- **Atrial fibrillation** (increased heartbeat in the top chamber of the heart): some automated devices provide unreliable readings, and in such instances another type of device should be used (NICE 2011).
- **Previous stroke with residual damage to one side**: the patient's circulation may be affected or the arm is limited in movement or sensation.
- **Lymphoedema**: this is swelling that can be due to many causes, for example mastectomy with lymph node removal, and taking a BP reading could damage an area that is already swollen.
- **Arthritic limb**: the patient may have arthritis in the arm(s) resulting in correct positioning being problematic and causing discomfort and pain.
- **Circulatory problems**: where circulation in the arms is affected this may result in inaccurate readings.

To ensure accurate BP readings it is essential that the patient be prepared, the equipment be in good working order and the healthcare assistant be competent in the skill. Table 6.6 summarises the common operator and equipment problems when taking a BP reading.

Table 6.6 Common problems when taking a blood pressure reading.

Problem	Action to reduce inaccurate readings
Poor technique of the user (Wallymahmed 2008)	Ensure that, before undertaking the procedure, competency based training and assessment have been completed in line with local policy
Machine malfunction	Report to appropriate personnel (e.g. medical physics, servicing department or manufacturer). Do not use the machine
Equipment has tape applied to secure	Report and do not use the damaged piece of equipment
Use of an incorrectly sized cuff (Wallymahmed 2008)	This is essential for accurate readings and an appropriate sized cuff should be sought (see Table 6.5)
Failure to ensure that the mercury column is initially at zero (Wallymahmed 2008)	Always ensure that the mercury column is initially at zero before commencing the procedure
Patient has tight clothing on	This will give an inaccurate reading and clothing needs to be removed
The arm is not correctly supported	If the arm is unsupported the muscles may contract, leading to a rise in diastolic blood pressure (Wallymahmed 2008). Incorrect positioning during the procedure can lead to an error rate as high as 10% (Jevon and Ewens 2007)
Blood pressure cuff comes off when reading taken	This can be due to the wrong size of cuff and the arm circumference should be re-measured and the correct cuff used
	In other instances, the Velcro on the cuff may be worn and ineffective and will need to be replaced
Cannot 'hear' blood pressure sounds	Ensure that all equipment is working. Palpate pulse and ensure that the stethoscope is at the correct pulse point. Seek assistance if unsure.
Patient complains that it is sore to take blood pressure	Do not pump cuff up too high unless patient has hypertension. Use estimated systolic value (see Table 6.3) or previous readings to act as a reference
Movement causes noise and inaccurate readings	Ask the patient to remain still or if the patient cannot do this, ask colleague to assist you
Rounding up readings to the nearest 5 or 10 mmHg (Wallymahmed 2008)	Document the exact reading that is obtained

Table 6.7 Competency framework: recording a blood pressure.

(BP)	First assessment/reassessment					Date/competent/ signature
Steps	**Demonstration**					
	Date/sign 1	Date/sign 2	Date/sign 3	Date/sign 4	Date/sign 5	
Blood pressure						
1 Describe what is blood pressure and the relationship with the heart						
2 State sites for recording blood pressure with rationale						
3 State examples of inappropriate sites for a healthcare assistant						
4 State the normal range for blood pressure readings						
5 Describe systolic and diastolic pressure						
6 Describe some factors affecting blood pressure						
7 Describe the procedure for manual, aneroid and automated devices, including choice of sites						
8 Describe maintenance of all pieces of equipment, including reporting faults						

(BP)

Recording blood pressure	First assessment/reassessment Demonstration					Date/competent/ signature
	Date/sign 1	Date/sign 2	Date/sign 3	Date/sign 4	Date/sign 5	
9 Describe the procedure for dealing with mercury spillage (if applicable)						
10 State when to report/ask for assistance						
11 Collect all equipment						
12 Demonstrate correct identification of patient, effective explanation and communication in relation to blood pressure recording						
13 Demonstrate accurate recording using: (a) automatic blood pressure machine, (b) mercury sphygmomanometer and/or (c) aneroid sphygmomanometer						
14 Demonstrate correct documentation of the recording						
15 Demonstrate tidying away of equipment including cleaning						

Summary

An understanding of how the body controls blood pressure can help link theory to practice. It is essential that BP be taken with equipment on which the healthcare assistant has completed competency based training because the recordings can affect patient management. Abnormal or unusual recordings for the patient should always be reported to ensure prompt management where necessary.

Blood pressure measurement is an area of healthcare assistant practice with the potential to make a real difference to the patient's quality of life and lifespan (Thornett 2007). Table 6.7 is an example of a competency framework for blood pressure measurement.

CASE STUDY 6.1

Mrs Wooley has come to the well woman clinic for a check up. As part of the process you are asked to take her observations. In your surgery you use an automatic machine and her blood pressure reading is 145/95 and you also notice her pulse is irregular. What might be causing this high reading and what actions would you take regarding her observations?

CASE STUDY 6.2

Mr Jones has lung cancer and is admitted for pain control and dehydration. He is emaciated (thin) and frail, and has an intravenous infusion running. His blood pressure is being taken with a mercury sphygmomanometer and a standard size adult cuff is being used. The readings are not what you would expect given his condition. What actions would you take to ensure that the readings are correct?

Self-assessment

Assessment	Aspects	Achieved ✓
Patient	*Have you considered all aspects of this section?* What blood pressure actually measures in the patient What the systolic and diastolic pressure represent The factors that affect blood pressure The role of the cardiac cycle	
Procedure	*Have you considered all aspects of this section?* Selecting equipment Suitable sites Patient information Documenting and reporting concerns	**Achieved ✓**

References

British Hypertension Society (2004) Guidelines for management of hypertension: report of the fourth working party of the British Hypertension Society, 2004 – BHS IV. *Journal of Human Hypertension* 18: 139–185.

British Hypertension Society (2006) Fact File 01/2006. Blood Pressure Measurement. Available at: www.bhsoc.org/bhf&uscore;factfiles/bhf&uscore;factfile&uscore;jan&uscore;2006.doc (accessed 1 March 2008).

Clancy J and McVicar A. (2009) *Physiology and Anatomy for Nurse and Healthcare Practitioners: A Homeostatic Approach,* 3rd edn. London: Arnold Hodder.

Dougherty L and Lister S (eds) (2011) *The Royal Marsden Hospital Manual of Clinical Nursing Procedures,* 8th edn. Oxford: Blackwell Publishing.

Dickinson H O, Beyer F R, Ford G A et al. (2008) Relaxation therapies for the management of primary hypertension in adults: a Cochrane review. *Journal of Human Hypertension* 22: 809–820.

Dieterle T (2012) Blood pressure measurement – an overview. *Swiss Medical Weekly* 142 (13517): 4–9.

ERPHO (2008) Modelled Estimates and Projections of Hypertension for PCTs in England. Available at: www.erpho.org.uk/viewResource. aspx?id=17905 (accessed December 2015).

Herminda R, Ayala D, Mojon A and Fernandez J (2011) Influence of time of day of blood pressure lowering treatment on cardiovascular risk in hypertensive patietns with type 2 diabetes. *Diabetes Care* 34(6): 1270–1276.

Hypertension Influence Team (2007) Let's Do it Well. Nurse Learning Pack. Available at: www.bhsoc.org/pdfs/hit.pdf (accessed 16 October 2008).

Jevon P and Ewens B (2007) *Monitoring the Critically Ill Patient: Essential Clinical Skills for Nurses,* 2nd edn. London: Blackwell.

Jevon P and Holmes J (2007) Blood pressure measurement. Part 3: lying and standing blood pressure. *Nursing Times* 103(20): 24–25.

Joint British Societies (2005) Joint British Societies' guidelines on prevention of cardiovascular disease in clinical practice. *Heart* 91(suppl 5): v1–52.

Loscalzo J, Fauci A and Braunwald E (2008) *Harrisons Principles of Internal Medicine.* New York: McGraw Hill.

Maddex S (2009) In: Baillie L (ed.) *Developing Practical Nursing Skills,* 3rd edn. London: Hodder Education, pp. 134–141.

Marieb E M and Hoehn K (2010) *Human Anatomy and Physiology,* 8th edn. San Francisco: Pearson Education.

MRHA (2009) Mercury in Medical Devices. Available at: http://www.mhra.gov.uk/Safetyinformation/Generalsafetyinformationandadvice/Product-specificinformationandadvice/Product-specificinformationandadvice–M–T/Mercuryinmedicaldevices/index.htm (accessed 18 July 2012).

NICE (2011) *CG127. Hypertension: Clinical Management of Primary Hypertension in Adults.* London: NICE.

NHS Lothian (2008) *Observations Chart.* Edinburgh: NHS Lothian.

O'Brien E, Asmar R and Beilin L et al. (2003) European Society of Hypertension recommendations for conventional, ambulatory and home blood pressure measurement. *Journal of Hypertension* 21: 821–848.

SCENIHR (2009) *Mercury Sphygmomanometers in Healthcare and the Feasibility of Alternatives.* London: SCENIHR.

Sathyapalan T, Aye M and Atkin, S. (2011) Postural hypotension. *British Medical Journal* 3128: 1–3342.

Thibodeau G A and Patton K T (2007) *Anatomy and Physiology*, 6th edn. St Louis, MO: Elsevier Mosby.

Thornett A (2007) New skills for healthcare assistants: taking a blood pressure. *British Journal of Healthcare Assistants* 1(3): 133–135.

Tortora G J and Derrickson B (2011) *Principles of Anatomy and Physiology*, 13th edn. Hoboken, NJ: Wiley & Sons.

Uzun G, Karagoz H, Mutluoglu M, et al. (2012) Non invasive blood pressure cuff induced lower extremity wound in a diabetic patient. *European Review For Medical and Pharmacological Sciences* 16(5): 707–708.

Valler-Jones T and Wedgbury K (2005) Measuring blood pressure using the mercury sphygmomanometer. *British Journal of Nursing* 14: 145–150.

Wallymahmed M (2008) Blood pressure measurement. *Nursing Standard* 22(19): 45–48.

Waugh A and Grant A (2010) *Ross and Wilson Anatomy and Physiology in Health and Illness*, 11th edn. Edinburgh: Churchill Livingstone.

Williams B, Poulter N R, Brown M J, et al. (2004) British Hypertension Society Guidelines. Guidelines for management of hypertension: report of the fourth working party of the British Hypertension Society 2004 (BHS IV). *Journal of Human Hypertension* 18: 139–185.

CHAPTER 7

Temperature

LEARNING OBJECTIVES

- Identify the normal temperature range and describe how body temperature is controlled
- List the factors that affect heat production and heat loss
- Identify the symptoms and causes of increased and decreased temperature
- Describe the different devices that record temperature and how they work
- Describe how to take and record an accurate temperature

Aim of this chapter

The aim of this chapter is review the principles and practice surrounding temperature measurement and its related physiology.

What is temperature?

Body temperature is the balance between heat loss and heat production (Clancy and McVicar 2009). To ensure that a constant temperature is maintained, a fine balance between heat produced in the body and heat lost to the environment is essential (Waugh and Grant 2010). The body's core temperature is the optimum temperature for the body's organs to function, and the range varies between 36 °C and 37.5 °C (Tortora and Derrickson 2011). The shell temperature is the temperature near the body surface (Tortora and Derrickson 2011). Figure 7.1 shows the body temperature at different sites.

Reasons for measuring temperature

- To determine a baseline (a reading against which future readings can be compared) on admission to hospital (Dougherty and Lister 2011).

Clinical Skills for Healthcare Assistants and Assistant Practitioners, Second Edition.
Angela Whelan and Elaine Hughes.
© 2016 John Wiley & Sons, Ltd. Published 2016 by John Wiley & Sons, Ltd.

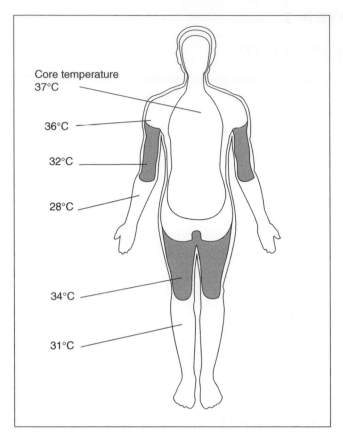

Figure 7.1 Body temperature at different sites on the body. (Adapted from Torrance and Semple 1998.)

- To monitor fluctuations in temperature (Dougherty and Lister 2011).
- To identify changes in a patient's condition so treatment can be planned accordingly (Dougherty and Lister 2011).
- To ensure patient safety (McCallum and Higgins 2012).
- To identify potential disease or infection (Jevon 2010).

Normal limits

In normal health, despite changes to external temperature, the body is able to maintain a core temperature around 37 °C (Tortora and Derrickson 2011). However, an individual's temperature can safely range from 36 °C to 37.6 °C without homeostasis being affected (Clancy and McVicar 2009). Because treatments can be based upon temperature recordings, it is essential that readings are accurate and reported as necessary.

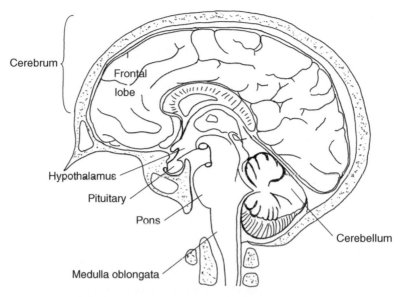

Figure 7.2 Location of the hypothalamus and medulla oblongata within the brain.

Relevant anatomy and physiology

Temperature is controlled by a temperature-regulating centre in the hypothalamus, which is situated in the brain. It is responsive to the temperature of circulating blood and the vasomotor centre in the medulla oblongata, which controls the diameter of blood vessels. This controls heat loss and gain (Waugh and Grant 2010). Figure 7.2 shows the location of the hypothalamus and medulla oblongata within the brain.

The body also has thermoreceptors (sensors) in the skin and mucous membranes that send signals to the hypothalamus stimulating the production or loss of heat. This results in the body being able to regulate temperature. It is therefore vital that our body temperature be kept within fairly strict limits. This is done via a negative feedback system and is known as homeostasis or the 'constant internal environment' (Clancy and McVicar 2009) (see Figure 7.5 later in text).

Related aspects and terminology

In order to understand temperature regulation, both heat production and loss need to be understood.

Heat production

All living cells produce heat during metabolism: in muscles when they are active and continuously by the liver. It can also depend on the body's metabolic rate (the rate at which the body uses energy). Factors that affect heat production are included in Table 7.1.

THINK ABOUT IT

What effect do you think prolonged exposure to either a hot, humid desert environment or a cold, snowy, freezing climate would have on body temperature?

Table 7.1 Factors affecting heat production.

Factor	Rationale
Metabolic rate	The basal metabolic rate produces heat, which in turn directly affects the body's temperature (Clancy and McVicar 2009)
Exercise	Exercise is known to increase the metabolic rate. Furthermore, during strenuous activity the basal rate can increase by up to 15 times, increasing up to 20 times for elite athletes (Tortora and Derrickson 2011). Immobility and age can have the opposite effect, with individuals needing to add layers of clothes for warmth (Turnball and Petty 2013; Sund-Levander and Grodzinsky 2010)
Sweat gland activity	Reduced sweat gland activity preserves heat that would normally be lost by evaporation (see heat loss)
Goosebumps/ shivering	Goosebumps occur when the muscles surrounding the hair follicles contract, causing the raising of the hair to trap a layer of air around the body and prevent heat loss. If this is ineffective, shivering often follows Shivering involves intense, muscular contraction and relaxation cycles. This physiological response to cold produces heat which directly increases body temperature (Clancy and McVicar 2009)
Hormones/disease	The main hormones relating to temperature control are those from the thyroid, predominantly thyroxine (T4). In the case of an overactive thyroid, where there is increased hormone production, individuals may have a higher than normal body temperature. An underactive thyroid results in the opposite with a reduced metabolic rate and a reduced temperature (Mulryan 2010) In times of stress, adrenaline and other hormones may be released, which can also increase the metabolic rate and produce heat (Tortora and Derrickson 2011). Other conditions that affect temperature include hypoglycaemia (low glucose level in blood) and adrenal insufficiency (adrenal glands are situated on top of the kidneys)
Infection	The body responds to infection by releasing pyrogens that change the hypothalamus reset point, having the effect of increasing body temperature (Clancy and McVicar 2009). For every degree centigrade increase in body temperature, the metabolism increases by around 10% (Tortora and Derrickson 2011)

(continued overleaf)

Table 7.1 (*continued*)

Factor	Rationale
Eating	Eating and digesting food can increase the metabolic rate up to 10–20%, with a higher increase for protein-based meals than that for carbohydrates and lipids (Tortora and Derrickson 2011)
Age	Neonates have an underdeveloped thermocentre in the brain and require intervention to ensure that heat loss is minimised, e.g. extra clothing, including a hat to reduce heat loss from the head. In low birth weight neonates, current practice advocates placing the infant into polythene bags to prevent rapid heat loss (Turnball and Petty 2013). In children the metabolic rate (in relation to their size) is double that of an older person, due to growth (Tortora and Derrickson 2011). In older people the metabolic rate is lower and there is a decreasing incline to sweating, which contributes to the body temperature generally being lower (Sund-Levander and Grodzinsky 2010)
Gender	Metabolic rates tend to be higher in males than females, which in turn increases the temperature (Tortora and Derrickson 2011)
Body shape	Larger individuals will have a higher basal rate due to an increase in surface area, therefore increasing the body temperature (Tortora and Derrickson 2011)
Pregnancy/ breast-feeding	Pregnancy and breast-feeding increase the basal metabolic rate and can have a direct influence on temperature (Tortora and Derrickson 2011)
Menstruation	Immediately prior to ovulation the body's temperature can reduce by up to 0.5 °C due to a reduction in progesterone. Following ovulation temperature returns to normal (Clancy and McVicar 2009).
Medications/ alcohol	Some medications can increase the basal rate and temperature, e.g. amphetamines (Tortora and Derrickson 2011). Antidepressants, sedatives and tranquillisers have the opposite effect and can reduce the body temperature Alcohol does not promote heat production and may suppress the body's warning of low or high temperatures due to altered consciousness and awareness
Environmental factors	In hot climates, a reduction in the basal metabolic rate occurs and the body reduces heat production in an effort to cool the body. Heat loss through sweating also occurs (Clancy and McVicar 2009)
Time of day	The body's natural variance, which causes hourly fluctuations, is known as the circadian rhythm. This is influenced by sleep patterns (e.g. day/night shift workers) with the higher recording of temperature in the hours after awakening and before retiring. This has implication for the basal metabolic rate which reduces during sleep (Clancy and McVicar 2009)

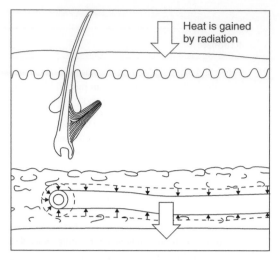

Figure 7.3 Heat production and heat gain from the skin.

When looking after patients, many factors may influence metabolic rate and temperature control. The skin can gain heat by radiation, for example through sunlight; this heat is then absorbed deep down into the subcutaneous layers and blood vessels (Clancy and McVicar 2009). Figure 7.3 shows how the skin controls heat production and heat gain.

Heat loss

Most heat loss from the body occurs through the skin (Figure 7.4), although small amounts are lost in expired air, urine and faeces (Waugh and Grant 2010). Heat is lost from the skin when heat is conducted to the skin surface. It is then lost by radiation, or mixed with sweat to be lost by evaporation.

The methods of heat loss are evaporation, conduction, radiation and convection, and each is described in turn.

Evaporation

Evaporation is the conversion of a liquid into a vapour. In the human body, evaporation of water requires heat energy to be used, causing heat to be lost primarily from the skin (Tortora and Derrickson 2011). An increase in temperature stimulates the sweat glands, which secrete sweat on the surface of the body via ducts. The evaporating sweat then cools the skin and the body loses heat (Waugh and Grant 2010).

THINK ABOUT IT

Can you think of a time when your body sweated or shivered? How did this make you feel?

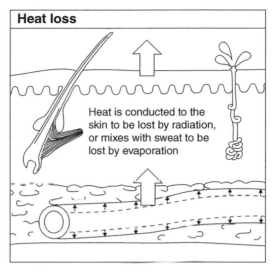

Figure 7.4 Heat loss from the skin.

Evaporation is of particular importance in high environmental temperatures when it is the only method that cools the body (Tortora and Derrickson 2011). Loss of heat by evaporation can also occur from the deeper layers of the skin to the surface of the body, from mucous membranes and during breathing. Here the individual is unaware that evaporation is occurring, and this is known as insensible loss (Waugh and Grant 2010). Insensible loss is often used when calculating fluid balance charts to ensure that all fluid loss is considered (see Chapter 14).

Conduction
This is the transfer of heat to any substance in direct contact with the body (Tortora and Derrickson 2011). It accounts for a relatively small amount of heat loss and examples include clothes or jewellery taking up heat from the skin. Hot and cold drinks as well as hot and cold baths can also cause the body to conduct (Tortora and Derrickson 2011).

Radiation
Radiation is the transfer of heat via infrared rays between a warmer and a cooler object without physical contact, for example the sun. In cool environments the body loses a greater percentage of heat loss from the skin by this method than through conduction and evaporation combined (Clancy and McVicar 2009). In hot environments no heat is lost by this route, but may be gained by heat radiating to the skin (Tortora and Derrickson 2011).

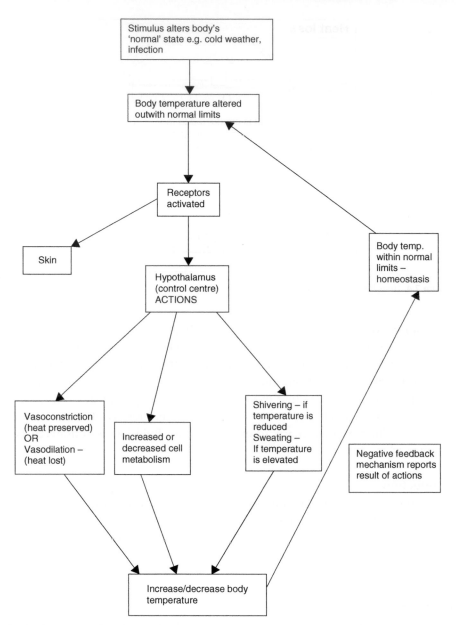

Figure 7.5 Negative feedback mechanism to control body temperature. (Adapted from Tortora and Derrickson (2011) and Dougherty and Lister (2011).)

Convection

This is movement of heat away from a surface by movement of heated air or particles (Tortora and Derrickson 2011). A cool fan or convection heater would fulfil this purpose by circulating and moving the air. Another example would be getting out of a hot bath, which would have provided heat to the body, and then the heat being quickly lost via a cool breeze from an open window (Tortora and Derrickson 2011).

THINK ABOUT IT

What nursing actions are taken to promote heat loss due to an increase in temperature in a patient and how do they work? Are there any particular patients you would take care with when reducing temperature?

Temperature control is essential for the well-being of the human body and this maintenance is done by constantly checking, and if necessary altering, systems. This cycle is called a negative feedback mechanism and is shown in Figure 7.5.

Terminology

- *Core temperature*: the temperature deep within the body supplying the major organs (Clancy and McVicar 2009).
- *Shell temperature*: the temperature near the body surface, including the skin and the subcutaneous layers (Tortora and Derrickson 2011).
- *Hypothermia*: lowering of the body's core temperature to 35 °C or lower (Maddex 2009).
- *Pyrexia*: a temperature >37.5–38.9 °C (Dougherty and Lister 2011).
- *Hyperthermia*: a core temperature >40.0 °C (Dougherty and Lister 2011).

Hypothermia

This is when the body's temperature is <35 °C and mechanisms to increase heat production are ineffective (Maddex 2009). The body's metabolic rate is reduced in an attempt to try to preserve heat (Clancy and McVicar 2009). The causes of hypothermia are shown in Box 7.1.

Box 7.1 Summary of causes of hypothermia

- Renal dialysis due to heat loss from the blood leaving the body and dialysate entering (Ronco and Ricci 2008).
- Anaesthesia (Tanner 2011).
- Burns as the body is unable to regulate surface temperature (Clancy and McVicar 2009).
- Extreme or overwhelming cold, for example exposure to a cold environment (Clancy and McVicar 2009)
- Low metabolic rate, especially in older people and in hypothyroidism (Clancy and McVicar 2009).
- Rapid blood transfusion (Vasiliki 2011).

- Metabolic conditions, such as hypoglycaemia (low blood sugar) and adrenal insufficiency (Dougherty and Lister 2011).
- Medications that alter the perception of cold, increase heat loss by vasodilatation or inhibit heat generation, for example alcohol, paracetamol, antidepressants (Dougherty and Lister 2011).

Patients may shiver due to being cold as the body attempts to increase its metabolic rate and therefore produce heat (Clancy and McVicar 2009). In these cases a warming blanket may be sufficient to raise the temperature, or in extreme cases warmed fluids may be used to raise core temperature (Mains 2008). If the temperature continues to drop, shivering is replaced by muscle rigidity and cramps, and blood pressure and heart rate begin to slow (Clancy and McVicar 2009). In extreme hypothermia, confusion, loss of consciousness or cardiac problems can occur, leading to death if the temperature falls to <25 °C (Clancy and McVicar 2009).

Pyrexia

The term pyrexia relates to an increase in the body's core temperature (Dougherty and Lister 2011). Patients with pyrexia often appear flushed, and as the body attempts to lose heat they can feel hot to the touch. Pyrexia can be divided into three grades and these are shown in Table 7.2.

Leach (2009) suggests that in half of patients that have a high temperature this is related to an infection that is either bacterial or viral in origin. Where there is an increase in temperature but no infection evident, the causes for the increase in temperature are known as non-infective causes of pyrexia and hyperthermia (Dougherty and Lister 2011). Causes of non-infective pyrexia and hyperthermia are shown in Box 7.2. Occasionally people who have very high temperatures will

Table 7.2 Grades of pyrexia.

Grade	Temperature (°C)	Details
Low grade	37 to 38	Indicates an inflammatory response as a result of mild infection, allergy or disturbance of body tissue. Can also be due to trauma, surgery, malignancy or blood clots (thrombosis)
Moderate-to-high grade	38–40	Caused by a wound or other infections (e.g. respiratory or urinary tract)
Hyperpyrexia	≥40	Bacteraemia (the presence of bacteria in the blood), damage to the hypothalamus or high environmental temperatures

Source: Adapted from Dougherty (2011). Reproduced with permission of Wiley Blackwell.

feel cold and begin to shiver, and this is known as a 'rigor'. The reason for this is that the hypothalamus becomes confused and resets itself to a higher point. The body then attempts to heat itself to meet this point by shivering in the same way it does when it is cold. When this reset point is met it is then that the patient stops shivering and begins to feel hot. This increase in body temperature due to infection is the body's own response of killing any bacteria in the body (Clancy and McVicar 2009).

Box 7.2 Non-infective causes of pyrexia/hyperthermia

- Alcohol withdrawal.
- Medications (including recreational drugs such as ecstasy).
- Allergic drug or transfusion reaction.
- Reaction to vaccines (common in neonates and children).
- Exercise.
- Gout.
- Trauma.
- Heat stroke or heat exhaustion.
- Hyperthyroidism (overactive thyroid), this causes an increase in metabolic rate.
- Malignancy (cancer).
- Status epilepticus (constant fitting).
- Stroke/heart attack (myocardial infarction)
- Central nervous system damage.
- Vasculitis (inflammation of a blood vessel).
- Surgery.
- Environmental factors – hot and humid surroundings/too many layers of clothing.
(Adapted from Dougherty and Lister 2011.)

Often patients with high temperatures will be given medication to reduce their temperature (antipyrexial medication) and a fan (to promote air circulation), or be sponged with cool, slightly warm water (tepid sponging), which will aim to cool the surface of the skin. The evidence for these routine interventions is limited, and it is suggested that giving antipyretics for high temperatures prevents the body's own defence mechanisms from working effectively as well as masking symptoms (Leach 2009). Care should also be taken when using fans and they should not be used in the chill phase as this can cause an increase in temperature due to shivering (Jevon 2010). However, if the patient is feeling hot provision of a fan with indirect air circulation across the skin can be beneficial in terms of patient comfort. Tepid sponging can have similar effects to fan cooling and cause patients to shiver. NICE (2007b) also recommend that tepid sponging should not be carried out on children as there are no proven benefits. If the temperature continues to rise, dehydration can occur as a result of loss of fluid through sweating, and convulsions can occur (particularly common in the under-5 age group). Following this, body proteins (enzymes), which are involved in chemical reactions, are disrupted, affecting the chemical reaction in the body, leading to death at 44–45 °C (Tortora and Derrickson 2011).

Taking a temperature reading

There are various methods of taking a temperature reading and each is discussed in turn. The equipment that you use will often depend on whether it is suitable for the patient and its availability in the clinical area. Recommended good practice is that the same site and method are used where possible and that this information is documented for future reference (Sund-Levander and Grodzinsky 2010). A summary of the advantages and disadvantages of each method is shown in Table 7.3. However, it should be noted that no one method or site is viewed as best, with many authors disagreeing about the accuracy of different methods and sites (Farnell et al. 2005; El-Radhi and Patel 2006; Mackechnie and Simpson 2006; DeVrim et al. 2007; Sund-Levander and Grodzinsky 2010).

Table 7.3 Summary of the advantages and disadvantages of different methods.

	Advantages	Disadvantages
Mercury	Can be reused for groups of patients	Mercury is actively discouraged due to the health and safety risk
		Risks of cross-infection with poor cleaning techniques
		Can be inaccurate if used incorrectly
Electronic	Quick, easy to use	Cost implications re-disposables
	Disposable cover for each measurement, promoting infection control	Machine requires maintenance
		When using the machine with an oral probe, because of the weight of the probe it needs to be held in place
Tympanic	Quick, accurate and easy to use	Cost implications re-disposables
	Disposable cover for each measurement, promoting infection control	Machine requires maintenance and calibration
		Not suitable for children under 4 weeks
		Can be used only in the ear for tympanic membrane use
Chemical	Totally non-invasive	Cost implications re-disposables
	Disposable for each patient	Requires storage at below 30 °C (Maddex 2009)
Temporal artery	Quick	
	Can be used on all age groups	Has been shown to be inaccurate compared to other methods of temperature measurement

The main methods are the following:

* Mercury thermometer – oral/axilla or rectal.
* Tympanic thermometer.
* Electronic thermometer.
* Chemical (dots).
* Temporal artery.

Mercury thermometer

Mercury thermometers have been withdrawn from sale since 2009 due to the risks of environmental contamination with spilt mercury. However, mercury thermometers still within use in the workplace and in a good state of repair can be used where there is no other alternative (MHRA 2013). There are different types of mercury thermometer available, namely oral (for oral or axillary use) or rectal (for rectal use, often with a red bulb to distinguish between oral and rectal) and a low reading thermometer (for hypothermic patients), which can be used at any site, but has a lower range starting at 24 °C.

Tympanic thermometers

Tympanic thermometers operate by sensing body heat through infrared energy given off by the tympanic membrane in the ear (Mains 2008). The only site for this method is the ear canal and DeVrim et al. (2007) report that, as the tympanic membrane and the hypothalamus share a common blood supply, it is a valid indicator of core temperature. Ear canal size, presence of wax, operator technique and the patient's position can potentially affect the accuracy of the readings; however, the literature surrounding this is inconclusive (Sund-Levander and Grodzinsky 2010; Mains 2008).

In addition, maintenance of the machines is essential and it is particularly important that they are calibrated correctly, because failure to do so results in the reading being unreliable, with measurements continually becoming less accurate as more readings are taken (Mackechnie and Simpson 2006). The thermometer can calculate the temperature at the tympanic membrane, but can also convert it into the reading at the skin surface, oral or core by using the 'mode' button. To ensure that accurate readings are obtained it is essential that healthcare assistants understand this function. Models and manufacturers do vary, so check locally with regard to the model used in practice.

Electronic thermometer

This is an electronic or digital machine with a probe, which can be used orally, rectally or in the axilla. Sahib El-Radhi (2013) suggests that digital thermometers record a temperature in less than a minute, which is generally indicated by an audible beep, making this a much quicker method of temperature measurement. They also have plastic sheaths to cover the probes that are aimed at reducing

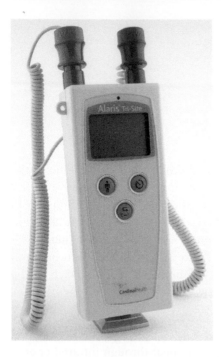

Figure 7.6 Electronic thermometer. Produced with kind permission from Cardinal Health.

the risk of infection; however, the thermometer should still be decontaminated between each patient use. Maintenance and knowledge of how to use the machine is essential to ensure accurate temperature measurement. Figure 7.6 shows an electronic thermometer.

Chemical thermometer

These are thin plastic strips that have 50 small dots of thermosensitive chemicals, which change colour with increasing temperature (Maddex 2009). They should be stored at below 30 °C and can be used orally or in the axilla (Maddex 2009). It is essential to ensure that they are placed correctly; where the axillary route is being used, the dots must placed next to the inner part of the body, in contact with it. For either oral or axilla use it is essential that the thermometer be left in place for one minute orally and three minutes for axillary (Sahib El-Radhi 2013). They are disposable for each patient and non-invasive and can therefore reduce the risk of cross-infection.

Temporal artery thermometer

This is a hand-held non-contact thermometer that takes a reading after the probe has been scanned along the forehead. The machine uses an 'arterial heat balance method' to take a reading by measuring the temperature of the skin surface over the artery and the ambient temperature, and then calculating the arterial temperature. However, sweat produced during fever can cause this type of thermometer to give inaccurate results, as can changes in the ambient room temperature (Sahib El-Radhi 2013). A study undertaken by Hamilton et al. (2013) compared the results of tympanic and temporal artery temperature measurements. Here it was found that the incidence of temporal thermometers misclassifying pyrexial patients as having a normal temperature were about three times higher than tympanic. Therefore this method of temperature measurement may have implications for the diagnosis and treatment of patients. In summary, there are many methods of taking a temperature recording. However, all equipment must be used as intended by the manufacturer, including correct placement and timing, otherwise inaccurate recordings will be obtained.

Route

The choices of sites for temperature measurement are oral, rectal, axilla, tympanic membrane and temporal artery. A summary of the advantages and disadvantages of each site is given in Table 7.4.

When choosing the site for recording temperature, factors such as previous sites, the equipment available and an assessment of the patient should all be considered. The procedure to obtain recordings is given next.

Taking a temperature reading

First, taking a temperature reading using a mercury thermometer is discussed at oral, rectal or axillary sites. The equipment required is shown in Box 7.3.

Box 7.3 Equipment needed to take a temperature recording with a mercury thermometer

- Vessel containing thermometer.
- Alcohol swabs.
- Tissue (for rectal use).
- Lubricant (for rectal use).
- Watch that is capable of timing in minutes.

The procedure for taking a temperature reading using a mercury or electronic thermometer device is shown in Table 7.5, taking a tympanic temperature reading is shown in Table 7.6 and temporal artery thermometer reading is shown in Table 7.7.

THINK ABOUT IT

Which methods and sites do you think would be suitable for the following patients: a frail, thin older patient; an unconscious patient; a baby of 11 months; and a child aged 10 years? What are the reasons for your choices?

Table 7.4 Summary of the advantages and disadvantages of different sites for measuring body temperature.

Sites	Advantages	Disadvantages
Oral: requires the probe tip to be placed in the mouth in the sublingual pocket, which is under the tongue (Mains 2008)	Easily accessible, no undressing required	Sublingual pocket must be used or inaccurate results will be obtained
		The patient cannot talk while the procedure is being performed and it is not suitable for breathless patients because it is important that the lips close around the thermometer (Sund-Levander and Grodzinsky 2010)
		It is also unsuitable for patients who have disease or pain/discomfort in the oral mucosa because the thermometer may cause further pain or discomfort
		Not suitable for children under 5, confused or unconscious patients, because they may bite the probe or be unable to hold in place
		When timing the duration, the thermometer must remain in place for an accurate reading; this is a source for error because it is often not left in situ for long enough, giving inaccurate readings
		When using mercury thermometer, if the glass breaks this causes a hazard (MHRA 2013)
		This route is unsuitable for patients who have recently had a hot or cold food or drink, or smoked (Mains 2008).
Rectal: involves placement of the probe 4 cm into the rectum in adults	Useful if the patient has peripheral shut-down (poor circulation at extremities)	Invasive and can be embarrassing for patients Not suitable for neonates because of incidence of rectal perforation (DeVrim et al. 2007)

(*continued overleaf*)

Table 7.4 (*continued*)

Sites	Advantages	Disadvantages
Sund-Levander and Grodzinsky 2010)		The presence of soft stools can alter recordings (Sund-Levander and Grodzinsky 2010)
	Useful only if other sites are not possible	Not suitable if any rectal disease or irritation is evident (Sund-Levander and Grodzinsky 2010)
Tympanic: the probe is inserted into the ear canal (see Table 7.3)	Non invasive Very quick – takes 3 seconds Suitable for most adults and children (Mains 2008) Value not influenced by food, drink or smoking	Correct placement not always achieved Localised temperature can affect results, e.g. cool air or placement against a pillow (which will generate heat) before measurement can affect results
Axilla: where the thermometer is placed under the arm	Non-invasive	Often not left in for sufficient time when using mercury thermometers
	Patient can talk while in place	Vasoconstriction (blood vessels narrow) or chilled skin give inaccurate readings (Sund-Levander and Grodzinsky 2010)
		Can prove difficult to hold in place for the required duration, especially for children, confused patients and the elderly
Temporal artery: requires the device to be 'stroked' across the centre of the forehead from the midline to the lateral hairline and then placed behind the earlobe, in the soft depression below the mastoid	Non-invasive Quick Value unaffected by eating, drinking or smoking	Correct placement will require some education Limited research available currently

The temperature recorded at different sites will give various different readings, rectal measurements giving the highest because it is deeper in the body, followed by tympanic, with oral methods recording the lowest value. Table 7.8 summarises the variance in temperature dependent on the site.

Documentation

The temperature recording must be documented in either the patient's case notes or on an observation chart depending upon the area of practice.

Table 7.5 Procedure for taking a temperature reading using either a mercury or electronic thermometer.

Action	Rationale
1. Explain the procedure to the patient fully, including reason for test and to gain verbal consent	Patient fully understands why test is being performed and the procedure, and has agreed to participate
2. Check whether the patient has had food or drink or has smoked in past 20–30 minutes. *Oral only*	To ensure accurate reading
3. Wipe thermometer with alcohol swab. Check that mercury is at base of thermometer Place cover over an electronic probe	Prevent cross-infection To ensure accurate reading
4. Place the thermometer	To ensure correct positioning of the thermometer for accurate reading
For oral: place the bulb of the thermometer in patients' mouths under the tongue in the sublingual pocket and ask them to close their lips around it	
For axillary: place the bulb fully under the arm of the patient with the arm across the chest to hold it in place	
For rectal: lubricate the thermometer with lubricating jelly; place 4 cm into the rectum (Sund-Levander and Grodzinsky 2010)	
5. Leave in place for 3–5 min Electronic thermometer will beep.	To ensure accurate reading
6. Remove the thermometer If rectal site is used immediately wipe both the patient's rectum and the thermometer with tissue Document and/or report reading	Patient comfort Report abnormal findings immediately to nurse in charge as further care may require planning. Documentation provides a legal record
7. Wipe with alcohol – start at the end held by the nurse and wipe in a rotating manner towards the bulb end	Prevent cross-infection
Shake the thermometer so that the mercury returns to the base	Thermometer ready for use next time
Remove the plastic cover on an electronic probe and dispose in clinical waste	
Replace probe in correct position for storage (electronic)	

Table 7.6 Procedure for taking a temperature reading using a tympanic thermometer.

Action	Rationale
1. Explain the procedure to the patient fully, including the reason for test and to gain verbal consent	Patient fully understands why test is being performed and procedure, and has agreed to participate.
	Note that not suitable for children under 4 weeks old (NICE 2007b) and the correct size probe should be used for accurate readings (Mains 2008)
2. Ensure that the patient is not positioned in a draught or that the ear has been against a pillow	May affect readings
3. Do not use ears that have been reported as sore	May affect placement and accurate readings
4. Apply a new probe cover each time the machine is used	As per manufacturer's instructions
	Prevent cross-infection
	Provide accurate readings
5. Position thermometer as per manufacturer's instructions	Optimal reading
6. Scan the ear, and then listen for audible beep	Confirms reading has been taken.
	A measurement may not be the same in the left and right ear due to physiological differences so record which ear the reading has been taken from
7. If reading is not valid, repeat	Wait at least 2 min before repeating a measurement in the same ear to reduce an artificially low reading from 'draw down', caused by placing the probe tip into the ear canal and reducing its internal temperature
8. Report any abnormal findings	To plan further management

Temperature recordings on an observation chart are usually documented in a graph (Figure 7.7). In Acute Hospital Trusts temperature measurements are part of the Early Warning Scoring system (track and trigger systems) recommended by NICE (2007a). A baseline recording, often done on admission to hospital, will act as a reference for what is 'normal' for that patient. As temperature can vary due to the site, documenting the site where the temperature is taken from, as well as the actual reading, is recommended (Jevon 2010).

Abnormalities should always be reported to the nurse in charge, so further management can be planned where necessary. However, the reading should also be taken together with how the patient looks and feels: for example is the patient

Table 7.7 Procedure for taking a temperature reading using a temporal artery thermometer.

Action	Rationale
1. Explain the procedure to the patient fully, including reason for test, and gain verbal consent	Patient fully understands why test is being performed and procedure, and has agreed to participate
2. Run or 'stroke' the scanner across the centre of the forehead from the midline to the lateral hairline, depressing the button constantly throughout. A disposable cover may be used in some models	To record an accurate temporal artery temperature Prevention of cross-infection
3. Touch behind the ear lobe, in the soft depression below the mastoid	To account for any differences in the temperature in the temporal artery due to sweat (the temperature would be lower)
4. Release the button and read the temperature from the display window	To view reading
5. Report any abnormal findings	To plan further management. Patient safety
6. Dispose of cover if being used or clean as per manufacturer's instructions	Prevent contamination
	Ready for use

Table 7.8 Variance in temperature range dependent on site.

Body site	Normal temperature range (°C)
Oral	36.9–37.1
Tympanic	36.9–37.1
Rectal	37.0–37.5
Axilla	36.5–37.0

(Adapted from Clancy and McVicar (2009).)

feeling hot/clammy, are they red in the face, hot or cold to the touch, shivering or is the body rigid? This helps ensure that inaccuracies are identified and, if necessary, checked by another method or route.

Common problems

Problems relating to thermometry can be split into three areas: the patient, the equipment and the technique.

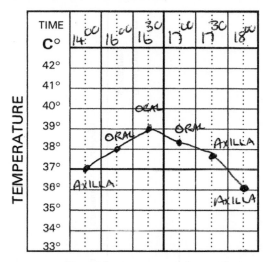

Figure 7.7 TPR (temperature, pulse and respiratory rate) chart with temperature recordings. Source: NHS Lothian 2008. Reproduced with permission of NHS Lothian.

The patient

Specific routes have disadvantages and limitations as mentioned in Table 7.4. If there is any doubt as to where exactly the thermometer should be placed, for example the sublingual pocket, further advice should be sought. Where possible the patient should also be actively involved in using any specific routes that may improve patient comfort, for example the rectal route would not be a preference for most people unless it was specifically indicated.

The equipment

As with all pieces of equipment the thermometer should be clean, in good working order and serviced (where applicable). Only dedicated disposables should be used and multiple uses of, for example, probe covers should never occur.

The technique

The specific technique in relation to both the type of thermometer and the route should be fully understood before commencing the procedure. Competency based training should also be undertaken in line with local policy.

Summary

It does not matter which route or site is used to record temperature, the most important thing is that it is accurate and that understanding of the variables of the different sites and external factors are taken into account. How the patient looks

Table 7.9 Thermometry competency: practical assessment form

Competency: record temperature	First assessment/reassessment					Date/competent signature
Steps	Demonstration					
	Date/sign	Date/sign	Date/sign	Date/sign	Date/sign	
	1	2	3	4	5	
Recording temperature						
1 State normal range for body temperature (°C)						
2 Define the terms pyrexia and hypothermia						
3 State different sites for recording temperature						
4 Describe different types of thermometers used and rationale						
5 Describe the common problems with each type						
6 Describe how you would prepare a patient for each method and gain consent						

Steps	Demonstration					Date/competent signature
	Date/sign 1	Date/sign 2	Date/sign 3	Date/sign 4	Date/sign 5	
Recording temperature						
7 Describe the procedures for the models of thermometer being used in your practice						
8 Identify and justify the use of documentation						
9 State when to ask for assistance/report findings						
10 Describe safe disposal and cleaning of the equipment following use						
11 State when to ask for assistance/report findings						

Supervisors/Assessor(s):

and feels should also be taken into consideration when assessing the patient's temperature, thus ensuring that the recording obtained represents true clinical symptoms. Table 7.9 gives an example of a competency framework for recording temperature.

CASE STUDY 7.1

Archie is an active 12-month-old boy. His temperature is taken with a tympanic thermometer and shows that it is within the normal range. However, he is very hot and clammy.
   You suspect the reading may be incorrect. Why?

CASE STUDY 7.2

Mrs Jones had abdominal surgery two days ago. She has a temperature of 39.5 °C. What actions do you think you should take and what are the possible causes of the increased temperature (pyrexia)?

Self-assessment		
Assessment	**Aspects**	**Achieved ✓**
Patient	*Have you considered all aspects of this section?* Why is temperature recorded? What mechanism does the body have to control temperature? Give some causes of increased/decreased temperature List some factors that affect heat loss and gain in the body	
Procedure	*Have you considered all aspects of this section?* Describe the different methods of recording temperature List the sites and rationale for each Documentation	**Achieved ✓**

References

Clancy J and McVicar A (2009) *Physiology and Anatomy: A Homeostatic Approach*, 3rd edn. London: Hodder Arnold.

DeVrim I, Kara A, Ceyhan M, et al. (2007) Measurement accuracy of fever by tympanic and axillary thermometry. *Pediatric Emergency* 23(1): 16–19.

Dougherty L and Lister S (eds) (2011) *The Royal Marsden Hospital Manual of Clinical Nursing Procedures*, 8th edn. Oxford: Blackwell Publishing.

El-Radhi A S and Patel S (2006) An evaluation of tympanic thermometry in a paediatric emergency department. *Emergency Medicine Journal* 23: 40–41.

Farnell S, Maxwell L, Tan S, et al. (2005) Temperature measurement: comparison of non-invasive methods used in adult critical care. *Journal of Clinical Nursing* 14: 632–639

Hamilton P A, Marcos L S and Secic M (2013) Performance of infrared ear and forehead thermometers: a comparative study in 205 febrile and afebrile children. *Journal of Clinical Nursing* doi: 10.1111/jocn.12060 (last accessed 9 May 2013).

Maddex S (2009) Measuring vital signs. In: Baillie L (ed.) *Developing Practical Nursing Skills*, 3rd edn. London: Hodder Education, pp. 116–157.

Jevon, P (2010) How to ensure patient observations lead to effective management of patients with pyrexia. *Nursing Times* 106(1): 16–18.

Leach R (2009) *Acute and Critical Care Medicine at a Glance*. Oxford: Wiley-Blackwell.

Mains, J A (2008) Measuring temperature. *Nursing Standard* 22(39): 44–47.

Mackechine C and Simpson R (2006) Traceable calibration for blood pressure and temperature monitoring. *Nursing Standard* 21(11): 42–47.

McCallum L and Higgins D (2012) Measuring body temperature. *Nursing Times* 108(45): 20–22.

Mulryan C (2010) Disorders of the thyroid function. *British Journal of Healthcare Assistants* 4(5): 218–222.

MRHA (2013) Mercury in medical devices. Available at: http://www.mhra.gov.uk/Safetyinformation/Generalsafetyinformationandadvice/Product-specificinformationandadvice/Product-specificinformationandadvice%E2%80%93M%E2%80%93T/Mercuryinmedicaldevices/index.htm (accessed 9 May 2013).

NHS Lothian (2008) *Observations Chart*. Edinburgh: NHS Lothian.

NICE (2007a) *CG50, Acutely Ill Patients In Hospital*. London: NICE.

NICE (2007b) *CG47 Feverish Illness in Children: Assessment and Management of Children Younger than Five Years of Age*. London: NICE.

Ronco C and Ricci Z (2008) Renal replacement therapies: physiological review. *Intensive Care Medicine* 34: 2139–2146.

Sahib El-Radhi A (2013) Temperature measurement: The right thermometer and site. *British Journal of Nursing* 22(4): 208–211.

Sund-Levander M and Grodzinsky E (2010) What is the evidence base for the assessment and evaluation of body temperature? *Nursing Times* 106(1): 10–13.

Tanner J (2011) Inadvertant hypothermia and active warming for surgical patients. *British Journal of Nursing* 20(16): 966–968.

Torrance C and Semple M (1998) Practical procedures for nurses. Recording temperature 1, no 6.1. *Nursing Times* 94(2): insert 2p.

Tortora G J and Derrickson B (2011) *Principles of Anatomy and Physiology*, 13th edn. Hoboken, NJ: Wiley & Sons.

Turnball V and Petty J (2013) Evidence-based thermal care of low birthweight neonates. Part one. *Nursing Children and Young People* 25(2): 918–922.

Vasiliki K (2011) Enhancing transfusion safety: nurses role. *International Journal of Caring Sciences* 4(3): 114–119.

Waugh A and Grant A (2010) *Ross and Wilson Anatomy and Physiology in Health and Illness*, 11th edn. London: Churchill Livingstone.

CHAPTER 8

Pulse oximetry

LEARNING OBJECTIVES

- Describe how a pulse oximeter works and produces a reading
- State the reasons for measuring and recording oxygen saturations
- List the conditions and factors that can affect readings
- Identify suitable sites for the probe
- Describe how to take and record an oxygen saturation reading

---

Aim of this chapter

The aim of this chapter is to understand how pulse oximetry measures the oxygen saturation levels in blood, its significance and its application in practice.

What is an oxygen saturation reading?

Pulse oximetry is a non-invasive method of measuring the oxygen saturation of arterial blood. Oxygen saturation is expressed as the percentage of haemoglobin (a component of red blood cells, see relevant anatomy and physiology) that is saturated with oxygen (Maddex 2009; Collins 2009).

Who can perform the test?

Only individuals who are taught how to use the machine correctly and have obtained a clinical competency should undertake this clinical skill. Local guidelines and policies should also be followed. Abnormal findings, or a change in the patient's 'normal' reading, should be recorded and reported immediately to the nurse in charge.

Clinical Skills for Healthcare Assistants and Assistant Practitioners, Second Edition.
Angela Whelan and Elaine Hughes.
© 2016 John Wiley & Sons, Ltd. Published 2016 by John Wiley & Sons, Ltd.

Reasons for recording an oxygen saturation level

- As part of lung function assessment in patients with long-term pulmonary (lung) disease such as COPD (Chronic Obstructive Pulmonary Disease) (Peate 2007).
- To monitor unstable cardiac conditions (e.g. cardiac failure or heart attack) (Maddex 2009).
- When transporting patients who are unwell and require oxygenation assessment (NICE 2007).
- To monitor the effectiveness of oxygen therapy or respiratory medication such as nebulisers (Higginson and Jones 2009; Maddex 2009; Dougherty and Lister 2011)
- Before, during and after procedures that may require sedation/anaesthesia, or that may cause potential respiratory depression (WHO 2008; Maddex 2009).
- To reduce the need for frequent arterial blood sampling in acute care (BTS/SIGN 2012).

When measuring the oxygen saturation levels in a patient, the overall condition and other vital signs should also be considered. This then allows review of the entire clinical presentation and not just the value of the reading in isolation. Preston and Flynn (2010) suggest that nurses should undertake observations such as pulse oximetry on an individual basis and use this to provide safe care for their patients whilst following NICE (2007) guidelines.

Pulse oximetry is useful for identifying patients who have a reduced level of oxygen in their blood (hypoxaemia). This is particularly relevant in acute settings where supplementary oxygen may be prescribed to correct this and prevent further deterioration of the patient's condition (Jevon and Ewens 2012; Collins 2009). Monitoring of pulse oximetry can help the healthcare practitioner to identify at an early stage those patients who are at risk of becoming cyanotic (Maddex 2009). Cyanosis leads to a bluish discolouration around the lips, mucous membranes of the mouth and at the nail beds. However, cyanosis is a late sign of hypoxia where oxygen saturation will have fallen to around 80–85% before discolouration occurs (Jevon and Ewens 2012; Casey 2011). It is also important that healthcare practitioners observe their patients and do not just take their oxygen saturations, as restlessness, confusion and agitation can be early indicators of clinical deterioration (Jevon and Ewens 2012). Reduced oxygen in arterial blood (hypoxaemia) can still occur without reduced oxygen to the skin and membranes (cyanosis). This occurs where the concentration of haemoglobin is low or the capillaries do not receive enough blood, sometimes referred to as not being well perfused (Jevon and Ewens 2012).

THINK ABOUT IT

Have you seen a pulse oximeter used in your clinical area? If so can you remember why the oxygen saturation level was being measured for your patient?

Relevant anatomy and physiology

Haemoglobin is the oxygen-carrying part of red blood cells (Dougherty and Lister 2011). The red blood cells are specifically designed by having a biconcave shape, which is a round curved shape, to maximise the available surface area. Each haemoglobin molecule has four oxygen binding sites. When oxygen binds with haemoglobin it is referred to as oxyhaemoglobin, and when all haemoglobin sites have oxygen molecules attached they are described as fully saturated (WHO 2011).

The amount of haemoglobin that combines with oxygen can be influenced further by various factors, including blood pH, temperature and carbon dioxide levels (WHO 2011). When certain levels of these substances are present, the oxygen will be at its optimum, that is the best possible level for oxygen uptake. This is known as the oxygen dissociation curve. The oxygen saturation reading is a measure of the percentage of haemoglobin molecules saturated with oxygen, but does not indicate the actual number of red blood cells (Dougherty and Lister 2011).

Related aspects and terminology

- *Hypoxia*: diminished oxygen in tissues.
- *Cyanosis*: bluish or purple coloration of the skin and mucous membranes due to excess carbon dioxide and insufficient oxygen in the blood (Casey 2011).
- *Hypoxaemia*: insufficient oxygenation of blood (Maddex 2009).
- *Haemoglobin*: the pigment contained in red blood cells, which is used to carry oxygen (Collins 2009).
- *Oxyhaemoglobin*: haemoglobin combined with oxygen molecules (Maddex 2009).
- *Plethysmographic waveform*: the visual representation of the pulse wave on a pulse oximeter machine. This represents the quality of the pulse at the point where oxyhaemoglobin saturation is being measured (Jevon and Ewens 2012)

The mechanics of pulse oximetry

The Beer–Lambert Law states that the concentration of an unknown solute dissolved in a solvent can be determined by light absorption (Chan et al. 2013). Therefore, pulse oximetry works on the principle that blood saturated with oxygen is a different colour from blood depleted of oxygen (Dougherty and Lister 2011). Thus, oxygen saturation can be estimated over a period of time by measuring the difference between light absorption of full and empty capillaries (Collins 2009). To assist this process, the pulse oximeter probe consists of two light-emitting diodes (one red and one infrared) on one side of the probe.

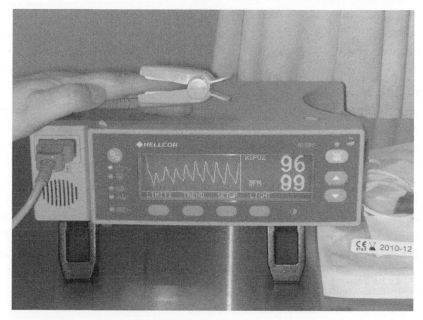

Figure 8.1 A pulse oximeter with probe in situ.

These transmit red and infrared light through body tissue, usually a fingertip or ear lobe, to a photodetector on the other side of the probe (Collins 2009). The amount of light that is absorbed by the red blood cells allows the microprocessor in the machine to determine the oxygen saturation of the patient (Jevon and Ewens 2012). Figure 8.1 shows an adult pulse oximetry probe. A pulsatile flow is required and the oximeter calculates this over a number of pulses (Maddex 2009; Chan et al. 2013). Therefore a good blood flow to the vessels is required for an accurate reading.

Advantages of pulse oximetry

Previously the only method of measuring the concentration of arterial blood would have been arterial blood gases. Sampling arterial blood either involves drawing blood from an arterial line, a line that is inserted into the main vessel of the heart (often used in the intensive care unit), or sampling from an artery using a needle. Sampling from an artery is a highly skilled procedure, mostly carried out by medical staff and nurses with additional training; carries complications of increased risk of infection and bruising; and is often painful (Maddex and Valler-Jones 2009). A sample from an arterial line is pain free for the patient but also carries the risk of infection. It is not expected that a healthcare assistant would undertake this procedure, but check local policy. The sample can either be sent to a lab for analysis or be tested in specialist areas where blood gas analysers are located. If the machine is within a unit or clinical area, it requires personnel to be trained in both its use and the interpretation of its findings. Therefore it can be seen that pulse oximetry is quick, generally reliable and cost effective and can be undertaken by a range of suitably trained healthcare personnel.

Limitations of pulse oximetry

As pulse oximetry measures only haemoglobin oxygen saturation and not haemoglobin concentration, the patient can still have a depleted amount of oxygen (hypoxia) despite a 'normal' pulse oximetry reading (Jevon and Ewens 2012). It should also be remembered that pulse oximetry does not provide an indication of the adequacy of ventilation, carbon dioxide retention, partial pressure of oxygen or respiratory rate (Casey 2011; Collins 2009; WHO 2011). However, it is still an invaluable monitoring tool in a variety of clinical settings as long as its uses and limitations are fully understood (Maddox 2009). The accuracy of the pulse oximiter is dependent upon the frequency of calibration, usually within +/- 2% for saturations >90%, with the accuracy falling at saturation levels lover than 80% (Casey 2011).

Equipment

Pulse oximeters are either non-invasive units or are fully integrated into a patient monitoring system, such as those found in critical care areas or electronic blood pressure machines. Some may record the pulse rate and this may be seen visually as a waveform. A pulse oximeter should not be used to take a pulse because the reading would give the rate of the pulse only and would not give important information such as the volume and rhythm. Therefore, use of a pulse oximeter is predominantly to measure haemoglobin oxygen saturation (WHO 2011).

Normal readings

Normal levels are usually between 95 and 100%, but depend on individual patients (Dougherty and Lister 2011; Collins 2009; WHO 2011). However, in the acutely ill patient this may vary between 94 and 98%, while a fall below 90% is classed as a clinical emergency (Jevon and Ewens 2012; WHO 2011). Alarms can be set depending on individual patients' clinical presentation, but guidance should be sought as to both the levels that should be set and whether local policy allows healthcare assistants to do this. It is essential always to record the oxygen therapy being received by the patient together with the readings, and to the clinical condition of the patient. A sustained trend of falling oxygen saturation levels is clinically important and should always be reported promptly (Dougherty and Lister 2011). Some conditions can affect readings, so the patient's medical history should be considered before carrying out the procedure (see Box 8.1 for possible factors).

Box 8.1 Factors affecting oxygen saturation readings

Poor circulation

This can be due to peripheral vascular disease or vasoconstriction (narrowing of blood vessels), low temperature (hypothermia) or low blood pressure (hypotension) (Dougherty and Lister 2011). All can give low readings due to the reduced blood flow. This results in a decreased pulsatile flow which is necessary for the pulse oximeter to calculate the reading (Preston and Flynn 2010). Arterial constriction or shock can also cause readings to be low (Chan et al. 2013). To ensure accurate readings it is recommended that the probe be placed where there is a good blood flow.

Carbon monoxide

The presence of carbon monoxide (CO) in blood can give falsely normal readings because the CO combines with O_2 to form carboxyhaemoglobin. This substance is bright red, similar to oxyhaemoglobin; as both compounds have a similar absorbence, this results in the pulse oximeter being unable to distinguish between oxygen and carbon monoxide in the red blood cells providing a 'normal' reading. This can be a result of expose to gas, cigarette smoking, exhaust fumes or exposure to smoke from house fires (Chan et al 2013; Casey 2011). In these instances pulse oximetry should not be relied upon (Jevon and Ewens 2012).

Tricuspid valve incompetence (heart valve failure)

Inaccurate readings are obtained due to the machine not being able to differentiate between arteriolar and venous pulsation (Casey 2011). Further advice should be sought as to whether pulse oximetry should be used.

Anaemia

High oxygen saturation can be recorded but inadequate oxygen is actually perfusing (getting into) the tissues due to the reduced number of haemoglobin molecules (Chan et al. 2013; Dougherty and Lister 2011). Advice should be sought to identify the appropriateness of pulse oximetry for these patients.

Atrial fibrillation

This is a fast heartbeat from the top chamber of the heart that interferes with the pulsatile signal (Maddex 2009). If this is an intermittent problem it may still be possible to obtain accurate readings, so further advice should be sought.

Parkinson's disease or seizures

An incorrect reading may be obtained due to the tremor associated with Parkinson's disease or the irregular movement caused by seizures or shivering (Dougherty and Lister 2011). Both conditions can cause interference and artefacts (disturbance) and therefore give inaccurate readings. However Chan et al. (2013) suggest that newer pulse oximeters have improved processing and can take account of movement and give accurate readings.

> **Altered red blood cell shape**
>
> As mentioned earlier, blood cells are biconcave in shape to promote oxygen uptake. Sickle cell disease and some medications (e.g. anaesthetic agents) alter the shape of red blood cells and will alter readings (Casey 2011; Chan et al. 2013). Therefore caution and further advice should be sought both in the interpretation of these readings and as to whether pulse oximetry is appropriate for these patients.

Using a pulse oximeter

Before performing the skill, ensure that you have received approved training and undertaken supervised practice in line with local policy. It is also advisable to consult the manufacturer's directions for the make and model in use (Dougherty and Lister 2011).

It is essential that the correct cable and probe be used with the appropriate machine (for accurate recordings. The machine should have been serviced in the past year (a PAT or medical devices sticker will be in place with a date), should be visibly clean and, when switched on successfully, should go through a series of self-tests with no error codes (see 'Common problems'). If an error code or abnormality is noted, report the fault and use another machine. Jevon and Ewens (2012) suggest that if there are problems getting a reliable trace or reading that the skin at the site where the probe is to be placed could be rubbed to improve circulation, using a different site to place the probe or changing the probe or the pulse oximiter itself for a different machine.

> **THINK ABOUT IT**
>
> Set up a pulse oximetry machine on yourself, rotating the site and type of probe where possible.
>   What reading would you expect to get and why?

Pulse oximetry probes

There are multiple sites where a probe can be placed, which depend on both the probe being used and the individual patient. The correct probe and its size for the site is essential in both children and adults. For infants, probes that attach to the palms and soles of the feet are available, and in a study by Das et al. (2010) it was found that in children with cyanotic heart disease the sensor on the sole of the foot is the most accurate of all probes.

In adults the probe is dependent on the site intended by the manufacturer, but possibilities include probes suitable for fingers or toes, and specialist ear probes. The cable should also be loose, so movement will not disrupt the sensor, and the clip should be attached to the shoulder of the patient. Finally, a headband is also available and this requires the cable to be looped around an ear and tucked in. This may not be available in every clinical area. To reduce the risk of hospital acquired infection, single-patient use probes are available in some clinical areas; however, the reusable probe has the advantage of being quick to use and cost effective (Chan et al. 2012).

If the pulse oximetry reading requires continuous monitoring, the patient's preference may be taken into account or, in the case of confused or agitated patients, a site that is out of vision may be best.

Whatever site is chosen, only an appropriate probe for the machine being used should be in place. Tape, to hold the probe in place, should not be used as this can cause pressure or thermal (heat) damage to the extremity (Dougherty and Lister 2011; Jevon and Ewens 2012). Where the site is used for continuous monitoring this should be checked and rotated at least 2-hourly to prevent any pressure damage resulting from prolonged use at any one site (MRHA 2010). Where the patient is unable to flex the fingers voluntarily, this may result in stiffness, and the site may need to be changed more frequently (Jevon and Ewens 2012).

The probe should be visually examined before use to ensure that it is not broken or dirty (Collins 2009). Replace the probe if it is faulty and always refer to the manufacturer's recommendations for cleaning. If it is proving difficult to obtain a trace, warm and rub the skin to improve the circulation (Jevon and Ewens 2012). Table 8.1 describes the procedure for recording an oxygen saturation level using a pulse oximeter.

Documentation

Ensure that any oxygen therapy that the patient is receiving is recorded together with the pulse oximetry reading. This can allow medical staff to make decisions about the continued use of supplementary oxygen therapy as prolonged unnecessary use of oxygen can be harmful. Likewise, avoid taking oxygen saturation levels when the patient has just been suctioned (a catheter inserted into the windpipe to remove secretions), because this will give a false reading (see Chapter 9).

Pulse oximetry recordings may be documented in the patient's case notes if the patient is in the community or on TPR/MEWS/NEWS charts if in hospital.

Common problems

Errors in pulse oximetry readings can be due to many different variables, some of which can be reduced to promote a more accurate trace. They have been split into three different areas, namely those caused by light transmission, pulse detection and actual use of the equipment.

Table 8.1 Procedure for recording an oxygen saturation level.

Action	Rationale
1. Explain the procedure to the patient and gain verbal consent. Document	The patient will fully understand the procedure and consent to participate
2. Check that the equipment has been serviced, is in good working order and clean, and has designated accessories (lead/probe)	The machine should be serviced as per local policy to ensure that an accurate reading is obtained A clean probe will prevent cross-infection Correct accessories essential for accurate readings
3. Ensure the patient is warm and comfortable	If the patient is cold they could have decreased peripheral blood flow that can reduce blood flow (and give a low reading) If the patient is shivering this can interfere with the signal If the patient is comfortable they will be more relaxed, especially if having continuous monitoring (Dougherty and Lister 2011)
4. Wash hands and put on a clean apron (Dougherty and Lister 2011)	Prevent cross-infection
5. Select a suitable site for the probe and place as per manufacturer's instructions	Ensures accuracy of reading
6. Switch the machine on and check function; should beep with each detected pulse or waveform (Dougherty and Lister 2011)	Accurate pulse detection Shows the patient that the procedure is painless and checks the machine
7. Record both the oxygen therapy (where applicable) and SpO_2 reading – reporting any abnormal readings. This may be a change for the patient or out with 'normal' limits	To provide a legal record of the measurement The nurse in charge may want to reset alarms/parameters to identify changes in recorded saturation levels (Collins 2009). If set incorrectly, alarms can be a nuisance if constantly activated
8. Remove the probe, if using for routine or intermittent observation (and when appropriate for continuous monitoring)	Patient comfort
When continuously monitoring, ensure that cable is positioned as safely as possible and probe secured if necessary	For health and safety round the bed space
Return to check probe is not causing any complications. Rotate site every 2 hours	To prevent damage to the patients skin (Jevon and Ewens 2012)
9. Clean the equipment, in line with local policy	Prevent cross-infection
Return to equipment store; plug in to recharge if appropriate.	To recharge the machine ready for use

Light transmission/absorption

As mentioned previously and shown in Figure 8.1, the finger probe consists of two parts, with one side receiving the light source and the other being a photodetector. If bright light, either artificial or sunlight, is picked up readings can be affected (WHO 2011). If the reading is an intermittent recording (i.e. not continuously in place), consider closing a curtain or switching off the fluorescent lights until the reading has been taken. In instances where the light is necessary for treatment, for example phototherapy to treat jaundiced babies or in operating theatres, the probe should be covered to ensure accurate readings (WHO 2011; Fouzas et al. 2011). Nail varnish also causes problems with transmission and patients who have nail varnish in place should be asked if they would mind removing it to obtain accurate readings (Dougherty and Lister 2011). There is some evidence to suggest that false nails interfere with the light source and may provide inaccurate readings (Fouzas et al. 2011).

Other factors that affect the transmission of light, and cause low readings, include the presence of dried blood on the skin, substances such as engine oil on the hands or heavily nicotine stained fingers (Collins 2009; Jevon and Ewens 2012). Chan et al. (2013) noted that intravenous dyes used in imaging affect light transmission, and individuals using pulse oximetry should seek advice about how long these agents are active for to enable measurements to be taken when they are no longer active.

Pulse detection

Jevon and Ewens (2011) and Dougherty and Lister (2011) discuss the fact that movement, including shivering, may cause interference in the signal or the probe to become dislodged. In some instances another site may produce a better trace, for example an ear or toe, and for intermittent readings supporting the probe in place may be beneficial.

Equipment use

As with all pieces of equipment, the pulse oximeter should have been serviced as recommended by the manufacturer and local policy. When the device is switched on it should perform a self-test and not display any error codes; this ensures the accuracy and reliability of the machine (Maddex 2009).

If the machine is dropped or broken, as with other pieces of equipment, suitably qualified staff should check it – local policy will dictate whether this is an in-house department or the manufacturer. The correct accessories, for example probes, should be used for each specific machine and the accessories checked to ensure that they are clean and for signs of damage.

Measuring oxygen saturation levels on the same arm as a BP cuff or venous line can disrupt the machine's ability to measure the pulse as the flow of blood allows the pulse oximiter to determine its reading (Jevon and Ewens 2012;

Table 8.2 Practical assessment form: competency framework for recording SpO_2.

Steps	First assessment/reassessment/demonstration					Date/competent signature
	Date/sign 1	Date/sign 2	Date/sign 3	Date/sign 4	Date/sign 5	
Recording oxygen saturation levels (SpO_2)						
1 State normal range for SpO_2 as a percentage						
2 State what oxygen saturation levels actually measure and the limitations						
3 Define the terms cyanosis and hypoxia						
4 State different sites for recording oxygen saturation						
5 List common causes of inaccurate recordings, caused by disease processes and the equipment						
6 Describe different types of models in use						
7 Describe appropriate sites and the reasons for these choices						
8 Describe how you would prepare a patient for obtaining an oxygen saturation reading and gaining consent						
9 Describe the correct procedure for recording oxygen saturation						
10 Describe safe disposal and cleaning of the equipment following use						
11 Identify and justify the use of documentation						
12 State when to ask for assistance/report findings						

Supervisors/Assessor(s):

Dougherty and Lister 2011). The pulse reading should match the patient's heart rate; if this is not the case it may indicate that not all pulsations are being detected and another machine should be sought as this can affect the accuracy of the reading

Summary

Pulse oximetry, when used appropriately, is a good way of accurately measuring oxygen saturation levels. Where the role of the healthcare assistant involves taking these readings it is essential that competency based training is undertaken in accordance with local policies and procedures for the specific device that is in use. Table 8.2 provides a competency framework for recording SpO$_2$ levels.

CASE STUDY 8.1

Mrs Semple is a frail 86-year-old woman who has been admitted to hospital with hypothermia (low temperature). She is shivering and requires her oxygen saturation levels to be monitored.

What equipment would you consider for her and what factors would affect your decision? What might affect the readings of the pulse oximeter?

Describe some of the reassurances and special precautions that should be taken for her.

CASE STUDY 8.2

Baby Ben is aged 8 months and has been admitted with a respiratory problem (suspected pneumonia). He is to be started on a pulse oximeter for continuous monitoring.

What factors affect the equipment and site choices for him? What special precautions should also be taken for him to ensure that no harm comes to him during his treatment?

Self-assessment

Assessment	Aspects	Achieved ✓
Patient	*Have you considered all aspects of this section?* The purpose of the red and infrared lights used to measure oxygen saturation The diseases that can affect pulse oximetry readings Advantages and disadvantages of pulse oximetry The indications for pulse oximetry use	
Procedure	*Have you considered all aspects of this section?* What the normal limits for pulse oximetry are The possible sites and types of probe available Documentation of readings	✓

References

BTS/SIGN (2012) British Guidelines on the Management of Asthma. Available at: http://www .sign.ac.uk/pdf/sign101.pdf (last accessed 20 May 2013).

Casey G (2011) Pulse oximetry: What are we really measuring? *Kai Tiaki Nursing New Zealand* 17(3): 24–29.

Chan E, Chan M and Chan M (2013) Pulse oximetry: Understanding its basic principles facilitates appreciation of its limitations. *Respiratory Medicine* 107: 789–799.

Collins T (2009) Pulse oximetry. In: Smith S, Price A and Challiner A (eds) *Ward-Based Critical Care*. M&K Publishing: Keswick.

Das J, Aggarwal A and Aggarwal N (2010) Pulse oximeter accuracy and precision at five different sensor locations in infants and children with cyanotic heart disease. *Indian Journal of Anaesthesiology* 54(6): 531–534.

Dougherty L and Lister S (eds) (2011) *The Royal Marsden Hospital Manual of Clinical Nursing Procedures*, 8th edn. Oxford: Blackwell Publishing.

Fouzas S, Pirifitis K and Anthracopoulos M (2011) Pulse oximetry in paediatric practice. *Paediatrics* 128: 740–752.

Higginson R and Jones B (2009) Respiratory assessment in critically ill patients: airway and breathing. *British Journal of Nursing* 18(8): 456–461.

Jevon P and Ewens B (2012) *Monitoring the Critically Ill Patient*, 3rd edn. Oxford: Blackwell Publishing.

Maddex S (2009) Measuring vital signs. In: Baillie L (ed.) *Developing Practical Adult Nursing Skills*. London: Hodder Arnold, Chapter 4.

Maddex S and Valler-Jones T (2009) Assessing physical health and responding to sudden deterioration. In: Baillie L (ed.) *Developing Practical Skills*, 3rd edn. London: Hodder Arnold.

MRHA (2010) *Top Tips for Pulse Oximetry*. MRHA: London.

NICE (2007) *Acutely Ill Patients in Hospital*. London: NICE.

Pete I (2007) Caring for the person with chronic obstructive pulmonary disease, part 2. *British Journal of Healthcare Assistants* 4(7): 347–349.

Preston R and Flynn D (2010) Observations in acute care: evidence -based approach to patient safety. *British Journal of Nursing*: doi 10.12968/bjon.2010.19.7.47446.

WHO (2008) Surgical Safety Checklist. Available at: http://who.int/patientsafety/safesurgery/ ss_checklist/en/ (accessed 20 May 2013).

WHO (2011) *Pulse Oximetry Training Manual*. WHO: Geneva.

CHAPTER 9

Respiratory care

LEARNING OBJECTIVES

- Discuss the anatomy and physiology of respiration
- Identify the reasons for recording a respiratory rate and accurately perform this skill
- List the reasons for measuring peak flow and discuss how to safely carry out the procedure
- Discuss suctioning techniques and safety aspects
- List the terms related to respiratory care
- Discuss the role of the healthcare assistant in respiratory care

---

Aim of this chapter

The aim of this chapter is to identify the anatomy and physiology relating to respiration, and explore the recording of a respiratory rate and a peak flow. Suctioning techniques will also be discussed.

What is respiratory care?

The respiratory system is made up of the nose, pharynx, larynx, trachea, bronchi and lungs (Tortora and Derrickson 2011) (Figure 9.1).

If there is a problem at any point in the system this may result in the patient feeling breathless. This chapter describes the role of a healthcare assistant in assessing and assisting a breathless patient through the observation, recording and reporting of respiratory rate and/or peak flow.

The treatments commonly associated with respiratory care, such as oxygen therapy or nebulisers, are explored briefly in Chapter 15; however, this may not be part of a healthcare assistant's accepted role and your workplace policy should be checked.

Clinical Skills for Healthcare Assistants and Assistant Practitioners, Second Edition.
Angela Whelan and Elaine Hughes.
© 2016 John Wiley & Sons, Ltd. Published 2016 by John Wiley & Sons, Ltd.

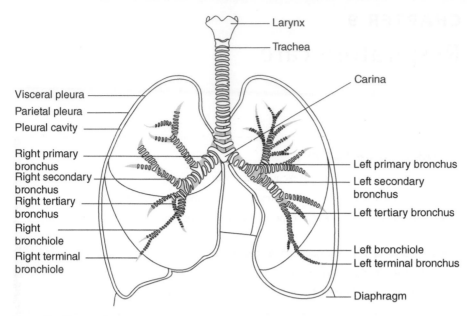

Figure 9.1 The respiratory system.

Relevant anatomy and physiology

The main function of the respiratory system is to supply the body with oxygen and remove carbon dioxide through the process of inspiration (breathing in) and expiration (breathing out) (Maddex 2009).

The lungs are the organs of respiration and are situated in the thoracic cavity. Therefore breathing can be defined as air moving in and out of the lungs and their associated structures. Air enters through the mouth and nose, and passes via the pharynx (throat), larynx (voice box), trachea (windpipe), bronchi and bronchioles into the air sacs called alveoli (Tortora and Derrickson 2011). Gas exchange takes place in the alveoli, which have been likened to a bunch of grapes. Their surface area is approximately 70 m^2 in an adult, and if spread out flat are equivalent to the surface area of a football pitch (Tortora and Derrickson 2011). The respiratory system is in two sections: the upper respiratory system refers to the nose, pharynx and associated structures; whereas the lower respiratory system refers to the larynx, trachea, bronchi and lungs (Tortora and Derrickson 2011).

Upper respiratory system

The nose has two parts: external and internal (Tortora and Derrickson 2011):
1 External: a supporting framework of bone and cartilage, covered with muscle and skin and lined by mucous membrane.

2 Internal: the nasal cavity is split by the nasal septum, which divides into a right and left side.

When air enters the nostrils it passes through the vestibule (just inside the nostrils), which is lined by skin, containing coarse hairs that filter out large dust particles. Air that is passed through the nose is filtered, but also warmed and moistened (humidified).

The pharynx (throat)

This is a funnel-shaped tube about 13 cm long, which lies behind the nasal and oral cavity, above the larynx and just in front of the cervical vertebrae. The pharynx functions as a passageway for air and food, provides a resonating chamber for speech sounds, and houses the tonsils, which help eliminate foreign invaders (Tortora and Derrickson 2011).

Lower respiratory system

Larynx (voice box)

This is a short passageway that connects the pharynx with the trachea, and the wall of the larynx is made of cartilage (Tortora and Derrickson 2011). When small particles, such as dust, smoke, food or liquids, pass into the larynx a cough reflex occurs to expel the material.

Normally, the epiglottis (a large leaf-shaped piece of elastic cartilage) is able to move up and down like a trap door (leaf portion), so during swallowing the larynx rises and allows the free edge of the epiglottis to move up and down and form a lid; therefore liquids and foods are routed into the oesophagus and kept out of the larynx and lungs.

Trachea (windpipe)

This is a tubular passage for air, about 12 cm long and 2.5 cm in width (Tortora and Derrickson 2011). It is found in front of the oesophagus, and extends from the larynx to the bronchi, which then split into a right and left primary bronchus.

Bronchi

When the trachea divides, a right primary bronchus (windpipe) goes into the right lung and a left primary bronchus goes into the left lung. The right main bronchus is more vertical, shorter and wider than the left, so any aspirated object, for example foodstuffs, is more likely to enter and lodge in the right primary bronchus. On entering the lungs, the primary bronchi divide to form smaller bronchi. This extensive branching from the trachea resembles a tree trunk with its branches and is commonly called the bronchial tree (Tortora and Derrickson 2011).

Lungs

These are a pair of cone-shaped organs lying in the thoracic (chest) cavity, separated from each other by the heart. The lungs have two layers of serous membranes called the pleural membrane which encloses and protects each lung. Between these membranes is a small space called the pleural cavity that contains a lubricating fluid secreted by the membranes. This fluid reduces friction between the membranes. Each lung is subdivided into lobes. The right lung has three lobes while the left lung has two (Tortora and Derrickson 2011).

The alveoli and gaseous exchange

Within the lungs are alveoli where gaseous exchange takes place; it is estimated that the lungs contain 300 million alveoli. A chemical called surfactant is secreted within the alveoli which prevents the surfaces within them from sticking to each other during the expiration phase (Clancy and McVicar 2009).

Breathing is regulated in the brain and has both conscious and unconscious control. Conscious control is when a patient takes an extra breath or a deeper inspiration, whereas most breathing is unconscious – we just do it without thought. The regulation of breathing is managed by the respiratory centre, which responds to the gas levels in the blood, usually oxygen and carbon dioxide and also hydrogen. The centre monitors gas levels, and in normal respiration is driven by the increase in the carbon dioxide level, which triggers nerve impulses down to the respiratory muscles and stimulates respiration (Tortora and Derrickson 2011).

In patients with a chronic lung disease, for example chronic obstructive pulmonary disease (COPD), over time the body adapts to a constantly elevated level of carbon dioxide (CO_2) and therefore the respiratory centre switches to respond to a drop in the oxygen (O_2) level. This is one reason why any acutely ill respiratory patient needs careful observation and monitoring of blood gases, and accurately and carefully titrated (dosed) O_2 therapy. Too high a level of O_2 would remove the respiratory drive in these patients, when the respiratory centre fails to trigger the respiratory muscles and the patient stops breathing (Clancy and McVicar 2009).

To aid breathing we have both principle and accessory muscles of respiration (Figure 9.2). The principle muscles consist of the diaphragm situated under the lungs and the intercostal muscles between the ribs. The accessory muscles consist of the abdominal muscles and the muscles above the ribcage into the shoulder and neck (Clancy and McVicar 2009). It is the expansion of these muscles that help breathless patients make their breathing more effective (Clancy and McVicar).

Breathing can be affected by many factors: disease – infection, lung cancer, asthma; emotional state – stress, fear leading to hyperventilation (overbreathing); position – cramped or slouched will restrict breathing; trauma – accident to the brain or chest, or surgery; and exercise.

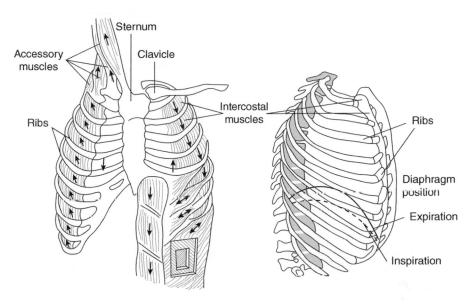

Figure 9.2 Muscles of respiration.

Recording a respiratory rate

Why and when a respiratory rate is observed, assessed and recorded

- On admission and before procedures – to provide a baseline record to compare later recordings (NICE 2007).
- When a patient's condition changes, for example feeling unwell, becomes breathless, complaining of pain or injury.
- To monitor response to treatments/medications, for example oxygen, morphine, inhalers.
- Before specified medications for baseline, for example blood administration.
- To monitor changes in oxygenation or respiration, for example someone with asthma.

What do you observe?

Massey and Meredith (2010), and Dougherty and Lister (2011) identify the importance of observing rate, depth, pattern, sound, regularity/rhythm and colour when assessing respirations.

Rate

When assessing the respiratory rate, you need to know the expected normal rate for a person's age group (Dougherty and Lister 2011; Cook and Montgomery 2010). The baseline rate on admission or before procedures/medications will

Table 9.1 Children's respiratory rate and age.

Age (years)	Respiratory rate (breaths/min)
Newborn	30–60
<1	30–45
1–2	25–35
2–5	25–30
5–12	20–25
>12	15–25

Adapted from Syers (2008); Cook and Montgomery (2010).

allow comparison. However, the respiratory rate varies according to age, size (build) and gender, and other demands, such as exercise; discussed in more detail below (Wild and Peate 2012).

The normal adult respiratory rate is 12–18 breaths/min (Dougherty and Lister 2011), while Maddex (2009) suggests this can vary with age, gender and size (Table 9.1).

Stress, fear, anxiety and exercise will increase the respiratory rate and this is normal. Let us consider a patient on admission; they may be anxious, have rushed to get to the appointment on time, or be in pain, and these factors may have affected the respiratory rate. Therefore this recording may not be a true baseline.

Both high and low respiratory rate should raise concern and be recorded and reported immediately to the nurse in charge (Wild and Peate 2012). The nurse should be aware of normal and abnormal ranges in order to act on their findings and ensure patient safety. A raised respiratory rate (tachypnoea) in an adult would therefore be over 20 breaths/min and a decreased respiratory rate (bradypnoea) is considered if the rate is below 8–10 breaths/min (Massey and Meredith 2010; Dougherty and Lister 2011).

We have noted that some factors, such as stress and exercise, can increase the rate, however some respirator conditions such as asthma, COPD and cardiac tamponade can also cause patients to have an increased respiratory rate (Massey and Meredith 2010; Wild and Peate 2012).

Bradypnoea can be caused by certain conditions, such as a brain tumour, or treatments, like morphine, which are known to depress (reduce) the respiratory rate and this is the reason why a patient newly started on any opioid (i.e. morphine) will have their respiration monitored. A rate of 10 or below must always be reported promptly (Massey and Meredith 2010; Wild and Peate 2012).

THINK ABOUT IT

Mrs Winifred Johnson is 57 years old and has been admitted for a bronchoscopy to investigate her persistent cough.

You are asked to record her observations and you measure her respiratory rate at 30 breaths/min.

What factors might you need to consider?

What action might you take?

Depth

Observation of the depth of breathing is useful as this can give an indication of ventilation (Maddex 2009).

Deep rapid breaths (hyperventilation) are often associated with anxiety or panic attacks. If prolonged, a patient will start to feel dizzy and faint; this is a result of a drop in the CO_2 level, and you can help by encouraging the patient to breathe slowly in and out of a paper bag (this allows the patient to re-breathe the exhaled CO_2 and so stabilises them). Slow shallow breaths (hypoventilation) can occur with some drugs, such as morphine, and will also lead to poor gas exchange and insufficient oxygen. Dougherty and Lister (2011) state that normal breathing is effortless, automatic and regular. The depth is the volume of air moving in with each respiration, and in an adult this is about 500 ml (Maddex 2009).

Pattern

As noted before, normal breathing is effortless, so, if a patient is having difficulty breathing (dyspnoea), you might observe irregular, noisy breaths and also possibly the use of the accessory muscles of respiration (neck and abdominal muscles). Changes in the pattern of respiration are often found in disorders of the respiratory centre in the brain (Dougherty and Lister (2011).

Therefore, assessment should include the pattern of breathing, for example mouth breathing, when a patient tries to gulp air in. This happens because there is less resistance to air flow through the mouth than the nose: noses can often block, as with a common cold, but this can cause the mouth to become dry and so oral hygiene is essential to help keep the mouth moist.

People with asthma, caused by narrowing of the airways, cannot 'shift' air and in some cases you might observe minimal movement of breathing, that is little rise or fall in the chest, which is serious and must be reported promptly. In general, you would observe the chest rise and fall to measure the respiratory rate and, to prevent a patient altering the respiratory rate, you can continue to hold the wrist as though still counting the radial pulse rate. This ensures that the respiratory rate is not altered consciously.

Sound

As noted earlier, breathing should be quiet, so, if it can be heard, there may be a problem (Maddex 2009).

A loud harsh, almost rasping sound (stridor), usually heard on inspiration, is frequently due to a partial or blocked larynx (airway) from injury, foreign body or illness, for example a tumour, and must be reported immediately (Wild and Peate 2012).

A wheeze, characterised by a noisy, high-pitched sound (Maddex 2009), usually on expiration, is usually found in people with asthma (during an asthmatic attack) and is caused by swelling, which leads to narrowing of the airways. Patients with chronic bronchitis and emphysema may also have a wheeze.

A 'rattly' chest is caused by the presence of fluid (e.g. sputum, blood) in the upper airway. Snoring, especially in the unconscious patient, may be due to a partial obstruction of the airway by the tongue airway (Wild and Peate 2012). Prompt checking and action are required here. Finally whooping cough causes a distinctive whoop sound, usually when coughing, and is most commonly found in children.

Regularity/rhythm

This might be considered similar to pattern, so breathing should be regular and rhythmic and any period without breathing (apnoea) must be reported immediately. Massey and Meredith (2010) and Wild and Peate (2012) describe Cheyne–Stokes respirations as a 'pattern' of breathing where the patient has periods of apnoea alternating with periods of overbreathing (hyperpnoea); it is often associated with left ventricular failure (heart failure), brain injury or the latter stages of dying.

Colour

As well as assessing rate, depth, pattern, sound and regularity, you should also be observing the patient's colour, to identify any abnormality. If patients are not getting enough oxygen they become cyanosed, which manifests as a bluish dusky colour of the mucous membranes, and can be observed on the skin and nailbeds. It is often most noticeable around the lips, earlobes, mouth and fingertips. In dark-skinned patients it is most noticeable in the lips, the mucous membranes of the mouth and nailbeds, which become dusky in colour (Wild and Peate 2012). This is also why we ask patients to remove makeup, especially before procedures such as surgery. The patient's condition will probably be poor by the time that you observe cyanosis, but it is one aspect that you should always consider whenever checking a patient's pulse and respiratory rate.

How to measure and record a respiratory rate accurately

Although gaining consent is an important part of any procedure, it is important not to let your patient know when you are actually counting their respirations. This can affect the accuracy of the rate that is recorded, as often breathing patterns alter when people are being watched (Smith and Roberts 2011; Nicol et al. 2012). In order to count a patient's respirations they should be comfortable and in a position that is easy to count the rise and fall of their chest. Respiratory rate should be counted over a full minute and the use of a watch with a second hand will improve the accuracy of this (Nicol et al. 2012). How often you record will depend on the patient's condition, treatment and monitoring requirements (NICE 2007). A patient with acute asthma might need the respiratory rate measured every 15 minutes, so always follow your local policies and practice. A patient who is stable will have measurements gradually reduced, maybe from 4-hourly to twice a day, which is a minimum amount in an acute area. Respiratory measurement in community settings is likely to be monitored less frequently and should be based on individual patient's needs. Any changes, however, would need to be quickly monitored, recorded and reported.

Respiratory rate is a measurement that simply records the number of times a person breathes in a minute. However, measuring and recording a peak expiratory flow rate (PEFR) can give valuable information about the patient's lung capacity.

Measuring and recording a peak expiratory flow rate

This is achieved by use of a meter called a peak flow meter; this simple device can be a very useful tool to monitor a patient's maximum expiratory force, and is very commonly used for monitoring asthma. It provides a simple, measurable, repeatable and objective measurement of airway function (Dougherty and Lister 2011).

The peak flow measures, in litres per minute, the maximum flow rate on forced expiration that a patient can blow out when starting from full inhalation. This measure allows monitoring of a patient with any lung disease; it is easy, quick and cheap, but technique is crucial to ensure accuracy (Maddex and Valler-Jones 2009; Dougherty and Lister 2011). It allows monitoring of ongoing treatments and can be very useful for someone who has difficulty recognising that their condition is worsening, for example asthma. Peak flow is also used for children and, in the same way as adults, gender and height considerations will

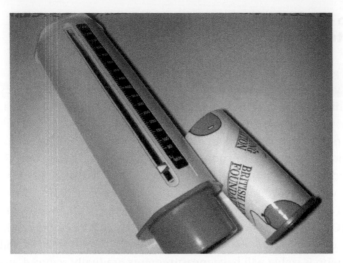

Figure 9.3 Peak flow meter with disposable one-way mouthpiece. Source: Photograph by I Lavery.

affect the readings (Ford et al. 2010; Lewis 2008). Due to age and understanding considerations, the nurse must always be certain that the child has understood the instructions to ensure a reliable reading.

To measure a peak flow, a meter is commonly used (Figure 9.3) and this comes with a disposable mouthpiece for each patient. Peak flow meters can be dispensed on prescription for home monitoring; in clinics or hospitals some may be used for multiple patients, but are always used with a disposable one-way mouthpiece. For infection control purposes, always follow your local policy regarding cleaning the device between patients (Dougherty and Lister 2011).

The patient should be sitting or standing upright, to allow full chest expansion. An exploration of the differences in measurements of various seating arrangements (lying, sitting and standing) determined that patients were able to produce higher scores when standing. However it should be noted that in acute areas it is not always possible for patients to stand because of their general condition (Wallace et al. 2013). Dougherty and Lister (2011) state that the patient must first be given information about the procedure so they can give consent and understand it. This is important to encourage compliance and prevents misunderstanding to ensure an accurate reading is obtained. With children, Lewis (2008) suggests that the nurse can demonstrate the technique to the patient first, and this technique may also be useful with adults whose technique is poor. Booker (2007) proposes that the nurse demonstrate the technique first to help the patient understand the procedure. The nurse must ensure that their hands are washed and an apron is put on before assembling the meter to follow infection control procedures. Box 9.1 outlines the technical aspects.

The frequency will depend on each patient's condition. For maintenance (to monitor ongoing treatment), the patient may measure the peak flow once in the morning, or in some cases twice daily and so also record an evening peak flow.

> **Box 9.1** Technique
>
> - Patient holds the meter level, and ensures their fingers don't obstruct the scale.
> - Flow indicator is set to zero/lowest reading on the scale.
> - With the mouthpiece fitted securely, the patient should take a deep breath, clamp the lips tightly round the mouthpiece and then blow out as hard and fast as possible, like blowing out candles.
> - Check the flow indicator position and record the score, for example 370 l/min.
> - It is recommended to do the best of three, so a further two attempts are made, ensuring that indicator is zeroed each time, then recording the best score
>
> Adapted from Dougherty and Lister (2011); Nicol et al. (2012); Maddex and Valler-Jones (2009).

During any acute episode of illness the frequency would increase, so that any treatments and their effectiveness, such as nebuliser therapy, would be monitored. In some cases measurements are taken pre-treatment, for example for asthma and nebuliser treatment, and then again 30 min after treatment (this monitors the effectiveness of any treatment). However it should also be noted that for any patient who cannot talk in full sentences or for whom use of the device will cause exacerbation of their condition, peak flow should not be recorded as this puts excessive strain on the respiratory system when already stressed (BTS/SIGN 2011; Dougherty and Lister 2011)

Normal peak flow measure

A peak flow measurement will vary depending on gender, age and height (Dougherty and Lister 2011):

- Gender: adults usually achieve 400–700 l/min, but males achieve higher readings and elderly women may range from 300 l/min.
- Age: children would be lower, and height is a factor in normal ranges. The normal range in children is 100–400 l/min.
- Height: this increases the lung capacity and so increases the peak flow scoring.

Other variations are due to timings; morning readings tend to be lower, with highest readings usually in the early evening, hence the usual twice daily readings for people with asthma to monitor and compare scores. Scores are plotted and trends can be spotted early, as one lower score may not be meaningful. However, it is best to report this remembering that other recordings will be monitored as well, such as temperature, pulse and blood pressure, and these can support findings. In people with asthma the pulse rate will increase, and if due to an infection they may also have a raised temperature.

Other circumstances can affect readings, for example cold air, animal hair acting as a trigger (allergies); and again, by keeping a record, these trends can be observed and identified.

Regular monitoring can therefore allow the patient to manage their breathing/condition, such as asthma, and respond quickly to any deterioration:

- If the rate falls below 80% of individual's best level, then refer to doctor as they would likely increase preventative treatment, such as an inhaler.
- If the reading falls below 50% of their usual reading, alert medical staff immediately (BTS/SIGN 2011).

Again, if in doubt refer to a professional colleague. Ask yourself – was the patient relaxed and rested? If the patient has just got back from the toilet, with maybe more demands on their breathing, they may be tired resulting in a lower reading, so wait 5 minutes and repeat.

THINK ABOUT IT

Jenny Wilkinson is a 15 year old with asthma; you are supervising her peak flow measurement and notice that her technique is poor.

Explain how this might affect her readings and what advice you might give her to help improve her technique.

Performing suctioning

Suctioning techniques are now considered; depending on your local policy it may be an accepted role with supervised training, *so please check before undertaking any aspect of a suctioning role*.

Dixon (2010) and Nicol et al. (2012) discuss methods of suctioning relevant to this book: oropharyngeal and nasopharyngeal suctioning.

Oropharyngeal

This is oral suction, which is used to help a patient clear the airway when too weak to cough (expectorate) sputum from the pharynx. Other indications include:

- Unconscious or semi-conscious patient, for example after surgery.
- No gag reflex, for example drug overdose, alcohol poisoning or stroke.
- Oral surgery or trauma.

Nasopharyngeal

This may be indicated when the oral suction catheter cannot pass to the back of the pharynx, as a result of teeth clenching, dental/oral surgery or trauma, or if the patient cannot tolerate a 'sucker' at the back of the pharynx, because it can often induce gagging. It is particularly useful for patients with a lot of secretions at the back of the throat who are unable to cough and expectorate (Nicol et al. 2012; Dixon 2010; Carey and Kelsey 2008).

Suction requires skillful practice, because some patients may be at risk of hypoxia (low oxygen level), causing cardiac arrhythmias (irregularities) if suctioning occurs for more than 10 seconds (Dougherty and Lister 2011).

Table 9.2 Assessment for suctioning.

Assessment	Rationale
Patient's airway	Check if obstructed? Any obvious secretions, e.g. vomit?
Patient's knowledge	Have they had this before? Offer explanations to reassure
Risk factors	Does the patient have: Impaired cough or swallowing? Impaired gag reflex? Decreased level of consciousness?

Adapted from Dougherty and Lister (2011); Maddex and Valler-Jones (2009).

Dougherty and Lister (2011) and Maddex and Valler-Jones (2009) describe three assessment aspects for suctioning (Table 9.2).

Having confirmed the need for suction, the following procedure should be followed:

1 Assemble the necessary equipment, for example a Yankauer (suction catheter) and suction tubing of appropriate size, suction machine (if not wall mounted), gloves, apron, sterile water with container, and clinical waste bag.
2 Wash your hands and apply non-sterile gloves to minimise risk of transmitting infection.
3 Turn on suction to appropriate level for your patient (Table 9.3).
4 Connect one end of plastic suction tubing to the machine and the other to the suction piece, for example a Yankauer (rigid short plastic tube). Test working by applying the Yankauer to a container with water and ensure that it sucks water.
5 Remove any oxygen mask if present on patient.
6 Insert the Yankauer catheter into the mouth, along the gum line to the pharynx; move the catheter gently around the mouth until all the secretions are cleared. This may take several repeated attempts. Also, if possible, encourage the patient to cough and check if there are any more secretions. Remember to take only a few seconds, and as Dougherty and Lister (2011) advise no more than 10 seconds per attempt to ensure that oxygen levels do not drop too low (hypoxia).
7 Replace the patient's oxygen mask, if present, after each suctioning and allow the patient time to recover breath between suctions, if required.
8 Clear the tubing by sucking more water, until tubing is clear of secretions, for example, sputum.
9 Switch off the suction.

Table 9.3 Suction pressures.

Wall-mounted suction (mmHg)		
Adult	Child	Infant
100–120	80–100	60–80

Adapted from Dixon (2010); Dougherty and Lister (2011); Carey and Kelsey (2008).

10 Dispose of the tubing and Yankauer as per local policy, and gloves and apron into clinical waste.

11 Wash your hands.

12 Ensure that patient is comfortable; check respiratory rate and colour to ensure that patient is stable before leaving.

13 Ensure that the procedure is documented in patient records as per local policy.

14 Ensure monitoring after the procedure to check that the patient does not develop any unexpected side-effects, such as increasing breathlessness (Dougherty and Lister 2011).

Care of suction equipment is also important to prevent cross-infection. Many practice areas use plastic disposable suction units, so the entire suctioning equipment is disposed of after each use to minimise the risk of cross-infection. However, in some areas glass bottles may still exist and you need to follow your local guidelines for changing and disinfecting these bottles, which usually occurs every 24 hours (Nicol et al. 2012). *Please check local equipment and guidance.*

You must be guided by your local policy and be assessed as competent to carry out both forms of suctioning. Please refer to your employer for guidance.

THINK ABOUT IT

Miss Barbara Jones, 34 years old, has returned from knee surgery. You observe that she is still very drowsy and is sounding chesty. If you were considering suctioning as an option, how would you assess her? Is suctioning appropriate here?

Related aspects and terminology

- *Apnoea*: cessation (stopping) of breathing.
- *Cyanosis*: due to low oxygen levels and presents as a dusky bluish colour of the mucous membranes, for example lips, nailbeds.
- *Tachypnoea*: raised respiratory rate, usually if rate above 20 breaths/min.
- *Bradypnoea*: decreased respiratory rate, if rate below 10 breaths/min.
- *Dyspnoea*: difficulty breathing, patient struggles to get air in so they might open their mouth and gulp air in, and heave shoulders up in an effort to get more air.
- *Hyperventilation*: deep rapid breaths.

- *Hypoventilation*: slow shallow breaths, often associated with drugs, such as morphine, an opioid that acts on the respiratory centre.
- *Cheyne–Stoke respirations*: often seen in patients with heart failure, in palliative patients before death or with brain injured patients, it leads to a gradual increase in the depth of respirations, in turn leading to hyperventilation, followed by a gradual decrease in depth, and then a period of apnoea of 15–20 seconds, before the cycle starts again.

Common problems

Respiratory rate measurement

Nicol et al. (2012) suggest that any activity before taking respiratory rates should be recorded and that the patient should be unaware of the measurement as they can alter their breathing patterns leading to an inaccurate reading. The position of the patient is also important as this can aid lung expansion, which can give a more accurate measurement.

Peak flow measurement

Dougherty and Lister (2011) and Maddex and Valler-Jones (2009) suggest the following problems should be monitored as these can affect the accuracy of the reading:

- Poor seal between lips and mouthpiece, so air leaks out.
- Forgetting to zero indicator between peak flow measures, leading to an inaccurate reading.
- Obstructing indicator with fingers, so blocking the movement of indicator.
- Poor position for recording, for example lying down, so hindering breathing.
- Failure to take maximum inhalation.
- Holding the breath at maximum inhalation for longer than two seconds, thus delaying blowing into the meter.
- Blocking the mouthpiece with tongue or teeth.

BTS/SIGN (2011) suggests that for those who are acutely breathless and cannot speak in full sentences, peak flow measurement should be avoided because of the exertion required. Therefore, you will need to decide, using your observational skills, if the patient is fit physically and able mentally to undertake this procedure. As noted before, a peak flow measure is simple and quick, but a wrong reading may have a serious effect if any treatment is based on a peak flow result.

Suctioning

Problems with suctioning might relate to faulty or poorly maintained equipment, or poor suctioning technique. The suction is part of the workplace emergency equipment and should be checked daily to ensure it is working correctly. When suctioning, observe the patient and time taken to suction, as each attempt should take no longer than 10 seconds with time taken to allow the patient to recover between each attempt (Dougherty and Lister 2011). If the patient is becoming distressed or tired, stop and, if they are on oxygen therapy, replace the mask or nasal cannula and allow the patient to rest, before considering further attempts.

Tables 9.4–9.6 are competency frameworks for recording a respiratory rate and PEFR and for suctioning.

Please ensure that you have undertaken supervised practice, in your clinical area and follow your local workplace policy.

Summary

In this chapter the skills of recording a respiratory rate, measuring a peak flow and suctioning technique were explored. Observation and communication are essential skills, as well as effective recording and reporting.

CASE STUDY 9.1

Melanie Jones is a 14-year-old girl admitted with an acute asthmatic attack. This is her first admission to hospital and she is very frightened.

What factors should you consider when admitting her and recording her respiratory rate?

Discuss what you might expect, in terms of her rate, depth, pattern, sound, regularity and colour.

CASE STUDY 9.2

Mr Adjit Singh, is a 24-year-old man and is 6 foot tall. He attends your clinic in the community as he has been using his reliever inhaler more regularly recently. You are asked to start monitoring his peak flow rate and educate him in self-monitoring at home; when you approach him, he tells you that he has never done this before.

Describe how you would explain the procedure to him and how he should carry out the procedure and document the results at home.

His best score is 245 l/min. Describe your actions.

CASE STUDY 9.3

Jane Sackler is a 78-year-old woman admitted with dense stroke and has developed a chest infection. She is very frail and is finding it hard to spit the sputum from her mouth and you are worried about maintaining her airway. She becomes very distressed and you can see thick sputum in her mouth.

Discuss possible actions that may aid her breathing.

If you are asked to undertake oropharyngeal suctioning, consider whether you are trained and competent in this procedure.

If yes, describe your actions in undertaking suctioning on Miss Sackler.

Table 9.4 Competency framework: recording a respiratory rate.

Steps	First assessment/reassessment					Date/competent signature
	Demonstration/supervised practice					
Recording a respiratory rate	Date/sign 1	Date/sign 2	Date/sign 3	Date/sign 4	Date/sign 5	
1 Identify need for respiratory check						
2 Ensure that patient is in best position (e.g. upright)						
3 Consider if patient is rested, so true baseline						
4 Explain to patient, reassure, get consent						
5 Have watch with second hand ready						
6 Note time and start counting for appropriate time						
7 Observe rise and fall of chest,						
8 Note depth of breaths						
9 Observe pattern of breathing						
10 Note sounds of breathing						
11 Consider how regular/rhythmic breathing is						
12 Observe patient's colour						
13 Record rate on appropriate chart, note any abnormalities, e.g. irregular, noisy breaths						
14 Report any abnormalities promptly and appropriately						

Supervisors/Assessor(s):

Table 9.5 Competency framework: recording a peak expiratory flow rate (PEFR).

Steps	First assessment/reassessment					Date/competent signature
	Demonstration/supervised practice					
Recording a PEFR	Date/sign 1	Date/sign 2	Date/sign 3	Date/sign 4	Date/sign 5	
1 Patient is upright, sitting or standing						
2 Patient is ready for procedure, so rested and consented						
3 Ensure that patient is able to undertake procedure, check understanding						
4 Peak flow assembled with clean mouthpiece secure						
5 Ensure that patient holds device level and fingers (nurse/patient) don't obstruct scale						
6 Flow indicator set to zero reading on scale						
7 Ensure that patient follows correct technique						
8 Check flow indicator position, record score						
9 Ensure that patient performs three, and record best score						
10 Check and compare with previous scores						
11 Report score and any variances promptly						
12 Store peak flow meter correctly, cleaning or disposing of mouthpiece as per local policy						

Supervisors/Assessor(s):

Table 9.6 Competency framework: suctioning.

Steps	First assessment/reassessment					Date/competent signature
	Demonstration/supervised practice					
Suctioning	Date/sign 1	Date/sign 2	Date/sign 3	Date/sign 4	Date/sign 5	
1 Undertake risk assessment pre-procedure						
2 Assemble the necessary equipment						
3 Wash hands and apply non-sterile gloves						
4 Turn on suction to required level						
5 Connect and test equipment, by ensuring that the catheter is sucking sterile water						
6 Remove oxygen mask, if present on patient						
7 Commence suctioning correctly, noting time and patient comfort						
8 Replace patient's oxygen mask, if present, and allow time to recover breath between suctions, if required						
9 Clear the tubing by sucking sterile water, until tubing is clear of secretions						
10 Switch off the suction						
11 Dispose of equipment as appropriate						
12 Remove gloves and wash hands						
13 Ensure patient comfort, and check respiratory rate and colour after procedure						
14 Ensure that documented in patient records						
15 Ensure that monitoring after procedure is in place, e.g. pulse and respiratory checks						
16 Report outcome to appropriate person						

Supervisors/Assessor(s):

Self-assessment		
Assessment	**Aspects**	**Achieved ✓**
Respiration	*Have you considered all aspects of this section?*	
	Patient assessment: rate, depth, pattern, sound, regularity/rhythm and colour	
	Recording the results	
	Reporting concerns or results	
	Problem solving	
Peak flow	*Have you considered all aspects of this section?*	
	Measuring a peak flow – technique aspects	
	Cleansing/disinfection of equipment	
	Recording the results	
	Reporting concerns or results	
	Problem solving	
Suctioning	*Have you considered all aspects of this section?*	
	Assessment of patient – risk assessment	
	Procedure	
	Maintenance and cleansing of equipment	
	Recording the results	
	Reporting concerns or results	
	Problem solving	

References

Booker R (2007) Peak expiratory flow measurement. *Nursing Standard* 21(39): 42–43.

BTS/SIGN (2011) *British Guidelines on the Management of Asthma*. London: BTS/SIGN.

Carey M and Kelsey J (2009) Suctioning. In: Kelsey J and McEwing G (eds) *Clinical Skills in Child Health Practice*. Edinburgh: Elsevier.

Cook K and Montomery H (2010) Assessment. In: Trigg E and Aslam Mohammed T (eds) *Practices in Children's Nursing: Guidelines for Hospital and Community*. Edinburgh: Elsevier Ltd.

Clancy J and McVicar A (2009) *Physiology and Anatomy for Nurses and Healthcare Practitioners: A Homeostatic Approach*, 3rd edn. London: Hodder Arnold.

Dixon M (2010) Suctioning. In: Trigg E and Aslam Mohammed T (eds) *Practices in Children's Nursing: Guidelines for Hospital and Community*. Edinburgh: Elsevier Ltd.

Dougherty L and Lister S (eds) (2011) *The Royal Marsden Hospital Manual of Clinical Nursing Procedures*, 8th edn. Oxford: Blackwell Publishing.

Lewis G (2008) Peak flow monitoring. In: Kelsey J and McEwing G (eds) *Clinical Skills in Child Health Practice*. Edinburgh: Elsevier.

Massey D and Meredith T. (2010) Respiratory assessment 1: why do it and how to do it? *British Journal of Cardiac Nursing* 5(11): 537–541.

Maddex S (2009) Measuring vital signs. In: Baille L (ed.) *Developing Practical Adult Nursing Skills*, 3rd edn. London: Hodder Arnold.

Maddex S and Valler-Jones T (2009) Assessing physical health and responding to sudden deterioration. In: Baille L (ed.) *Developing Practical Adult Nursing Skills*, 3rd edn. London: Hodder Arnold.

National Institute for Health and Clinical Excellence (NICE) (2007) CG50. Acutely Ill Patients in Hospital: *Recognition of and Response to Acute Illness in Adults in Hospital*. London: NICE.

Nicol M, Bavin C, Cronin P, et al. (2012) *Essential Nursing Skills*. London: Mosby.

Smith J and Roberts R (2011) *Vital Signs for Nurses: An Introduction to Clinical Observations*. Oxford: Wiley-Blackwell.

Syers S (2008) Interpretation of observations. In: Kelsey J and McEwing G (eds) *Clinical Skills in Child Health Practice*. Edinburgh: Elsevier

Tortora G J and Derrickson B (2011) *Principles of Anatomy and Physiology*, 13th edn. Hoboken, NJ: John Wiley & Sons Inc.

Ford L, Maddox C, Moore E and Sales R (2010) The safe management of medicines in children. In: Trigg E and Aslam Mohammed T (eds) *Practices in Children's Nursing: Guidelines for Hospital and Community*. Edinburgh: Elsevier Ltd.

Wallace J, George C M, Tolley E, et al. (2013) Peak expiratory flow in bed? A comparison of 3 positions. *Respiratory Care* 58(3): 494–497.

Wild K and Peate I (2012) Clinical observations 5/6: breathing/respiratory rate. *British Journal of Healthcare Assistants* 6(9): 438–441.

Addendum

Wright meter cleaning information

Reproduced with kind permission from Clement Clarke International.

How to disinfect the Mini-Wright Standard Peak Flow Meter, the AFS Low Range Mini Peak Flow meter and the Mini-Wright Digital

The Mini-Wright Peak Flow Meter was designed as a portable device to help healthcare professionals monitor lung function; to minimise the risk of cross-infection, it has an integral one-way valve that prevents the patient from breathing in any of the previous patient's exhaled breath that could remain in the meter (the Mini-Wright Digital does not have a one-way valve).

The importance of peak flow monitoring results in many patients receiving their own personal meter for home monitoring of lung function, by prescription or recommended purchase. Doctor's surgeries and hospitals may also wish to issue peak flow meters on a loan basis and therefore need a means of reprocessing each device before reissue. The following instructions have been prepared to facilitate multiple-patient use.

Note that we would recommend that, if the last user was diagnosed or suspected of having a serious communicable disease, the meter should be disposed of.

Devices used for multiple patients may need to be replaced more often than those used by only one person.

Frequency of disinfecting the Mini-Wright range of peak flow meters

The following recommendations for disinfecting peak flow meter frequencies are presented as a guide only. In practice, the person responsible for the clinical well-being of the patient should consider the specific circumstances of the next patient and the risk posed by cross-infection.

Mouthpiece type	Disposable one-way cardboard mouthpieces (single use device[a])	Disposable bacterial filters (single-use device[a])	Disposable cardboard mouthpieces (single-use device[a])	Sterilisable plastic mouthpieces
Frequency	WEEKLY	WEEKLY	Between patients	Between patients

[a]Single use device means 'do not reuse' (EN 980:2003). Clement Clarke International Ltd consider that multiple measurements being made by the same patient in one consultation can be considered as 'single use' as long as the mouthpiece/filter is not damaged between measurements. This interpretation cannot be applied to all devices marked as 'single use'.

Reprocessing: sterilisable plastic mouthpiece

- Clean using an automatic dishwasher (2 min pre-wash, 3 min detergent wash, dry).
- Autoclave in saturated steam (max. 134–137°C) for 3 minutes (refer to autoclave manufacturer's instructions for details of cycles available).
- Alternatively, the method below can be used to disinfect the mouthpiece.

Cleaning and disinfection

1 Inspect the unit for signs of damage or wear; if any is evident replace meter.
2 Prepare a solution of detergent in accordance with the manufacturer instructions in a container large enough for the peak flow meter(s) to be totally submerged.
3 Agitate the meter while in the solution to ensure that any trapped air is expelled. Do not use any mechanical aids such as brushes or cloths.
4 Rinse and dry as recommended.
5 Prepare a quantity of your chosen disinfectant in a suitable container.
6 Immerse the peak flow meter; again agitate the meter to ensure that air is expelled and leave it in the solution for the recommended time.
7 Rinse as stated, shake gently to remove any excess water and allow to dry naturally; do not use hot air or a drying cupboard.

Detergents

The following detergents have been tested for compatibility with Clement Clarke International Ltd's peak flow meters.

Name	Solution strength	Comments
Lancerzyme	40 ml in 5 litres of water	Enzymatic cleaner
Cidezyme		Enzymatic cleaner
Hospec		

Disinfectants

The following disinfectants have been tested for compatibility with Clement Clarke International Ltd's peak flow meters.

Chemical type	Examples	Solution strength	Comments
Chlorine dioxide generator	Tristel one day	20 ml in 1 litre water	Safety data sheet and further information available from www.tristel.com
ortho-Phthalaldehyde	Cidex OPA	Undiluted	
Sodium hypochlorite (NaOCL)	Milton	1000 p.p.m.	Ensure thorough rinsing, as corrosion of the metal parts will occur if exposed to chlorine for long periods.
Sodium dichloroisocyanurate (NaDCC)	Presept, Actichlor, Sanichlor, Haz-Tab	1000 p.p.m.	
Hydrogen peroxide and peroxygen compounds	Pera Safe	1.62% w/v	

Clement Clarke International Ltd accepts no liability for damage caused to products if the above procedure and recommended solutions are not used.

It is the user's responsibility to choose which of the recommended solutions are used within their establishment or hospital and we stress that the infection control nurse/department should be consulted when making the choice.

It is the responsibility of the user to keep up to date with the latest information from the relevant disinfectant manufacturer concerning instructions, effects, concentrations and immersion times.

If your preferred cleaner/disinfectant is not on the recommended list, please contact our customer service advisers on 01279 414969 or fax 01279 456 304 or email resp@clement-clarke.com.

Reference

Medical Healthcare product Regulatory Agency (MHRA). *Chemical disinfection in hospitals – PHLS, Sterilization, disinfection and cleaning of medical device equipment (MAC Manual)*. London: MHRA.

CHAPTER 10

Urinalysis and faecal occult blood testing

LEARNING OBJECTIVES

- Identify the importance of urinalysis in practice
- Describe how to undertake urinalysis testing
- Discuss the importance of faecal occult blood testing and how this is performed

Aim of this chapter

The aim of this chapter is to describe how to undertake urinalysis and faecal occult blood tests (FOBt) and to discuss why these are performed within the clinical environment.

Reasons for performing urinalysis and FOB tests

Urinalysis is a simple non-invasive clinical procedure. It is quick, cost-effective and easy method of screening that can give clues as to the health status of the person and can be carried out by the healthcare worker or the patient at home (Foxley 2010). For this reason it is suggested that healthcare practitioners should not only be able to perform the task but interpret the results as well (Mulryan 2011).

Faecal occult (hidden) blood tests (FOBt) involve the testing of a specimen of faeces to identify whether there is any blood present that is not visible to the naked eye, which is referred to as malaena. It is useful in helping to diagnose many gastrointestinal conditions that may cause bleeding, for example colorectal (bowel) cancer or peptic ulcers (Baillie and Busuttil Leaver 2009). The procedure is simple and non-invasive and requires a small sample of uncontaminated faeces to smear onto a specimen card or place into a pot for the lab; it is also quick and easy for patients and healthcare workers to carry out. FOBt is a key part of the NHS National Bowel Cancer Screening Programme

Clinical Skills for Healthcare Assistants and Assistant Practitioners, Second Edition.
Angela Whelan and Elaine Hughes.
© 2016 John Wiley & Sons, Ltd. Published 2016 by John Wiley & Sons, Ltd.

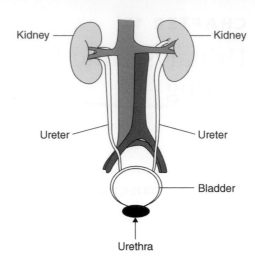

Figure 10.1 Urinary system.

(Public Health England 2013). This national programme focuses on adults aged 60–69 and encourages self-collection of FOBt samples; it is thought to have reduced bowel cancer deaths by 16% since the programme commenced in 2006 (Moss et al. 2012).

Relevant anatomy and physiology

In normal health, the urinary system has two kidneys, two ureters, one urinary bladder and one urethra (Tortora and Derrickson 2011) (Figure 10.1). The kidneys are located in the lumbar area and are described as bean-shaped organs. The kidneys are highly vascular and receive approximately 180 litres of blood per day via the renal arteries, and their main purpose is to filter the blood, reabsorb the required solutes and remove waste products and water for excretion via the formed urine (Clancy and McVicar 2009).

The kidneys are connected to the bladder by the ureters and are hollow tubes of length approximately 25–30 cm (10–12 inches). The formed urine passes through the ureters for storage in the bladder.

The urinary bladder is a hollow muscular organ lying in the pelvic cavity; in males directly anterior (in front) to the rectum, and in females anterior to the vagina and inferior to (below) the uterus (Tortora and Derrickson 2011).

The urethra is a hollow muscular tube that transfers the urine from the bladder to the external sphincter and is approximately 4 cm in females and 20 cm in males. The short length of the female urethra can predispose women to urinary tract infections (Clancy and McVicar 2009; Tortora and Derrickson 2011).

It is worth briefly reviewing the process of digestion, because from this we get the formation of faeces. Food is consumed via the mouth and transported to the stomach via the oesophagus. It is in the stomach that the first digestion of food

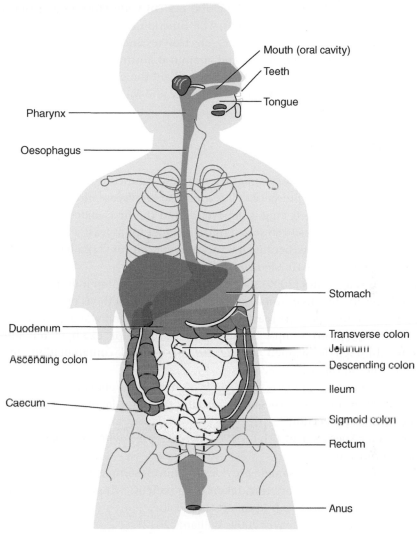

Right lateral view of head and neck and
anterior view of chest, abdomen, and pelvis

Figure 10.2 Digestive system.

begins that will enable the nutrients to be absorbed within the small intestine
(Tortora and Derrickson 2011)) (Figure 10.2).

The small intestine begins at the pyloric sphincter (circular muscle that con-
stricts an opening) at the exit of the stomach and coils round the abdominal
cavity, before opening into the large intestine. The small intestine is 2.5 cm in
diameter and can vary from around 3 m to 6.5 m long (Tortora and Derrickson 2011; Clancy and McVicar 2009). The small intestine is divided into three
sections: duodenum, jejunum and ileum; most digestion occurs within these
three sections while absorption of nutrients occurs at the end of the ileum.

The large intestine is 1.5–2 m long and 6.5 cm wide (Tortora and Derrickson 2011; Clancy and McVicar 2009). The function of the large intestine is to complete the absorption process (water, electrolytes and vitamins), manufacture certain vitamins such as vitamin K and vitamin B, form faeces, produce gases as a by-product of carbohydrate metabolism and aid the expulsion of faeces from the body (Tortora and Derrickson 2011; Clancy and McVicar 2009).

Urinalysis testing

Elimination of urine is an essential normal bodily function and urinalysis is a useful tool to assess the presence of infection and for disease monitoring (Foxley 2010). Timing of urine testing is important, and the first voided sample (early morning urine) that has been stored in the bladder for at least 4 hours provides the most accurate results, because it is the most concentrated (Baillie and Busuttil Leaver 2009; Foxley 2010; Siemens Diagnostics 2009).

Siemens Diagnostics (2009) state that specimen collection must be in a clean, dry and preservative-free container. There are several methods of specimen collection depending upon the reason for the test and the individual patient:

1 A random (clean) sample at any time of day, for example on admission, although in women it may contain vaginal contamination during menstruation (monthly bleeding).
2 An early morning sample – first sample after sleep (as above).
3 A midstream urine (MSU) sample, usually taken for laboratory sampling so needs careful collection.
4 A catheter specimen of urine (CSU) sample, used when the patient has a catheter in situ.
5 A suprapubic catheter sample provides the purest sample, but is rarely used.
6 A urostomy specimen of urine, taken from patients who have urinary diversions and wear stoma bags to collect their urine.
  (Baillie and Busuttil Leaver 2009; Williams 2012)

A urine sample must be tested within 4 hours of collection or bacteria can multiply affecting the accuracy test results. Where this testing period cannot be adhered to urine should be refrigerated and allowed to return to room temperature before testing. For the most accurate results, always test urine immediately after collection (Baillie and Busuttil Leaver 2009; Williams 2012; Foxley 2010).

THINK ABOUT IT

How are you going to collect a specimen of urine from a patient on admission?

Before testing the urine using reagent test strips, there are useful observations that you can undertake, including the colour of the urine, the smell (odour) and the clarity (Baillie and Busuttil Leaver 2009; Siemens Diagnostics 2009).

Baillie and Busuttil Leaver (2009) and Dougherty and Lister (2011) describe urine as typically clear, pale to deep yellow in colour and slightly acidic (pH 6), although they add that the pH can change as a result of metabolic processes or diet (e.g. beetroot). Foxley (2010) suggested that some laxatives could change urine to an orange bright yellow, whereas diet and medications, for example rhubarb and antibiotics, can change urine to a red/orange colour.

The composition of urine can change dramatically as a result of disease and may contain red blood cells, proteins, glucose, bile or white blood cells. The presence of these abnormalities in the urine can be an indicator of illness (Dougherty and Lister 2011).

Dougherty and Lister (2011) state that freshly voided urine smells faintly aromatic, and Foxley (2010) suggests that urine can develop an ammonia smell if it is left standing. There should not be a strong odour to urine, which can signify the presence of bacteria (Baillie and Busuttil Leaver 2009). Foxley (2010) suggests the smell and clarity of the urine should be observed as this can also indicate illness. Infected urine can be described as having a 'fishy' smell, whereas acetone excreted by patients with diabetic ketoacidosis gives urine a sweet smell. Clancy and McVicar (2009) also state that certain foods in the diet can affect the odour of urine, such as asparagus and sugar-puffs.

Urine that is cloudy or has sediment (debris) can indicate the presence of infection, therefore observation is important (Foxley 2010). Cloudy urine is caused by suspended particles, such as white and red cells, which will settle on standing to leave a deposit, while frothy urine contains protein (Mulryan 2011).

Baillie and Busuttil Leaver (2009) identify the importance of ensuring that any patient providing a sample of urine for testing gets the following information. The procedure for catheter samples can be found in Chapter 11:

- An explanation of the reason for testing.
- Instruction in the method of collection.
- Provision of suitable equipment, for example a container for the specimen.
- An appropriate environment, for example privacy and space.

There is a lack of agreement in the literature as to best practice concerning cleaning around the urethral meatus. In two studies (Lifschitz and Kramer 2000; Unlu et al. 2007) there was found to be little difference in cleansing with soap and water, not cleansing or cleansing with a chlorhexidine solution. Therefore the individual nurse must look towards their own workplace policies for guidance. When obtaining a MSU from a male, patients should first wash their hands, then retract the foreskin and cleanse the meatus with soap and water, or as per local policy. To collect the sample the patient passes the first part of the urine stream (15–30 ml) into the toilet, and then collects the next part (50–100 ml) in a clean dry container, and finally finishes emptying the bladder into the toilet. The container cap must be replaced immediately and the hands washed.

For females, again patients wash their hands, then clean the vulval and urethral meatus with soap and water, or as per local policy, then separate the labia (this might be difficult for some patients, e.g. a patient with arthritis) and continue as above.

Jasper (2008) and Maddox and Pearson (2010) suggest there are several methods to collect samples from children or infants:

1 Adhesive urine bags, which attach to the perineal area; however, this is the least favoured method because it carries a risk of contamination from the perineum and rectum.
2 Urine collection pads: these need to be checked every 10 minutes for the sample or replaced after 30 minutes if the infant has not voided to prevent contamination of the sample.
3 'Clean catch' where the child or infant is sat over a sterile container and urine collected as they pass urine.
4 MSU sample: most reliable for testing; however, not always possible in young children. Females should be encouraged to part the labia and males should retract the foreskin and then pass urine into a sterile container.
5 Catherter specimen of urine: used if the child has a catheter in situ. The sample is always taken from the specimen collection port to avoid contamination.
6 Suprapubic bladder aspiration would be performed only in urgent situations because it carries the risk of bladder puncture and is not suitable in children aged under 2 years.

Once the sample has been collected and you have observed, and recorded, the colour and noted the presence, if any, of odour, or if the urine is cloudy, you proceed to test the urine. Reagent test strips allow testing of a range of factors: leucocytes (white cells), nitrites, urobilinogen, protein, pH, blood, specific gravity, ketones, bilirubin and glucose (Baillie and Busuttil Leaver 2009). Check the strips in your area and check which substances are tested (Table 10.1). (Figure 10.3 is an example of a recording slip.)

Procedure for testing

1 Check that reagent strips are correctly stored and have not expired (discussed later).
2 Explain and discuss the procedure with the patient (discussed earlier).
3 Wash hands using the Ayliffe technique and put gloves on.
4 Obtain fresh sample of urine from the patient.
5 Dip reagent strip fully into the urine, remove immediately and allow any excess urine to drain away ensuring the chemicals are not mixed.
6 Wait the specified time interval for each square as noted per bottle.
7 Read and record your findings as per local policy.
8 Dispose of urine in sluice or toilet and test strip and gloves into the clinical waste.
9 Wash your hands.
10 Report findings and results as per local policy.

Table 10.1 Significance of substances in the urine.

Substance	Causes
Glucose: not normally detected in urine	Diabetes mellitus, acute pancreatitis, pregnancy, glycosuria
Bilirubin (stale urine may give a false positive)	Liver cell damage: viral/drug induced, hepatitis, paracetamol overdose, cirrhosis; Biliary tract obstruction – gallstones, cancer of pancreas
Ketones	Due to excessive breakdown of body fat – fasting, specially with fever/vomiting, some high protein diets, diabetic ketoacidosis, starvation/excessive dieting
Specific gravity: normal 1.001–1.035	High: concentrated urine due to dehydration or chronic renal failure Low: high fluid intake, renal disease
Blood: haematuria	Kidney disorders: urinary tract infection (UTI), stones, tumour, severe burns, transfusion reaction, trauma
pH: normal 4.5–8.00	High: stale urine, UTI, Low diabetic ketoacidosis, starvation
Protein: test may not be sensitive to presence of all proteins	UTI, fever, pre-eclampsia, heart failure, high-protein diet, severe hypertension, glomerulonephritis, diabetes and contamination of the sample In men may be due to sperm after sex
Urobilinogen: normally present in urine, stale samples can give false positives	Increased secretion: viral hepatitis, cirrhosis, blood disorders such as sickle cell anemia or thalassemia Decreased secretion – biliary tract obstruction caused by gallstones, pancreas cancer, medicines, e.g. neomycin
Nitrite: not usually found in urine	UTI
Leucocytes	Renal or bladder infection

UTI, urinary tract infection.
Adapted from Baillie and Busittil Leaver (2009), Foxley (2010).

11 Ensure that the patient is comfortable, and where appropriate given results; please discuss this role locally before proceeding. Rigby and Gray (2005) noted the debate over the reliability of urinalysis, and suggest that reports are only 85% reliable, so its use in screening is questionable. However NICE (2006) suggest that urinalysis should be completed on all women with incontinence to identify potential urinary tract infections. Therefore, it is important that the test is completed correctly to ensure that it is as accurate as possible.

Bayer
Diagnostics
MULTISTIX* 10 SG REPORT

Name _____ Date _____

Ward _____ Patient No. _____

TESTS   Please tick appropriate box for each test

LEUCOCYTES 2 minutes	NEG.	TRACE	SMALL +	MODERATE ++	LARGE +++

NITRITE 60 seconds	NEG.		POSITIVE (any degree of pink colour)		

UROBILINOGEN 60 seconds	Normal 3	16	µmol/l 33	66	131

PROTEIN 60 seconds	NEG.	g/L TRACE	0.30 +	1 ++	3 +++	≥ 20 ++++

pH 60 seconds	5.0	6.0	6.5	7.0	7.5	8.0	8.5

BLOOD 60 seconds	NEG.	NON HAEMOLYZED TRACE	HAEMOLYZED TRACE	SMALL +	MODERATE ++	LARGE +++

SPECIFIC GRAVITY 45 seconds	1.000	1.005	1.010	1.015	1.020	1.025	1.030

KETONE 40 seconds	NEG.	mmol/L TRACE 0.5	SMALL 1.5	MODERATE 4	8	LARGE 16

BILIRUBIN 30 seconds	NEG.			SMALL +	MODERATE ++	LARGE +++

GLUCOSE 30 seconds	NEG.	mmol/L 5.5 TRACE	14 +	28 ++	55 +++	≥111 ++++

*Trademark of Bayer Corporation, USA.   X800264   mpl

Figure 10.3 Example of a test recording slip. Source: Photograph by I Lavery.

THINK ABOUT IT

Emily Boyd, aged 54 years, has type 2 diabetes and is frequently treated for UTIs and fungal infections. She requires a urine test while she is in clinic. What aspects will you observe and test for?

From the test results, any action taken may depend on other results (e.g. blood tests); however, your action must be to report any abnormalities immediately. If the specimen is old and has been lying for a while, a fresh sample of urine should be obtained. Depending upon the results obtained further laboratory tests may follow, for example urine for microscopy, culture and sensitivity (Baillie and Busuttil Leaver 2009). Therefore accurate testing, recording and prompt reporting is essential. If in doubt, report.

Accurate testing leads us to consider storage of the reagent strips. Baillie and Busuttil Leaver (2009) suggest that healthcare workers should check that strips are in date, stored and used correctly. Incorrect handling of the test strips can affect the results. Mulryan (2011) and Siemens Diagnostics (2009) advise the following to increase reliability of the test results:

- Store reagent strips out of direct sunlight.
- Keep strips at a constant temperature, usually cool and dark, not in the fridge.
- Use strips according to manufacturer's guidance.
- Strips should be stored in the bottle supplied.
- Replace cap on the bottle as quickly as possible after each test.
- Never remove desiccant (some manufacturers place this in the lid).

Faecal occult blood testing

Faeces consist of the unabsorbed end products of digestion and contain fibre, some electrolytes, water and bile pigments, which give faeces their colour (Clancy and McVicar 2009). Nicol et al. (2012) states that normal stools are brown, soft and formed but should not have an offensive smell. Therefore when collecting a specimen for FOB testing, or any other stool specimen test, the colour, smell and consistency should be noted and recorded as part of the bowel assessment. The majority of clinical areas use the Bristol Stool Form Scale to classify faeces (see Addendum at end of chapter).

Baillie and Busuttil Leaver (2009) discussed smell as part of a bowel assessment. Fatty, offensive-smelling stools can indicate bowel disease, for example gallbladder disease. Stools that are covered with mucous and/or blood indicate disease such as ulcerative colitis. Black tarry stools can indicate digested blood and have a distinctive smell, often due to upper tract disorders, for example stomach ulcer. Finally, stools with fresh blood often indicate haemorrhoids. All these require prompt reporting.

There are different methods of FOBt sample collection. In many acute hospital settings the use of specimen pots with integral spatulas are used to send the sample to the lab. However in some areas sample cards may be used (Figure 10.4). There are two kinds of cards for FOBt collection, one aimed at healthcare workers with chemical additives and another aimed at patients as part of the National Bowel Cancer Screening Programme (Public Health England 2013). Ouyang et al. (2005) suggest that for 4 days before the first sample is taken and during the test period patients' diets should be modified as outlined below. However, in acute hospital settings, this may not be possible if specimens are urgently required. As gastrointestinal bleeding may be intermittent, three FOBts should be carried out on three different separate samples of faeces from the patient on different days, but do not need to be from consecutive samples (NHS Bowel Cancer Screening Programme 2013).

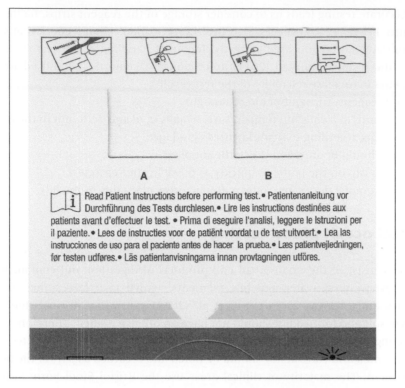

Figure 10.4 A faecal occult blood (FOB) specimen card. Source: Photograph by I Lavery.

Kyle and Prynn (2004) offered advice for patients before having an FOBt; this may be a useful guide for staff to discuss with each patient, and suggests that patients:

- eat a diet rich in roughage (helps stimulate bleeding if any lesions present);
- avoid alcohol and aspirin or other non-steroidal anti-inflammatory drugs, and vitamin C or iron tablets (could worsen bleeding or affect results);
- avoid fish with dark meat, for example salmon, tuna, sardines, mackerel;
- avoid red meat and blood products, for example black pudding, kidneys or liver;
- avoid tomatoes, cauliflower, horseradish, turnip, melon, bananas and soybeans;
- are asked if menstruating (if female), have diarrhoea or had a recent nose or throat bleed (as could affect result); if yes postpone the test;
- ask staff if they have any concerns or queries.

Ouyang et al. (2005) note that, with guaiac FOBt (cards for healthcare workers use and for patient self collection), false positives can occur with red meats and some fruits and vegetables, such as turnip, and also false negatives can occur with high doses of vitamin C. However, research by Bapuji et al. (2012) states that there is a difference between the advice given by health professional in relation to FOBt, which can affect patients' compliance with the test and preparation for it. This potentially can lead to incorrect results, which makes the advice of healthcare workers essential in the accurate diagnosis of bowel cancer.

> **THINK ABOUT IT**
>
> Wendy Williamson is to have FOB tests, and you have been asked to give her advice about the procedure and preparation. What advice might you offer?

Equipment for the FOB test using a guiac impregnated card
- Sample card (see Figure 10.4) and wooden stick.
- Chemical solution.
- Non-sterile gloves and apron.
- Container.

Once the patient has opened their bowels, take the container to the sluice and collect two samples from different parts of the faeces (in case of false readings); smear a small amount from each on the two sample windows indicated on the card by the foldaway section. Once smeared on, close the cover and turn the card over, and then follow the instructions for administering the chemical, taking care not to spill the chemical because this can cause some hazards, for example a chemical might cause a skin reaction (Control of Substances Hazardous to Health (COSHH) – HMSO 1999).

The test area should be observed for a change in colour. Ouyang et al. (2005) indicate that this is a blue colour change depending on whether blood is in the stool, and usually occurring within 1 minute. This can be further classified, so if pale blue it could indicate weakly positive, whereas strong blue indicates strongly positive.

Equipment needed for an FOB test using a specimen pot
- Gloves and apron.
- Labelled sterile specimen container with integral spatula (if not available then use a wooden tongue depressor).
- Labelled specimen bag.

Once the sample has been obtained from the patient (this should not be contaminated with urine), don gloves and apron and take a sample from the stool with the spatula or tongue depressor filling the pot around a third full. Close the lid tightly and remove your apron and gloves and wash your hands thoroughly. Ensure the specimen is labelled correctly and put it into a labelled laboratory bag. The sample should then be refrigerated if it is not being sent to the lab immediately (Nicol et al. 2012; Baillie and Busuttil Leaver 2009).

> **THINK ABOUT IT**
>
> What hazards might you encounter with an FOB test?

Related aspects and terminology

- *Jaundice*: yellow pigmentation of the whites of the eyes, skin or mucous membranes due to build-up of bilirubin.
- *Cirrhosis*: scarred liver, often due to chronic inflammation.
- *Diabetes mellitus*: a group of disorders that lead to an elevation of glucose in the blood; as glucose (sugar) levels increase, glucose appears in the urine.
- *Glycosuria*: presence of sugar in the urine.
- *Renal function*: function of the kidneys.
- *Haematuria*: presence of intact red blood cells in the urine.
- *Pre-eclampsia*: abnormal condition of pregnancy associated with high blood pressure and protein in the urine.
- *Suprapubic*: above the pubic bone.
- *Meatus*: passageway or opening at the external point of the canal.
- *Labia*: liplike structure.
- *Hypertension*: high blood pressure.
- *Acute pancreatitis*: inflammation of the pancreas.
  (Tortora and Derrickson 2011.)

Common problems

Urinalysis, if not tested on a fresh sample, as noted before, can lead to false results, so always ensure that freshly passed urine is tested or that refrigerated urine has been allowed to return to room temperature before testing.

In females, take care if the patient is menstruating, because this can lead to a false reading of haematuria.

Ensure that you handle the strips correctly, when in storage and when undertaking the test, otherwise this can also affect results.

FOB testing problems may be due to poor sampling (contaminated with urine or incorrect storage), in the case of guiaic test cards not smearing sufficient faeces on the test areas, insufficient chemical or reading the result too quickly (before it has time to change). Please check the type of test in your area and follow the manufacturer's instructions or hospital procedure concerning sample collection fully.

Summary

Urinalysis and FOB testing are quick and simple tests and allow for prompt results; however, they require safe and competent practice to ensure their accuracy. As discussed, there are risks with these procedures and the healthcare assistant should follow universal precautions to prevent the risk of cross infection. Tables 10.2 and 10.3 are competency frameworks for urinalysis and FOB testing.

CASE STUDY 10.1 URINALYSIS

Julie Forth is 68 years old and lives in a nursing home; over the past few days she has had a couple of episodes of incontinence and is complaining of abdominal discomfort and pain on passing urine. Her temperature is 38 and the Nursing Home staff tell you she is confused. She has been admitted with a suspected UTI.

What might you expect to find present in her urine?

CASE STUDY 10.2 FOB TEST

John Armour is 73 years old and has been admitted with weight loss and altered bowel habits.

Discuss why FOB will be requested, and outline how you will collect a sample of stool and test for the presence of occult blood.

Self-assessment

Assessment	Aspects	Achieved ✓
Urinalysis	*Have you considered all aspects of this section?*	
	Timing of collecting	
	Specimen collection procedure	
	Observation, e.g. colour, smell	
	Performing the test	
	Recording the results	
	Reporting concerns or results	
	Problem solving	
FOB testing	*Have you considered all aspects of this section?*	
	Assessment, e.g. colour, smell and consistency	
	FOB test procedure	
	Storage and handling of equipment	
	Patient education	
	Recording the results	
	Reporting concerns or results	
	Problem solving	

Table 10.2 Competency framework: urinalysis testing.

Steps	First assessment/reassessment					Date/competent signature
	Demonstration/Supervised practice					
Urinalysis testing	Date/sign 1	Date/sign 2	Date/sign 3	Date/sign 4	Date/sign 5	
1 Checked reagent strips are correctly stored and in date						
2 Explained procedure to the patient						
3 Washes hands, applied disposable gloves and apron						
4 Obtained fresh urine sample in clean container						
5 Dipped reagent strip fully into the urine, removed immediately, excess urine removed						
6 Held stick at an angle, to ensure no mixing						
7 Waited specified time interval for each square as noted per bottle						
8 Read and recorded findings						
9 Disposed of urine in sluice or toilet and test strip into clinical waste						
10 Disposed of gloves and apron, washes hands						
11 Reported findings and results						
12 Ensured patient is comfortable, where appropriate given results						

Supervisors/Assessor(s):

Table 10.3 Competency framework: faecal occult blood (FOB) testing.

Steps	First assessment/reassessment					Date/competent signature
	Demonstration/Supervised practice					
FOB testing (Guiaic cards)	Date/sign 1	Date/sign 2	Date/sign 3	Date/sign 4	Date/sign 5	
1 Washes hands, dons disposable apron and gloves						
2 Collected sample from the faeces						
3 Smeared a small amount on the test card						
4 Closed test area						
5 Administered the chemical, carefully						
6 Observed the test area for change of colour						
7 Disposed of gloves and apron, washes hands						
8 Disposed of card and protective clothing						
9 Recorded and reported results						

Supervisors/Assessor(s):

(continued overleaf)

Table 10.3 (*continued*)

Steps	First assessment/reassessment					Date/competent signature
	Demonstration/Supervised practice					
FOB testing (Specimen pot)	Date/sign 1	Date/sign 2	Date/sign 3	Date/sign 4	Date/sign 5	
1 Washes hands, dons disposable apron and gloves						
2 Collected sample from the faeces						
3 Fills sample pot using spatula or wooden tongue depressor to around a third full						
4 Tightly seals pot						
5 Disposes of gloves and apron, washes hands						
6 Ensures specimen pot and laboratory form is labeled correctly						
7 Stores specimen in refrigerator for collection or sends to laboratory immediately						
8 Records and reports completion of specimen collection						

Supervisors/Assessor(s):

References

Baillie L and Busuttil Leaver R (2009) Meeting elimination needs. In: Baillie L (ed.) *Developing Practical Nursing Skills*, 3rd edn. London: Hodder Education, pp. 321–393.

Bapuji, S. Lobchuk M M, McClement S E, et al. (2012) Fecal occult blood testing instructions and impact on patient adherence. *Cancer Epidemiology* 36: 258–264.

Clancy J and McVicar A (2009) *Physiology and Anatomy: A Homeostatic Approach*, 3rd edn. London: Hodder Arnold.

Dougherty L and Lister S (eds) (2011) *The Royal Marsden Hospital Manual of Clinical Nursing Procedures*, 8th edn. Oxford: Blackwell Publishing.

Foxley S (2010) Urinalysis: analysing urine and interpreting the results. *Journal of Renal Nursing* 2(3): 137–140.

HMSO (1999) Control of Substances Hazardous to Health (COSHH) No 437. Available at: www .hmso.gov.uk/is/si1999/19990437.htm (accessed 27 January 2007).

Jasper E (2008) Specimen collection. In: Kelsey J and McEwing G (eds) *Clinical Skills in Child Health Practice*. Edinburgh: Elsevier.

Kyle G and Prynn P (2004) Guidelines for patients undergoing faecal occult blood testing. *Nursing Times* 100(48): 62, 64.

Lifschitz E and Kramer L (2000) Outpatient urine culture. *Archives of Internal Medicine* 160: 2537–2340.

Maddox C and Pearson B (2010) Specimen collection. In: Trigg E and Mohammed T (eds) *Practices in Childrens Nursing: Guidelines for Hospital and Community*, 3rd edn. Edinburgh: Elsevier.

Moss S M, Campbell C, Melia J, et al. (2012) Performance measures in three rounds of the English bowel cancer screening pilot. *Gut* 61: 101–107.

Mulryan C (2011) Urine testing through the use of dipstick analysis. *British Journal of Healthcare Assistants* 5(5): 234–239.

Bowel Cancer Screening Programme (2013) *NHS Bowel Cancer Screening Programme: Information Leaflet*. London: NHS.

NICE (2006) CG40. *Urinary Incontinence*. London: NICE.

Nicol M, Bavin C, Kronin P, et al. (2012) *Essential Nursing Skills: Clinical Skills for Caring*. Edinburgh: Mosby.

Ouyang D L, Chen J, Getzenberg R H and Schoen R E (2005) Noninvasive testing for colorectal cancer: a review. *American Journal of Gastroenterology* 100: 1393–1403.

Public Health England (2013) National Bowel Cancer Screening Programme. Available at: http:// www.cancerscreening.nhs.uk/bowel/index.html (last accessed 15 May 2013).

Rigby D and Gray K (2005) Understanding urine testing. *Nursing Times* 101(12): 60–62.

Siemens Diagnostics (2009) *Your Practical Guide to Urine Analysis*. Camberley: Siemens Healthcare Diagnostics.

Tortora G J and Derrickson B (2011) *Principles of Anatomy and Physiology*, 12th edn. Hoboken, NJ: John Wiley & Sons Inc.

Unlu H, Çetinkaya Şardan Y and Ülker S (2007) Comparison of sampling methods for urine cultures. *Journal of Nursing Scholarship* 39(4): 325–329.

Williams J (2012) Stoma care: obtaining a urine specimen from a urostomy. *Gastrointestinal Nursing* 10(5): 11–12.

Addendum

Bristol Scoring Chart

Permission granted via Wikipedia site: http://en.wikipedia.org/wiki/Bristol_ Stool_Scale (accessed 3 March 2008).

THE BRISTOL STOOL FORM SCALE

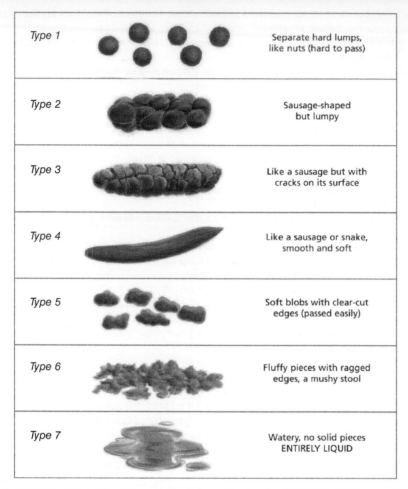

Type 1	Separate hard lumps, like nuts (hard to pass)
Type 2	Sausage-shaped but lumpy
Type 3	Like a sausage but with cracks on its surface
Type 4	Like a sausage or snake, smooth and soft
Type 5	Soft blobs with clear-cut edges (passed easily)
Type 6	Fluffy pieces with ragged edges, a mushy stool
Type 7	Watery, no solid pieces ENTIRELY LIQUID

Figure A10.1 The Bristol Stool Form Scale. Source: Used under CC-BY-SA 3.0 Unported https://creativecommons.org/licenses/by-sa/3.0/deed.en.

Figure A10.1 The Bristol Stool Chart or Scale is an aid for healthcare staff that classifies faeces into seven categories. It was developed by Dr S J Lewis and Dr K W Heaton at the University of Bristol, and was first published in 1997 in the *Scandinavian Journal of Gastroenterology* 32: 920–924.

CHAPTER 11

Urinary catheterisation and catheter care

LEARNING OBJECTIVES

- List the reasons for inserting a urinary catheter
- Discuss common catheters and the equipment associated with catheterisation
- Outline the procedure of urinary catheterisation
- Discuss the importance of catheter care and how to prevent and manage common problems associated with catheterisation

Aim of this chapter

The aim of this chapter is to discuss urinary catheterisation and catheter care in adults and children, and to review potential complications and their prevention or management. This chapter is aimed at supporting local training and supervision and focuses primarily on urinary catheterisation. Intermittent self-catheterisation is also discussed, because the healthcare assistant may need to assist a patient in this process or carry out this procedure.

Urinary catheterisation

A urinary (or urethral) catheter is a hollow tube that is inserted from the urethral orifice into the bladder. NHS Quality Improvement Scotland (NHS QIS 2004) described urinary catheterisation as a procedure to enable emptying of the bladder by insertion of a catheter, and ongoing care and maintenance are considered as catheter care. The Department of Health (DH 2001) stated that the use of indwelling catheters should be considered only after alternative methods have been explored, and these include intermittent catheterisation, use of medications, voiding programmes or incontinence pads with children (NICE 2012).

Mangnall and Watterson (2006) indicated that urinary catheterisation is one of the most common healthcare interventions, with around 25% of patients

Clinical Skills for Healthcare Assistants and Assistant Practitioners, Second Edition.
Angela Whelan and Elaine Hughes.
© 2016 John Wiley & Sons, Ltd. Published 2016 by John Wiley & Sons, Ltd.

in hospital requiring this procedure, so attention to infection control aspects is critical. Currently catheter-associated urinary tract infections (CAUTI) account for approximately 80% of all hospital acquired infections, which has ensured that the Department of Health has made this one of their focal points in their Harm Free Care agenda with the NHS Safety Thermometer by aiming to reduce the rates of infection by 50% (DH 2012; Foxley 2011). Leaver (2007) also noted that nurses insert at least 50% of all catheters and subsequently perform the majority of catheter care, so there is a need to ensure that they are at the forefront of good practice. This is supported by the RCN (2012), NICE (2012) and NHS QIS (2004) who discuss the importance of best practice in catheterisation and infection control.

Relevant anatomy and physiology

Chapter 10 should be referred to for details of the urinary system; however, a review of the relevant parts of the urinary system may be useful.

The bladder is a hollow muscular structure lying in the pelvic cavity; in males directly anterior (in front) of the rectum, whereas in females it is anterior to the vagina and inferior (below) to the uterus (Tortora and Derrickson 2011). The urethra is an opening leading from the bladder to the exterior of the body, made of epithelial cells, which is often described as a tube; in females it is about 4 cm (1.5 inches) long, and in males about 15–20 cm (6–8 inches) long (Tortora and Derrickson 2011) (Figures 11.1 and 11.2). For this reason catheters come in different lengths and are often referred to as male and female lengths.

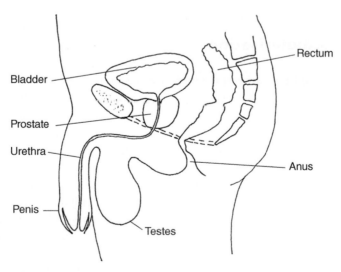

Figure 11.1 Male bladder and urethra.

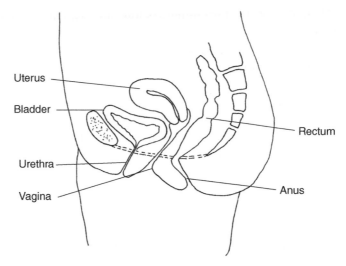

Figure 11.2 Female bladder and urethra.

Elimination of urine is an essential bodily function and, normally, day- and night-time bladder control is developed by age 6 years (Pellatt 2007). Bray and Saunders (2006) suggest that children are usually toilet trained between 2 and 1½ years, and girls generally achieve dryness before boys.

In the adult, the kidneys filter about 150 l/day, and concentrate this into urine producing a minimum of 0.5 ml/kg/hr (Hughes 2004), while in children the output is usually 1 ml/kg body weight per hour (Bray and Saunders 2006).

Reasons for urinary catheterisation and catheter care

Bray and Saunders (2006) suggest that the reasons for inserting a catheter in children are usually:

- Acute retention: with sudden onset often after surgery (after 12 hours), medication related, or after spinal or epidural anaesthesia; it can be an associated secondary complication due to acute constipation, spinal injury or obstruction at the urethral outflow.
- Post-operative urine monitoring: where a child is unwell after emergency surgery, trauma or injury, a catheter would be inserted to monitor fluid balance and measure specific gravity (see Chapter 10).
- Skin and wound integrity: a catheter is inserted after surgery to allow a wound to heal, and a catheter minimises the risk of infection, pain and discomfort for the child.

There are several reasons for catheterisation in adults that have been outlined by Dougherty and Lister (2011), Baillie and Busuttil Leaver (2009) and Foxley (2011), and which are outlined below:

- to empty bladder contents, for example before surgery, childbirth and some investigations;
- to accurately measure urinary output, especially if the patient is acutely ill;
- to determine residual urine;
- to allow bladder irrigation;
- to bypass an obstruction;
- to relieve urinary retention;
- to instil drugs into the bladder, for example cytotoxic drugs for bladder cancer or drugs for hyperactive bladders);
- to allow bladder function tests (e.g. urodynamics);
- to help bladder healing, for example after bladder, pelvic or urethral surgery;
- to maintain skin integrity in intractable incontinence where patients are at high risk;
- to avoid complications from insertion of radiotherapy (e.g. in gynaecological or prostate cancer).

Types of catheterisation

This chapter focuses on indwelling catheterisation, and also discusses intermittent catheterisation by both the healthcare assistant and the patient. The other option for draining urine from the bladder is via a suprapubic catheter, where a catheter is inserted above the pubic bone; as this would be carried out by trained personnel it is not outlined in this book.

Assessment considerations

NHS QIS (2004) suggested that intermittent catheterisation should be considered a first option, rather than inserting an indwelling catheter, and this would be done after a full patient assessment. Initial assessment would be to identify the reason for the bladder-emptying problem, which would include consideration of the holistic effects a catheter may have on the individual, such as impact on the patient's body image or sexuality. NHS QIS (2004) also indicated that catheterisation can be a challenge with children; older, frail, confused patients; or patients with a learning disability, and they will need additional consideration, especially around communication and consent.

The decision as to the type of catheter technique can then be made in consultation with the patient and carers or family if necessary. With older confused people or patients with a learning disability, consideration is also needed about their capacity to consent, briefly discussed in Chapters 1 and 4, as well as later in this chapter.

The materials, gauges, balloon sizes, tip design and lengths of catheters, and drainage systems, will now be discussed to assist in catheter selection.

Length of time the catheter is in place

Dougherty and Lister (2011) suggested the need to consider how long a catheter will be in situ, because this will affect the choice of material (Table 11.1). Therefore, Dougherty and Lister (2011) used the following time frames:

- Short term: 1–7 days.
- Short to medium term: 28 days.
- Medium to long term: 6 weeks–12 weeks.

Gauges (sizes)

Choose the smallest size suitable, because larger sizes can cause pain, discomfort, bypassing (urine leaks past catheter) and lead to abscess and stricture formation (Dougherty and Lister 2011; Bray and Saunders 2006).

Catheters are measured in Charrière (Ch) or French gauge (FG) which refers to the external circumference of the catheter. Each Ch is 0.3 mm and comes in a range of sizes for use with adults and pediatrics in varying lengths (Bailie and Busuttil Leaver 2009) (see Table 11.2 for paediatric sizes).

NHS QIS (2004), Dougherty and Lister (2011) and Nazarko (2010) all suggest that the smallest size catheter possible should be used to prevent trauma and complications. For both males and females a size 12 is usually suitable but the individual and the risk of encrustation leading to a blocked catheter in long-term use also need to be considered. The European Association of Urological Nurses (2012) suggests the following as a guide to catheter sizes in adults:

- size 10: clear urine, no debris, no grit (encrustation);
- size 12–14: clear urine, no debris, no grit, no haematuria;
- size 16: slightly cloudy urine, light haematuria with or without small clots, none or mild grit, none or mild debris;
- size 18: moderate to heavy grit, moderate to heavy debris; haematuria with moderate clots;
- size 20–24: used for heavy haematuria, need for flushing.

Materials

Catheters are manufactured from many different materials and selection of the material is based upon the purpose and length of time the catheter is likely to be in place. It is important to also consider patient comfort when choosing a catheter, the potential for the build up of encrustations in long-term catheterised patients and the potential of allergic reaction to the material (EAUN 2012). An outline of these materials can be found in Table 11.1.

Balloon sizes

Balloons are used to hold the indwelling catheter in place and are inflated once the catheter has been correctly inserted into the bladder (Baillie and Busuttil Leaver 2009). The volume in the balloon varies; in children the balloons are commonly filled with 3–5 ml of sterile water, and 5–10 ml for adults; however, some

Table 11.1 Catheter selection.

Length in situ	Type of material	Discussion
Short term	PVC with or without balloons	Rigid catheter with wide lumen, so allows rapid flow rate, used mainly for intermittent catheter or postoperatively. Due to rigidity it can cause some patients discomfort or pain, or bladder spasm
	Latex	Softest material, but causes surface friction which tends to allow encrustation formation. Also risk of patient allergy with latex, so ensure that this is checked with patient. Avoided where possible
	Teflon (PTFE)	Teflon is applied to latex to prevent the risk of latex allergy and reduce urethral irritation
Short to medium term	Silver alloy coating	Silver alloy coated latex. Evidence suggests that this material reduces bacterial growth in catheters in situ <7 days
Long term	100% silicone	Less likely to cause urethral irritation. Has a large inner lumen with reduced tendency to develop encrustations. Silicone can also allow balloon to deflate (water leaks out) and so catheter can fall out prematurely
	Hydrogel coated latex	These coat the catheter and cause the least irritation and as they become rehydrated they become smoother, and so reduce friction in the urethra. This reduces the risk of becoming contaminated with bacteria or encrusted
		NHS Quality Improvement Scotland (2004) note this type of material is unsuitable for patients with a latex allergy
	Hydrogel-coated silicone	Suitable for patients with latex allergy, however are rigid so can be uncomfortable for some patients
	Silicone elastomer coating	Latex catheters coated with silicone inside and out. Acts in a similar way to pure silicone with less incidence of encrustations
	Nitrofurazone coating	Bactericidal coating which reduces the frequency of asymptomatic bacteria in the urine within a week. Not for routine use

PVC, polyvinylchloride.
Adapted from Dougherty and Lister (2011) and NHS QIS (2004), and EAUN (2012)

Table 11.2 Paediatric catheter sizes.

Age (years)	Charrière (Ch) size
0–2	6
2–5	6–8
5–10	8–10
10–16	10–12

Reproduced from Bray and Saunders (2006) with permission.

balloons inflate to 30 ml, but these are used mainly after urological procedures. Dougherty and Lister (2011) noted that as the balloon sits at the base of the bladder neck in a sensitive area called the trigone this can cause irritation to the bladder wall, often causing bypassing and bladder spasms, while an over-filled balloon can cause damage to the neck of the bladder and too little fluid can also cause irritation. It is important that balloons are not repeatedly inflated and deflated as this can create asymmetry of the balloon causing the tip of the catheter to irritate the trigone. If a Foley-type catheter (catheter with a balloon) is inserted, always make sure that it is draining before inflating the balloon with sterile water as per manufacturer's guidelines. Water is used in case the balloon leaks, and therefore prevents irritation of the bladder (NHS QIS 2004).

Design of catheter tip
Dougherty and Lister (2011) describe tip designs; these can affect drainage:
- the Tiemann-tip is curved with one to three drainage eyes;
- the Whistle-tip has a lateral eye in the tip and eyes above the balloon to provide a large drainage area; helpful in drainage of debris or blood clots;
- the Roberts tip has an eye above and below the catheter to help drain residual urine.

Length of catheter
Authors note a variance, but all agree on three lengths (Dougherty and Lister 2011; NHS QIS 2004; Baillie and Busuttil Leaver 2009; Bray and Saunders 2006):
1 Paediatric: 30–31 cm
2 Female: 20–40 cm
3 Male or standard: 40–45 cm.

However, Baillie and Busuttil Leaver (2009) suggested that standard length is often used for women, particularly if the patient is obese or chair bound, because it allows easier access to the connector end and the drainage bag (NHS QIS 2004). The use of standard length catheters in females is now much more common since their withdrawal from some areas following a patient safety issue where female catheters had been incorrectly used for male catheterisation. Where female catheters are available these must be clearly labelled to ensure patient safety (NPSA 2009).

> **THINK ABOUT IT**
>
> Why are there different lengths of catheters (male and female)?

Drainage systems

A drainage bag allows periodic emptying, and so eliminates the need to discon-nect it from the catheter, reducing the risk of catheter associated urinary tract infections (CAUTIs) (Baillie and Busuttil Leaver 2009). Dougherty and Lister (2011) noted that the highest risk of infection is when emptying or changing the bag, hence NHS QIS (2004) suggested changing bags every 5–7 days.

Most drainage bags attach either to a stand on the floor or bed side, or to a patient's leg, and depend on the patient's condition and mobility and also their preference. Bags also vary in capacity and length of inlet tube and type of outlet tap, and this will also influence choice. Baillie and Busuttil Leaver (2009) suggest that outlet taps are usually of a lever type or push-across design; therefore, when assessing the patient for the right product for them the cognitive and physical capability of patients or carers should be considered. Bags can vary from 180 ml capacity in leg bags to 2 litres for overnight bags, while for some people the choice of a valve rather than a bag provides greater freedom (Baillie and Busuttil Leaver 2009; Gibney 2010; EAUN 2012). See Figure 11.3 for bag and outlet tap.

> **THINK ABOUT IT**
>
> When choosing a drainage bag, what could be some factors that you should consider?

When considering the use of catheter valves as an alternative to a closed drainage system, EAUN (2012) suggests that this is a good alternative for patients who have good manual dexterity and no cognitive impairment. However it should be contraindicated in those who have physiological problems, such as urinary tract infections, overactive bladder syndrome or renal impairment. Gibney (2010) provides a good algorithm to determine the suitability of patients for valve use. Bray and Saunders (2006) calculated the bladder volume in children using the formula: 30 × child's age + 30, so, for example, a 6 year old would have a calculated bladder volume of 210 ml. This formula is applicable until a child reaches age 12 years, and then one would expect the bladder volume to be that of an adult, which ranges from 300 ml to 500 ml (Bray and Saunders 2006). Therefore, for some patients a valve may offer more privacy and fewer restrictions to their mobility and lifestyle. Dougherty and Lister (2011) and Gibney (2010) also add that the use of a valve largely eliminates the need for bags and can be cost effective in long-term indwelling catheters, as the valve can be in place for 5–7 days.

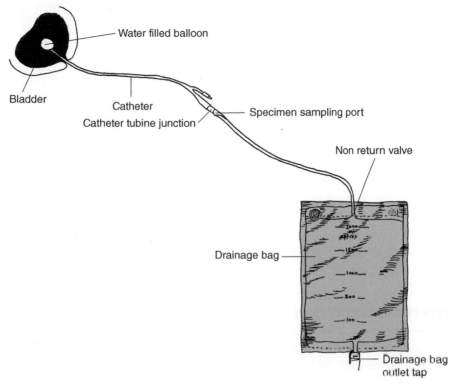

Figure 11.3 Catheter bag and outlet valve.

The use of closed drainage systems are commonplace, but to prevent CAUTI it is essential that effective aseptic non-touch techniques occur on insertion, emptying or removal, so care must be exercised at all times.

It is important that there is no tension on the catheter, so ensure that the bag, if attached to a stand, is in a good position, below the level of the waist and not caught in clothing or bedclothes. The same applies to a leg bag; here the use of adjustable straps or a 'sleeve or holster' is essential to secure the bag in a suitable position, remembering patient comfort, drainage and privacy (Baillie and Busuttil Leaver 2009; EAUN 2012; Fisher 2010).

Patient preparation for catheterisation

Dougherty and Lister (2011) discuss the importance of explaining the procedure to the patient and gaining their consent. It is essential that the patient is educated regarding their catheter and how to care for it before the procedure with regards to cleansing around the catheter and fluid consumption to reduce the risk of infection.

If possible, patients should be advised to wash their genital area first with unperfumed soap and water, and then men need to retract the foreskin (where present) and clean the area thoroughly and then replace the foreskin, whereas women need to wash from front to back to prevent contamination from the rectal area.

Lubricating gel should be used in both male and female catheterisation (Dougherty and Lister 2011; NICE 2012). Workplace policy should be followed with regards to the type of lubricant used, that is anaesthetic or aqueous, as there is debate over which is the best to use (Patel 2008); EAUN (2012) suggest that anesthetic gel should be used. However, it is important to note that when using anaesthetic gel the manufacturer's instructions should be adhered to with regards to the amount of time to wait before the gel takes full effect. Bray and Saunders (2006) suggested that local anaesthetic gel (e.g. 2% lidocaine) should be used with children because this also acts as a lubricant and ideally is applied 3–5 min before catheterisation. This may not, however, be achievable with younger children due to their anxiety.

Insertion technique

The catheterisation equipment required is: a sterile catheter pack preferably or sterile dressing pack with gallipot; two pairs of sterile gloves; catheter (recommend one of assessed size and one spare plus a smaller size); sterile sodium chloride or antiseptic solution as per local policy; sterile water and syringe as per age and balloon size; sterile single patient anaesthetic gel or lubricating gel; holder or leg straps; drainage bag (as appropriate); sterile receiver and waterproof protective sheet/pad (if not in catheter pack); sterile specimen container (often a sterile sample is sent to laboratory, depends on the reason for catheter insertion); apron; screens; and good lighting (may require portable or angled light).

The whole procedure must follow an aspetic non-touch technique, equipment used must be sterile and single use (Figures 11.4 and 11.5), and all packaging should be checked and verified intact and in date.

Table 11.3 describes the procedure for male or female catheterisation; however, in some clinical areas healthcare assistants may require additional training for male catheterisation because of technical aspects and the use of anaesthetic gel and, as this is an administration of a medicine, some clinical areas may not cover this role for healthcare assistants; as usual, *please check your local policy*. (See Figures 11.1 and 11.2 re male and female anatomy for catheterisation.)

Men, particularly the older age population, may suffer from an enlarged prostate gland. Tortora and Derrickson (2011) describe this as a single doughnut-shaped gland, which surrounds the urethra, so if it enlarges this can affect the flow of urine and also the ease with which the catheter is inserted. If a male patient reports pain or discomfort during the procedure, stop and always seek advice.

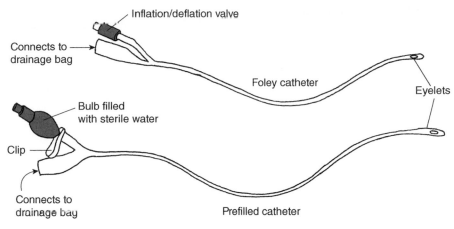

Figure 11.4 Catheter.

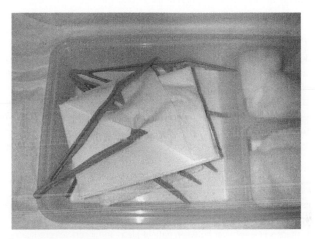

Figure 11.5 Sterile pack. Source: Photograph by I Lavery.

Bray and Saunders (2006) note that in children's insertion the usual aspects should be documented as for point 24 in Table 11.3, plus the catheter batch number, the inserter's name, the type of analgesia used, if any, and consent.

Intermittent catheterisation

Intermittent catheterisation can be undertaken by the patient, carer or healthcare professional, and the bladder must have sufficient capacity to store urine between catheterisations (NHS QIS 2004). Dougherty and Lister (2011) describe the procedure as the periodic removal of urine and, after the procedure, the catheter is removed, leaving the patient catheter free. The procedure is carried out (see Table 11.4 for the procedure) as often as the patient requires, usually four to five times a day.

When patients, commonly at home, carry out this procedure it is a clean procedure, whereas any healthcare assistant would carry it out as an aseptic

Table 11.3 Catheterisation procedure.

Step	Procedure
1	Approach the patient, explain procedure, and gain consent and cooperation
2	Help patient into a safe position, preferably flat on back, covered and screened for privacy
3	Wash hands, put on plastic apron, assemble equipment on clean trolley, take to the screened bedside/area
4	Place waterproof sheet under patient's buttocks – to protect the bed
5	Open catheter pack taking care not to touch inside – to protect sterile field
6	Open the catheter but leave in internal packing and drop onto sterile field
7	Draw up the required amount of sterile water with a sterile syringe
8	Pour sterile sodium chloride into sterile gallipot in pack, and open single use gel (lubricating or anaesthetic), set up drainage bag (on stand if being used)
9	The assistant now uncovers the patient and supports the legs, and knees bent up and apart
10	Open sterile gloves and wash hands or use alcohol rub to cleanse hands
11	Sterile gloves on, place sterile towels over patient's thighs and under buttocks
12	Males: wrap a sterile towel around the penis, and retract the foreskin to clean round the top of urethra with the sodium chloride or antiseptic solution as per workplace policy Females: cleanse the perineal area with sodium chloride, then, using non-dominant hand, separate the inner labia (lips) and cleanse the meatus (opening). Change sterile gloves ready for the clean part of the procedure
13	Males: insert the nozzle of the anaesthetic gel into the urethra, and squeeze the gel in, remove the nozzle and discard the tube, massage the gel along the urethra (penis) and wait 5 min Females: carefully locate the urethra and insert either lubricant or anaesthetic gel and wait 5 min
14	Males: grasp the penis behind the glans (acorn-shaped rim) and raise penis until extended and maintain this grasp till procedure finished – see below Females: expose the tip of the catheter by pulling off serrated end of internal wrapper (also for male catheterisation)
15	Males: place sterile receiver between patient's legs and insert selected catheter for 15–25 cm (6–9 inches) until urine flows, pulling back internal wrapper and ensuring that catheter end is in receiver Females: place sterile receiver between patient's legs and insert selected catheter for 5–7 cm (2–3 inches) until urine flows, pulling back internal wrapper and ensuring that catheter end is in receiver
16	Males: if resistance is felt, increase the traction on the penis slightly and ask the patient to strain gently as though passing urine and apply steady gentle pressure on the catheter; this may help insertion past bladder sphincter; if not, stop and seek advice Females: Bray and Saunders (2006) noted that occasionally a catheter may enter the vagina and so no urine drains. If this happens, leave this catheter in place as a marker, and recommence with new catheter, then remove the first one once the second catheter is correctly in situ
17	Males: advance catheter forward to ensure safely within the bladder to bifurcation (Y section) (Figure 11.4) Females: advance the catheter a further 5 cm; never force the catheter. If resistance is met stop and seek medical advice
18	Inflate balloon with sterile water as per manufacturer's instructions, and ensure that urine is still draining
19	Withdraw catheter slightly – balloon will hold in place
20	Attach free end to drainage system and ensure secured and no drag on catheter

Table 11.3 (*continued*)

Step	Procedure
21	Males: ensure that penis is clean and foreskin is retracted Females: ensure that genital area is clean
22	Dispose of equipment, per local policy
23	Check that patient is comfortable and has understood catheter education
24	Document procedure, noting catheter type, size and balloon volume inserted, along with date, time and drainage, and if any specimen sent or tested

Adapted from Dougherty and Lister (2011), Baillie and Busuttil Leaver (2009) and EAUN (2012).

Table 11.4 Intermittent self-catheterisation procedure.

Step	Procedure in males	Procedure in females
1	Wash hands using bactericidal soap and water, or bactericidal alcohol hand rub and dry thoroughly	Take up a comfortable position, dependent on mobility, e.g. sitting on toilet or standing with one foot up on toilet rim (see Step 10)
2	Stand in front of toilet, or low bench with a container if easier (see Step 10)	Spread the labia (lips) and wash the genitalia from front to back with soap and water, then dry
3	Clean the glans of the penis (head) with plain water, retract foreskin, if applicable, during the procedure	
4	Hold penis with left hand (if right handed) three fingers underneath and thumb on top, holding the penis straight out. Coat the end of the catheter with the lubricating gel	Insert the catheter, use lubricant gel if wish for comfort, and a mirror to help see genitalia
5	Pass the catheter gently with the right hand (or left if left handed); it can be felt as it passes the fingers holding the penis. There will be a change in feeling as catheter passes through the prostate gland into the bladder. It may be a little painful on the first few occasions only; if any resistance is felt, stop and seek medical advice immediately	Urine will drain as soon as the catheter reaches the bladder, so have the end positioned over the toilet or the container
6	Urine will drain as soon as the catheter enters the bladder, so have end positioned over toilet or container	
7	Withdraw the catheter slowly so that all the urine is drained and it should slide out easily	Remove the catheter slowly when urine has stopped draining; it should slide out easily
8	Wash catheter through if reusable and store in dry, clean container	
9	Wash hands again as Step 1	
10	If patient has a large abdomen, a mirror standing in front can assist observation and insertion	

Source: Adapted from Dougherty (2011). Reproduced with permission of Wiley Blackwell.

procedure. At certain times, such as during acute illness, the patient may not have the usual physical and manual dexterity to carry out the procedure themselves. Therefore the healthcare assistant may carry out the procedure for the patient, or may even teach a carer to undertake this for the patient if they prefer it (NHS QIS 2004).

Dougherty and Lister (2011) suggest patients who are suitable for intermittent self-catheterisation as the following:

- Those who can comprehend (understand) the technique.
- Those with a reasonable degree of manual dexterity (able to use hands).
- Those who are highly motivated.
- Those who have a willing partner (if suitable for both to participate).
- Those who can position themselves to attain reasonable access to the urethra, especially in females.

The benefits of intermittent catheterisation can include an improved quality of life, greater patient satisfaction, greater freedom to express sexuality and minimisation of urinary complications (Dougherty and Lister 2011).

There are two types of catheters used for intermittent self-catheterisation. One is a single use pre-lubricated catheter where the lubrication is activated in water; the other type is PVC and requires lubrication. This latter catheter can be used for up to 1 week before being discarded. NHS Quality Improvement Scotland (NHS QIS 2004) suggest intermittent catheter cleaning (PVC reusable catheters) should involve washing in warm soapy water, rinsing thoroughly and then leaving in a clean dry area to air dry, before storing in a clean dry container.

Catheter care

NHS QIS (2004) outlined the following aspects:

- Maintain a closed system, as much as possible.
- Empty drainage bags regularly (when bag two-thirds full); always ensure they are positioned below level of bladder (exception: a 'belly bag', see Figure 11.6) and change every 5–7 days.
- Body-worn bags, for example a 'belly bag' (Figure 11.6): change weekly (a 'belly bag' is worn round the waist and has 1000 cm^3 capacity and can be used with Foley-type catheters).
- Bedside-type drainage bags must be supported off the floor to reduce the risk of infection.
- A separate clean container is used for each individual when emptying the catheter; avoid contact with the drainage tap and container.
- Wear gloves to empty drainage bags and ensure new gloves and hands washed between patients – strict aseptic technique.
- Leg bags can be emptied directly into toilets.
- When overnight bag is required, a new single-use 2-litre bedside bag is used and emptied and discarded in the morning.

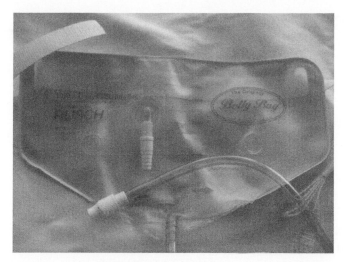

Figure 11.6 Belly bag. Source: Photograph by I Lavery.

- Encourage the patient to have a daily bath or shower and wash around the catheter with warm soapy water.
- Frequent vigorous meatal (genital area) cleansing with antiseptic solutions is not needed, and may even increase the risk of infection.
- Clean the outlet valve with a 70% isopropyl alcohol-impregnated swab and allow to dry thoroughly.
- Once urine is drained, re-clean as above.
- Record volume and document if necessary.
   (Adapted from Dougherty and Lister 2011; NHS QIS 2004; EAUN 2012)

Sampling

Breaking the closed system to obtain a sample increases the risk of catheter-related infection, so use of a drainage bag with a sample port (Figure 11.7) incorporated removes the need to break the closed system (NHS QIS 2004).

   Dougherty and Lister (2011) and NHS QIS (2004) described the steps in sampling as follows:
- Only take a sample for a valid reason, such as a suspected urinary infection.
- Wash hands, put on gloves and apron.
- Cleanse port with a 70% isopropyl alcohol-impregnated swab and allow to dry thoroughly.
- Take the sample from the bag sample port.
- Using a sterile syringe (and needle if necessary), aspirate the required amount of urine taking care not to touch the far side of the catheter tube to prevent contamination of the sample. Dougherty and Lister (2011) noted that, if there

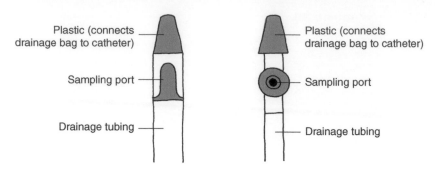

Figure 11.7 Sampling ports.

is no urine in tubing, it is possible to clamp the tubing below the sample port/cuff only until sufficient volume collects.

- Re-clean sample port with a 70% isopropyl alcohol-impregnated swab and allow to dry thoroughly.
- Place specimen into sterile container and label correctly.
- Dispose of needle and syringe.
- Wash hands again with bactericidal soap and water, and dry thoroughly.
- Unclamp tubing, if necessary.
- Consider recording volume, where applicable, for example if the patient is on a fluid balance chart.
- Send specimen and form promptly to laboratory, as per local policy.

Trigg and Mohammed (2010) suggest that the same procedure should be used for catheterised children. Tables 11.6–11.9 are competency frameworks for catheterisation procedures and sampling.

Removal of catheter

NHS QIS (2004) indicate removal of the catheter as soon as possible to reduce the risk of infection, depending on the patient's condition and the judgement of healthcare staff. Assessment of patients should consider whether they are physically and mentally able to cope with normal micturition (passing urine).

Kelleher (2002) suggested removal at 12 midnight, increasing the time before the patient would pass urine, leading to a greater initial volume and faster return to normal voiding (passing) of urine, which can decrease levels of anxiety. A Best Practice Statement from the Joanna Briggs Institute (JBI 2006) discussed the time of removal and noted that this is a balance between avoiding infection (early removal) and voiding (passing urine) problems (by later removal), and midnight removal may lead to shorter hospital stays.

The urine output must be monitored after removal, to ensure that the patient is passing urine and in adequate volumes (Baillie and Busuttil Leaver 2009).

Table 11.5 Problem solving.

Catheter problem	Possible reason	Possible solution
Urine not draining/blockage	Catheter in wrong position – not in bladder, maybe in vagina	Deflate balloon and gently reposition catheter forward
	Drainage bag in wrong position – above the level of the bladder	Check bag position – move to below bladder level
	Drainage tubing may be kinked	Check tubing and unkink
	Catheter blocked by debris	Prescribed flush, gently with saline preferably or sterile water
	Bladder spasm	Consider use of medication
Haematuria (presence of blood in urine)	Trauma post-catheterisation	Observe output and document severity of haematuria, report to nurse in charge and/or doctor
	Infection	
	Calculi (stones)	
	Cancer	Observe and report as above
	Prostatic enlargement	Encourage fluid intake and observe and report as above
Bypassing of urine around catheter	May indicate infection	Send sterile urine specimen if indicated.
	Bladder spasm/instability	Consider use of medication
	Constipation	Increase fluid and dietary fibre intake: 2–3 l in adults, 1500 ml for children over 5 years and 2000 ml for teenagers where clinically indicated
	Incorrect positioning of drainage system	Check drainage bag position
	Balloon volume incorrect	Check volume in balloon, remove if overinflated or add if less than specified volume
	Drainage bag more than two-thirds full	Regular emptying
Pain or discomfort	The eyes of the catheter may be blocked	Raise the drainage bag above the level of the bladder for 10–15 s only
	Maybe a sign of infection	Obtain sterile specimen of urine
	On removal, may indicate crusting	Ensure correct catheter size inserted in first place and the patient maintains daily cleaning of genital area and catheter
Catheter retaining balloon will not deflate	Valve port and balloon inflation channel may be compressed	Check no compression on tubing
	Faulty valve mechanism.	Aspirate balloon port slowly; if too fast can cause valve mechanism to collapse
		Can inject a small additional amount of sterile water in and then slowly aspirate again
		Do NOT cut catheter, if all fails, seek medical advice

Adapted from NHS Quality Improvement Scotland (QIS 2004), EAUN (2012) and Bray and Saunders (2006).

Table 11.6 Competency framework: indwelling catheterisation.

Steps	First assessment/reassessment					Date/competent signature
	Demonstration/supervised practice					
	Date/sign 1	Date/sign 2	Date/sign 3	Date/sign 4	Date/sign 5	
Indwelling catheterisation						
Procedure stages: male and female						
1 Patient approached, procedure explained, consent/cooperation gained						
2 Helped patient into safe position, covered and screened						
3 Washed hands, equipment assembled on clean trolley						
4 Placed waterproof sheet/pad under patient's buttocks						
5 Catheter pack opened protecting sterile field						
6 Catheter opened onto sterile field						
7 Appropriate volume of sterile water drawn up with sterile syringe						
8 Sterile sodium chloride prepared and single use gel opened						
9 Patient uncovered and legs supported in appropriate position						
10 Sterile gloves opened and hands washed as per policy						
11 Sterile gloves on, sterile towels placed over patient's thighs and under buttocks						

Male-specific aspects

	Date/sign 1	Date/sign 2	Date/sign 3	Date/sign 4	Date/sign 5
12 Sterile towel wrapped around penis, foreskin retracted, and top of urethra cleaned with sodium chloride or antiseptic solution, wash hands and change gloves					
13 Anaesthetic gel nozzle inserted into urethra, gel squeezed in, nozzle removed, discarded, massaged gel along penis, waited 5 min					
14 Penis grasped safely and raised until fully extended, for all procedure					
15 Sterile receiver placed between patient's legs, catheter tip exposed, then inserted smoothly and gently for 15–25 cm until urine flows					
16 Catheter advanced forward so safely within bladder, and urine is draining into receiver					
17 Balloon inflated with sterile water and ensured urine still draining					
18 Catheter withdrawn slightly to ensure secure in bladder					
19 Free end attached correctly and securely to selected drainage system					
20 Ensured penis clean and foreskin retracted at finish					

Indwelling catheterisation: female-specific aspects

	Date/sign 1	Date/sign 2	Date/sign 3	Date/sign 4	Date/sign 5
12 Perineal area cleansed with sodium chloride, inner labia separated and meatus cleansed too. Wash hands and change gloves					
13 Urethra located, lubricant or anaesthetic gel inserted, waited 5 min					

(continued overleaf)

Table 11.6 (*continued*)

Indwelling catheterisation: female-specific aspects	First assessment/reassessment				
	Date/sign 1	Date/sign 2	Date/sign 3	Date/sign 4	Date/sign 5
14 Tip of catheter exposed by pulling off serrated end of internal wrapper					
15 Sterile receiver placed between patient's legs, catheter inserted smoothly and gently for 5–7 cm until urine flows					
16 If no urine drained, checked if catheter in vagina, so left in place, recommenced with new catheter, then removed first once second is correctly in situ					
17 Advanced catheter a further 5 cm to ensure safely within the bladder and urine still draining into receiver					
18 Balloon inflated with sterile water and ensured urine still draining					
19 Catheter withdrawn slightly – to test secured in bladder					
20 Free end attached correctly and securely to drainage system and genital area is clean					

Male and female aspects	Date/sign 1	Date/sign 2	Date/sign 3	Date/sign 4	Date/sign 5
21 Disposed of equipment, per local policy, gloves removed and hands washed					
22 Checked patient is comfortable, has understood catheter education, allowed questions					
23 Procedure documented, noting catheter type, size and balloon volume inserted, along with date, time and drainage, and if any specimen sent or tested					

Supervisors/Assessor(s):

Table 11.7 Competency framework: intermittent catheterisation competency – patient/carer.

Steps	First assessment/reassessment					Date/competent signature
	Demonstration/supervised practice					
Supervised aspects for _learner_ patient/carer self-catheterisation	Date/sign 1	Date/sign 2	Date/sign 3	Date/sign 4	Date/sign 5	
1 Patient/carer washed hands using bactericidal soap and water, or bactericidal alcohol hand rub and dried thoroughly						
2 Took up a comfortable position, e.g. sat on toilet or stood with one foot up on toilet rim (female); or stood at toilet or low bench with a container (male)						
3 Genital area cleaned correctly: **Female:** spread labia and washed from front to back with soap and water, then dried **Male:** cleaned the head of penis with water, foreskin retracted during procedure						
4 **Male:** held penis with three fingers underneath and thumb on top, straight out, coated the end of the catheter with the lubricating/anaesthetic gel **Female:** inserted catheter, used lubricant or anaesthetic gel if wished, and a mirror to help see genitalia						
5 Passed catheter gently with one hand; in males it can be felt as it passes the fingers holding the penis. Urine drained and catheter end positioned over toilet or container						
6 Withdrawn catheter slowly once all the urine is drained						
7 If container, urine disposed in toilet and container cleaned/disposed						
8 Catheter washed correctly if re-usable and stored in clean container						
9 Hands washed again post procedure						

Supervisors/Assessor(s)

Table 11.8 Competency framework: intermittent catheterisation by healthcare assistant.

Steps	First assessment/reassessment					Date/competent signature
	Demonstration/supervised practice					
Intermittent catheterisation by healthcare assistant	Date/sign 1	Date/sign 2	Date/sign 3	Date/sign 4	Date/sign 5	
1 Hands washed using bactericidal soap and water, or bactericidal alcohol hand rub and dried thoroughly						
2 Patient assisted into a comfortable position						
3 **Females:** perineal area cleansed with sodium chloride then inner labia separated and meatus cleansed too						
Males: sterile towel wrapped around penis, foreskin retracted and top of urethra cleaned with sodium chloride or antiseptic solution						
4 Urethra located, lubricant or anaesthetic gel inserted, waited 5 min						
5 Sterile receiver placed between patient's legs, catheter inserted smoothly and gently for required distance; Males 15–25 cm and females 5–7 cm, until urine flows						
6 Catheter withdrawn slowly once all the urine is drained						
7 Catheter washed correctly if reusable and stored in dry clean container or if single use disposed of correctly as per local policy						
8 Procedure documented and volume recorded						
9 Patient left clean and comfortable						

Supervisors/Assessor(s):

Table 11.9 Competency framework: sampling competency.

Steps	First assessment/reassessment					Date/competent signature
	Demonstration/supervised practice					
Sampling competency	Date/sign 1	Date/sign 2	Date/sign 3	Date/sign 4	Date/sign 5	
1 Checked reason for sampling valid, e.g. suspected urinary infection						
2 Washed hands, put on gloves and apron						
3 Cleansed port with isopropyl alcohol 70% swab and allowed to dry thoroughly						
4 Used sterile syringe (and needle if necessary) aspirated the required amount of urine						
5 If no urine in tubing, clamped the tubing below the sample port/cuff until sufficient volume collected						
6 Re-cleaned sample port with isopropyl alcohol 70% impregnated swab and allowed to dry thoroughly						
7 Placed specimen into sterile container and labelled correctly						
8 Washed hands again with bactericidal soap and water and dried thoroughly						
9 Unclamped tubing, if necessary						
10 Recorded volume, if patient is on fluid balance chart						
11 Sent specimen and form promptly to laboratory, per local policy						

Supervisors/Assessor(s):

It may be recommended that a portable bladder scan be used to measure residual volumes in the first few days, because retention can often be a problem after a catheter is removed in patients who have had their catheter for some time (NHS QIS 2004). Bray and Saunders (2006) and EAUN (2012) noted that careful gentle removal must be ensured in case a catheter has become encrusted (possible in medium- to long-term catheters), while EAUN (2012) suggest that letting the balloon deflate naturally and not applying suction to it can reduce the ridge that can be left around the balloon and therefore decrease discomfort on removal.

Dougherty and Lister (2011), EAUN (2012) and Baillie and Busuttil Leaver (2009) outlined the procedure as follows:

- Explain the procedure to the patient and any possible after effects, for example urgency or discomfort as well as the need for a good fluid intake of around 2–3 litres a day where physically allowed.
- Wash hands and, wearing gloves, clean the meatal/urethral area with sodium chloride, females from front to back, males around urethral opening.
- Clean/change gloves, having previously checked volume of water in the balloon, use a syringe to withdraw the water and deflate the balloon.
- Ask the patient to breathe in and out and, on an exhalation, gently but quickly remove the catheter. Advise males that they may note some discomfort as the deflated balloon passes the prostate gland.
- Cleanse area; dry, remove and dispose of equipment as per local policy. If urine is present in drainage bag, empty before disposal in clinical waste and wash and dry hands.
- Document removal, volume in bag, and date and time; also whether any problems reported, for example patient discomfort.

Related aspects and terminology

Communication, consent and clinical holding

In adults this includes consideration of communication, consent and education and in children one may also need to consider the issue of holding (see Chapters 3 and 4 for more information on consent).

NHS QIS (2004) discussed patient consent and gender issues, and indicated key aspects in relation to catheterisation:

- Informed consent must be obtained first and is ongoing, so the patient may/can withdraw consent at any time.
- Patient's capacity is crucial (e.g. in Scotland, the Adults with Incapacity Act 2000 protects the interests of adults who are not capable of making a decision, e.g. learning difficulty or mental health problem).
- Ensure accurate documentation, which includes the process for consent, and indicates that the patient has understood and verbally consented to the procedure.

- Patients are entitled to request the procedure be carried out by a specific gender of healthcare worker, for example a male patient may wish a male nurse, to fit with their cultural/personal preferences.

Dingwall and McLafferty (2006) also considered patient preferences in relation to catheterisation because the patient may be embarrassed; in addition they considered the effect that a catheter may have on body image and sexuality, and found that this was noted more in males. However, as Rees and Mawson (2007) indicated, if the reason for an indwelling catheter is because of incontinence, this in itself can cause social embarrassment and isolation and so affect their quality of life. Thus, the option of a catheter may be seen here as advantageous. Incontinence affects 6 million people worldwide and in the UK 40 in 1000 people are affected (Rees and Mawson 2007).

Bray and Saunders (2006) stated that catheterisation in children is a sensitive issue that requires effective communication, sensitivity and diplomatic skills. They further noted that a child's rights can be ambiguous where procedures such as catheterisation are to be carried out, as a parent or healthcare professional can override a child's wishes. Bray and Saunders (2006) therefore discussed the need for healthcare workers to understand the child's level of understanding and, as catheterisation is an unpleasant procedure, ensure that the child is involved, so that they feel they have some control over the situation.

Parents should be encouraged to be present, because they can act as chaperones and relieve their child's anxiety by being there (Bray and Saunders 2006). If the child is strongly opposed, Bray and Saunders (2006) stated that this must be fully explored with the child before the procedure is undertaken. Therefore discussions must take place with the child and their parent(s) or carer(s), including the reason for catheterisation versus other options, such as a voiding programme or incontinence pad.

Education would include the reason for the initial catheterisation, how long the catheter might remain in place and how it will be secured and emptied, and patients can be encouraged to self-cleanse the genital area and catheter: a daily bath or shower with soap and water is adequate (NHS QIS 2004; Baillie and Busuttil Leaver 2009). Further education would include asking the patient to drink adequate fluids; this is good practice (maintaining healthy fluid levels), and would ensure good urine drainage and output and reduce the risk of urinary infections. Other aspects: advise the patient to ensure that the drainage bag (if used) is always kept below bladder level to achieve drainage and to observe that urine is draining (Baillie and Busuttil Leaver 2009), the exception to this would be if a patient was to use a belly bag which allows for discrete draining of urine.

Bray and Saunders (2006) talked about clinical holding – positioning a child for a medical procedure, so that it can be carried out in a safe and controlled manner and, where possible, with the consent of the child and the parent/carer. Holding must be seen as a last resort, so other options that should be considered first are use of a play specialist to help distract or guided imagery. Preparation can include acting out the procedure with a doll and playing with products that may be used (Bray and Saunders 2006). Finally, Bray and Saunders (2006) noted the use of pharmacological interventions (drugs) that may aid with relaxation and minimise discomfort, for example Entonox (this gas would be administered only under prescription by a registered children's nurse and/or doctor).

Terminology

- *Intermittent catheterisation*: catheter inserted routinely and not left in place.
- *Suprapubic*: above the pubic bone.
- *Acute retention*: sudden inability to pass urine (micturate).
- *Epidural anaesthesia*: anaesthetic drug is injected into spine to 'numb' lower body, often used in childbirth and if a patient is unable to tolerate a general anaesthetic, for example a patient with chronic bronchitis.
- *Residual urine*: volume left in bladder after voiding (passing urine).
- *Cytotoxic*: medicine therapy to destroy 'cancer' cells.
- *Bladder irrigation or instillation*: drug therapy inserted directly into the bladder.

Common problems

The most common problem is urinary infection, hence thorough asepsis at all times is necessary (Bray and Saunders 2006). EAUN (2012) suggest that for each day a catheter is in place then the risk of CAUTI is increased by 3–10%.

Another patient problem associated with catheterisation is bladder spasms, which often cause the urine to flow around the catheter. In instances such as this medication may be prescribed, and can include anticholinergic drugs (NHS QIS 2004). However Bray and Saunders (2006) noted that, in children, the use of oxybutynin or tolterodine has been found to be successful, but care is needed because these can cause side-effects and some may not be licensed for certain ages. *The administration of these to children would not necessarily be part of a healthcare assistant's role; please check your local policy.*

However, NHS QIS (2004), EAUN (2012) and Bray and Saunders (2006) identified other problems and these are shown in Table 11.5.

Summary

This chapter has outlined the skills necessary for inserting and removing urinary catheters, discussed intermittent catheterization and sampling, as well as ongoing catheter care. All require strict aseptic technique and competent practice. Also required are effective communication and documentation.

CASE STUDY 11.1

Mrs Fiona Wilson is 82 years old and lives in a nursing home; she was diagnosed with terminal cancer two years ago and her condition has steadily deteriorated and she now requires full assistance with her activities of daily living and spends most of her time sleeping in bed. She is now incontinent of urine and her skin is becoming excoriated.

What actions would you recommend and why?

CASE STUDY 11.2

Brian Fredericks, aged 32 years and wheelchair bound after a road traffic accident, is being discharged home in a few days. You are part of a team caring from him and he is being considered for intermittent self-catheterisation.

What might be the benefits for this young male?

How would you explain the technique?

Below there is a self-assessment checklist; however, you may also wish to review Skills for Health (2010) guidelines regarding the insertion of urethral catheters.

Self-assessment		
Assessment	**Aspects**	**Achieved ✓**
Indwelling catheterisation	*Have you considered all aspects of this section?*	
	Reasons for insertion or other options explored	
	Catheter material, gauge and length considered	
	Patient assessment carried out	
	Consent, communication and patient education	
	Procedure and infection control aspects	
	Recording the procedure	
	Reporting concerns or outcome	
	Problem solving	
	Disposal of equipment	
Sampling	*Have you considered all aspects of this section?*	**Achieved ✓**
	Procedure and infection control aspects	
	Process for dealing with sample	

(continued overleaf)

Assessment	Aspects	Achieved ✓
	If for testing refer to Chapter 10 If for laboratory purposes, is aware of local process for sending sample Recording the results Reporting concerns or results Problem solving Disposal of equipment	
Catheter care	*Have you considered all aspects of this section?* Procedure and infection control Reporting concerns or results Problem solving Disposal of equipment	**Achieved ✓**
Removal	*Have you considered all aspects of this section?* Procedure and infection control Reporting concerns or results Problem solving Disposal of equipment	**Achieved ✓**
Intermittent catheterisation	*Have you considered all aspects of this section?* Assessment – nurse or patient procedure? Procedure and infection control Self-catheterisation: patient education and clean technique and storage and cleaning of catheter Reporting concerns or results Problem solving Disposal of equipment Ordering of equipment	**Achieved ✓**

References

Baillie L and Busuttil Leaver R (2009) Meeting elimination needs. In: Baillie L (ed.) *Developing Practical Nursing Skills*, 3rd edn. London: Hodder Education, pp. 321–393.

Bray L and Saunders C (2006) Nursing management of paediatric urethral catheterisation. *Nursing Standard* 20(24): 51–60.

Department of Health (DH) (2001) Guidelines for preventing infections associated with the insertion and maintenance of short-term indwelling urethral catheters in acute care. *Journal of Hospital Infection* 47(suppl): S39–46.

Department of Health (DH) (2012) *The NHS Safety Thermometer Equality Analysis*. London: DH.

Dingwall L and McLafferty E (2006) Nurses' perceptions of indwelling urinary catheters in older people. *Nursing Standard* 21(14–16): 35–42.

Dougherty L and Lister S (eds) (2011) *The Royal Marsden Hospital Manual of Clinical Nursing Procedures*, 8th edn. Oxford: Blackwell Publishing.

European Association of Urological Nurses (EAUN) (2012) *Evidence-based Guidelines for Best Practice in Urological Health Care: Catheterisation & Indwelling Catheters in Adults*. EAUN: Arnhem.

Fisher J (2010) The importance of effective catheter securement. *British Journal of Nursing (Continence Care Supplement)* 19(18): S14–S18.

Foxley S (2011) Indwelling urinary catheters: accurate monitoring of urine output. *British Journal of Nursing* 20(9): 564–569.

Gibney L (2010) Offering patients a choice of urinary catheter drainage system. *British Journal of Nursing* 19(15): 954–958.

Hughes E (2004) Principles of post-operative care. *Nursing Standard* 19(5): 43–51.

Joanna Briggs Institute (JBI) (2006) *Best Practice: Removal of Short Term Indwelling Urethral Catheters*, vol 10. Adelaide: Blackwell Publishing.

Kelleher M (2002) Removal of urinary catheters: midnight vs 0600 hours. *British Journal of Nursing* 11(2): 84–90.

Leaver R B (2007) The evidence for urethral meatal cleansing. *Nursing Standard* 21(41): 39–42.

Mangnall J and Watterson L (2006) Principles of aseptic technique in urinary catheterisation. *Nursing Standard* 21(8): 49–56.

Nazarko L (2010) Effective evidence-based catheter management: an update. *British Journal of Nursing* 19(15): 948–953

NHS Quality Improvement Scotland (NHS QIS) (2004) *Best Practice Statement: Urinary Catheterisation and Catheter Care*. Edinburgh: NHS Quality Improvement Scotland.

National Institute for Health and Clinical Excellence (NICE) (2012) *Infection Control, Prevention of Healthcare-associated Infection in Primary and Community Care*. Clinical Guideline 139. London: NICE.

NPSA (2009) Female urinary catheters causing trauma to adult males: Rapid Response Report RRR02 Available at: http://www.nrls.npsa.nhs.uk/alerts/?entryid45=59897 (accessed December 2015).

Pellatt G C (2007) Anatomy and physiology of urinary elimination. Part 1. *British Journal of Nursing* 16: 406–410.

Patel A R, Jones J S and Babineau D (2008) Lidocaine 2% gel versus plain lubricating gel for pain reduction during flexible cystoscopy: a meta-analysis of prospective, randomised, controlled trials. *The Journal of Urology* 179(3): 986–990.

RCN (2012) Catheter Care: *RCN Guidance for Nurses*. RCN: London.

Rees J and Mawson T (2007) Guidelines on catheter use in patients with a hip fracture. *Nursing Times* 103(16): 30–31.

Skills for Health (2010) CC02 Insert and secure urethral catheters. Available at: https://tools.skillsforhealth.org.uk/competence/show/html/id/1008/ (accessed 9 December 2015).

Tortora G J and Derrickson B (2011) *Principles of Anatomy and Physiology*, 12th edn. Hoboken, NJ: John Wiley & Sons Inc.

Trigg E and Mohammed T (2010) *Practices in Children's Nursing*, 3rd edn. Churchill Livingston: Edinburgh.

CHAPTER 12

Venepuncture

LEARNING OBJECTIVES

- Discuss the anatomy and physiology relating to venepuncture
- Review skills and competence with regard to undertaking venepuncture
- Describe possible complications of venepuncture and how to manage them

Aim of this chapter

The aim of this chapter is to review the reasons for undertaking peripheral venepuncture (blood sampling) and the associated complications and risk prevention. *This may not, however, be a role that is expected of all healthcare assistants, so please check your local policy and access any approved training.*

Reasons for performing venepuncture

The term 'venepuncture' is used to describe the introduction of a needle into a vein to obtain a representative sample of the circulating blood for laboratory (haematological, biochemical or bacteriological) analysis, and is usually requested by a medical practitioner/doctor to diagnose or monitor a patient's condition and/or treatment.

Relevant anatomy and physiology

It is essential that healthcare assistants and assistant practitioners undertaking the technique have a good understanding of the anatomy and physiology of arteries, veins and associated nerves.

Blood vessels comprise a network of channels through which blood flows and they are active organs that, when functioning properly, assist the heart in

Clinical Skills for Healthcare Assistants and Assistant Practitioners, Second Edition.
Angela Whelan and Elaine Hughes.
© 2016 John Wiley & Sons, Ltd. Published 2016 by John Wiley & Sons, Ltd.

circulating the blood and influence the blood's constitution. The vessels that take blood away from the heart are arteries. The vessels that bring blood toward the heart are veins. Veins carry deoxygenated blood back to the heart and their pressure is significantly lower than in arteries. Arteries transport blood away from the heart under pressure and are larger vessels with more elastic tissue and muscle, although this does vary depending on the size of the vessel. Generally, arteries have veins of the same size running right alongside or near them, and they often have similar names (Norris and Siegfried 2011). Veins and arteries are different; both have three layers of tissue but vein walls are thinner, having less muscle and elastic tissue in the middle layer (tunica media) (Tortora and Derrickson 2014). Veins also have valves (which help blood return to the heart) that are common especially where blood return is against gravity, for example lower limbs. Care must be taken to avoid sites where veins meet (bifurcation) due to the presence of these valves, because these can be damaged.

For successful venepuncture, blood is sampled from a vein in the patient's arm. As arteries, veins and nerves can be in similar locations, care must be taken during the assessment and procedure to avoid arteries and nerves.

Common sites for venepuncture

The site most commonly chosen for taking a sample of venous blood is the area in the bend of the elbow, the antecubital fossa, where superficial veins (the median cubital vein, the basilica vein, the cephalic vein) are readily accessible (Bishop 2009). Preferred or first choice should be the median cubital vein (Figure 12.1).

The healthcare assistant and assistant practitioner needs to consider many aspects when selecting a vein and Table 12.1 gives some reasons for choice.

THINK ABOUT IT

What are two differences between a vein and an artery?

In summary, the healthcare assistant must, as part of good assessment practice, be able to see and feel (palpate) the vein.

Infection

Understanding infection control issues in venepuncture is essential to prevent complications due to poor practice (Hobson 2008). Venepuncture is the most common clinical practice that breaches the circulatory system, so healthcare assistants and assistant practitioners should consider their role in the prevention of infection (Box 12.1).

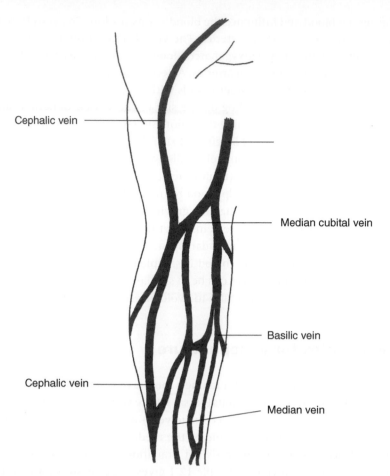

Figure 12.1 Common sites (upper arm).

Box 12.1 Predisposing infection risk factors and management

- Skin colonisation (surface bacterial spread) can allow bacteria to enter the circulatory system through the insertion of a needle, so ensure careful site selection and cleansing if there is evidence or concern of contamination.
- Remote infection (e.g. urinary tract infection) can also lead to a risk; the patient should be educated about not tampering with the site or sterile dressing, if used, and this should reduce the risk.
- Multi-use disinfectants can become colonised with bacteria very quickly, so use only single-use sachets when cleansing the site.
- Expired or damaged stock can be a source of infection; ensure that stock is in date and has been stored correctly, and is used for its intended purpose; single-use devices must be used (Medicines and Healthcare Products Regulatory Agency (MHPRA) 2013).
- Practitioner hands are the single most common way that bacteria are transferred onto devices (equipment), so ensure correct hand cleansing.

Adapted with permission from NHS Lothian (2007).

Table 12.1 Summarising possible considerations for vein choice.

Consideration	Explanation
Patient knowledge	Discussing past experience with the patient is always advisable. Patients can tell you of any previous difficulties and preferred sites (Bishop 2009) which may result in less discomfort for the patient (Ingram and Lavery 2009). You may also take consideration as to whether the patient is left or right handed.
Belonephobia – fear of needles	Patient anxiety is well documented; for some, fear of needles, however, goes beyond anxiety to phobia. Physical symptoms range from sweating to fainting and even death (Ellson 2008). It is important to use good communication skills and distraction therapy to help to relax your patient. Check with local policy for recommendations regarding use of a local anaesthetic cream to. Refer to a more experienced member of staff.
Feeling/palpate the vein	This helps to distinguish veins from arteries or tendons. To palpate a vein, place one or two fingertips over it and press lightly. Release the pressure to assess the veins elasticity and rebound filling (Bishop 2009). A vein suitable for venepuncture should feel round, bouncy and engorged as opposed to hard (tendon), bumpy and flat. Nerves are not palpatable and the patient will complain of a shooting 'electric shock' type of pain if a nerve is touched (Witt 2011).
Vein choice	Veins to avoid are those that appear sclerosed, fibrosed, oedematous, small, non-palpable, inflamed, bruised, sore and close to arteries, valves or nerves (Hobson 2015).
Visual appearance of skin	Skin should be assessed for dermatological conditions (e.g. psoriases), signs of infection; haematoma; oedema; injury/damage (e.g. burns, wounds) which could result in increased complications and/or discomfort for the patient.
Health factors – existing conditions may result in complications for example: Rheumatiod arthritis Parkinson's disease Cerebrovascular accident Arterioveous fistula for dialysis Intravenous infusion in place	The joint capsule, for example the elbow, may be inflamed and the tourniquet position may cause pain (Ingram and Lavery 2009). Tremors and movement may make venepuncture difficult, additional help maybe required (Witt 2011). Do not use the affected arm because sensation and circulation may be altered, and thus, if pain or injury occurs, may not be identified at an early stage (Ingram and Lavery 2009). An arteriovenous fistula is an artificial shunt, which is permanent fusion of a vein of artery for patients undergoing dialysis. This site must **not** be used – seek advice. Check local policy. Any samples of blood taken above an IV infusion may be contaminated (Witt 2011), otherwise this may alter blood results (Ingram and Lavery 2009). Devices may be turned off prior to blood tests, however, *remember to check your policy and always seek advice on any action taken.*

> **Box 12.2** Additional requirements (for vacuum system)
>
> - Blood culture set (aerobic and anaerobic bottles).
> - Three needles.
> - Two alcohol wipes.
> - 20 ml syringe and adaptor (Figure 12.7).

Hand hygiene

Transmission of microorganisms by the hands of healthcare workers is the most likely method of contributing to the spread of infections in hospitals (Loveday et al. 2014). The Royal College of Nurses (RCN 2013a) emphasise the need to be vigilant about hand hygiene. Standard infection control precautions, formerly known as universal precautions, underpin routine safe practice, protecting both staff and clients from microorganisms that may cause infection. By applying standard precautions at all times and to all patients, best practice becomes second nature and the risks of infection are minimised (RCN 2012). The WHO's Five Moments for Hand Hygiene (WHO 2014) defines the crucial times when healthcare workers should perform hand hygiene and has been adapted by the National Patient Safety Agency (NPSA) for application in the UK context to include:

1 Before contact.
2 Before aseptic task.
3 After body fluid exposure risk.
4 After patient contact.
5 After contact with patient surroundings.

The Five Moments approach to hand hygiene applies the most comprehensive evidence that aims to improve hand hygiene across the NHS. The approach supports coordinators in ensuring hand hygiene is performed at the right time (the Five Moments) in the right place (the point of care) using the appropriate method (soap and water hand washing or alcohol hand rub) using the correct technique. The RCN (2015) highlights the importance of reducing Healthcare Associated Infections (HCAIs), which is an essential part of the role of the HCA and AP when performing venepuncture. Please check your local policies and procedures.

An effective handwashing technique involves three stages: preparation, washing and rinsing, and drying. Preparation requires wetting hands under tepid running water before applying liquid soap or an antimicrobial preparation. The handwash solution must come into contact with all of the surfaces of the hand. The hands must be rubbed together vigorously for a minimum of 10–15 seconds, paying particular attention to the tips of the fingers, the thumbs and the areas between the fingers. Hands should be rinsed thoroughly before drying with good quality paper towels.

> **THINK ABOUT IT**
>
> Read the WHO's Five Moments for Hand Hygiene, thinking about your own actions. Think about the effects that not washing your hands can have on a single patient in one shift.

Aseptic (sterile) technique

Aseptic technique is a term used to describe a sterile process within nursing practice to minimise infections associated with invasive procedures (Hobson 2008). The National Institute for Health and Care Excellence (2012) assert that aseptic technique ensures only uncontaminated equipment and fluids come into contact with susceptible body sites. Using the principles of asepsis minimises the spread of organisms from one person to another and should therefore be used during any clinical procedure that bypasses the body's natural defences.

The use of aseptic technique should be used in line with local policy. The venepuncture site should be cleansed thoroughly with a cleaning agent, such as with a 70% isopropyl alcohol/2% chlorhexadine wipe (e.g. Clinell swab) or a 70% isopropyl alcohol wipe (e.g. street). It must then be left to dry. Povidine iodine must be used as an alternative if the patient is sensitive to chlorhexadine. It is recommended that the site is not re-palpated after cleansing, although this may be necessary if the patient's vein is difficult to find (Boyd 2013). Skills for Health (2015) have identified the importance of infection control in Standard 15 of the Care Certificate.

Health and safety

All staff who undertake venepuncture should be up to date with their hepatitis B vaccination and, as Bishop (2009) points out, should be aware of local policy and practice in order to protect themselves and others. Appropriate protective clothing such as gloves and aprons should be worn to minimise the risk of infection when undertaking the procedure (Hobson 2008). It is important to check if the patient has an allergy to latex in order to avoid wearing gloves that may cause a reaction. The Health and Safety Executive (HSE) report that natural rubber latex (NRL) proteins have the potential to cause asthma and urticaria. More serious allergic reactions, such as anaphylaxis, are also possible. NRL proteins are substances hazardous to health under COSHH (Control of Substances Hazardous to Health Regulations). Therefore, careful patient history must be taken into account when selecting gloves to avoid impacting patients who suffer with allergies and sensitivity to latex.

Environment

The environment must be visibly clean, free from dust and soilage. Hart (2011) maintains cleaning and disinfection programmes and protocols for environmental surfaces in patient care areas must be defined and areas fully monitored to ensure high standards of cleanliness are achieved. The trolley and equipment must be prepared in line with local policy to ensure good practice with adequate lighting to enable careful assessment of the patient and veins.

The patient needs to be prepared and made as comfortable as possible, which will go some way to reducing the level of anxiety experienced. If the patient is relaxed, effective interpersonal skills used and the arm supported, veins are likely to be dilated and access less painful and so there is greater likelihood of a positive patient experience (Dougherty 2011) (Table 12.2).

THINK ABOUT IT

Identify the common predisposing infection risk factors and describe how to prevent these risks in venepuncture practice.

Performing the skill: requirements and technique

Venepuncture equipment
For equipment using a vacuum system, see Figure 12.2 and examples below.

Examples of venepuncture equipment
- Tourniquet: consider the quick-release type.
- Non-sterile gloves.
- Apron.
- Alcohol wipe, for example 70% isopropyl alcohol.
- Bactericidal alcohol hand rub, for example Hibisol.
- Requisition forms and blood specimen bags.
- Blood specimen tubes: system as used by local organisation.
- Sterile needle: size (gauge) appropriate to the vein and sampling needs, using smallest where possible (RCN 2013b).
- Cotton-wool ball: non-sterile.
- Tray or trolley.
- Sterile hypoallergenic plaster.
- Sharps disposal bin.

Patient safety must be considered in relation to the patient's position when this procedure is being performed, so ensure that the arm is supported (Figure 12.3). Morris (2011) advocates that the practitioner anticipates if the patient may faint; in which case, lie them flat on a couch or the bed prior to commencing the procedure to ensure patient safety. When performing

Table 12.2 Guide to good venepuncture practice: vacuum system.

Action	Reason
1. Wash hands with liquid soap, and dry hands thoroughly followed by an alcohol hand rub, or wash with an approved antiseptic solution	To minimise the risk of healthcare-associated infection
2. Assemble the equipment required for the procedure on a trolley or a tray. Ensure that all equipment and disposables used are intact and within their expiry dates	Procedure is carried out safely, efficiently and without interruptions To maintain asepsis during the procedure
3. Identify the tests on the requisition form and select the appropriate blood collection tubes	To ensure correct sampling
4. Allow the patient time to ask questions and express concerns about the procedure	To obtain patient consent and cooperation
5. Identify the patient, check the addressograph label or written details on the requisition form and ensure that it corresponds with the details on the patient's identity wristband Check all details verbally by actively asking the patient to state their name and date of birth (DOB) Where a patient is unable to verbally state their name and DOB, good practice suggests that two staff check the identity bracelet against health records and requisition form(s)	To ensure the blood specimen is taken from the patient indicated on the request form To ensure all details are correct
6. Help the patient into a comfortable position either sitting in a chair or lying on the bed. The arm must be supported in an extended (straight) position	To enable the healthcare assistant to carry out the procedure with ease and maintain the patient's comfort
7. Prepare the area, e.g. provide adequate lighting, and heighten the bed, lower cot sides	To ensure a safe working environment

Source: Adapted from NHS Lothian 2007. Reproduced with permission of NHS Lothian.

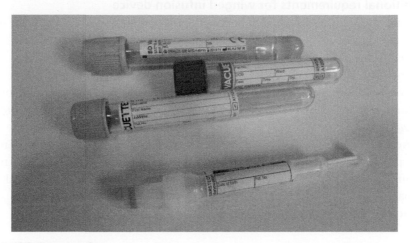

Figure 12.2 Vacuum tubes.

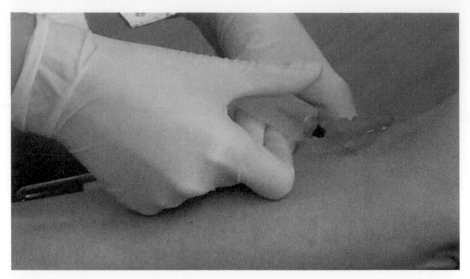

Figure 12.3 Insertion technique example.

venepuncture it is essential that the HCA or AP remains calm and talks to the patient in a supportive manner. The ability to perform this task confidently and competently not only reassures the patient but also helps to reduce the risk of avoidable complications occurring (Table 12.3).

Winged infusion device, for example the butterfly option

The option of using a winged infusion device may not be open to all healthcare assistants; *please check local policy and confirm if this practice is taught, supported and supervised before undertaking*. Refer to Table 12.4 for specific guidance on inserting a winged device.

Additional requirements for winged infusion device

- Butterfly 21 or 23 gauge, size depending on patient's vein, for example a 23 gauge for a frail elderly patient with small veins.
- Adaptor: see Figure 12.4.
- Tape for securing butterfly.

Some practice areas only use senior and experienced healthcare staff in blood culture sampling, *so again please check local policy and practice prior to undertaking this procedure, if an accepted role.*

According to Gilligan (2012), low contamination rates are because of training, practice, resources and professionalism. Ernst (2001) said that the most common cause of contamination occurred when a practitioner touched the prepared site, and suggested the use of mental markers, such as freckles, to reduce this urge.

Table 12.3 Specific actions and observations during the procedure.

Action	Reason
1. Wash hands with liquid soap, and dry hands thoroughly followed by an alcohol hand rub, or wash with an approved antiseptic solution	To minimise the risk of healthcare-associated infection
2. Identify the patient's own preferred site for the procedure based on their previous experience	To actively involve the patient in their treatment. To familiarise the healthcare assistant with the patient's medical history and factors that may influence choice of vein
3. Apply a tourniquet to the upper arm on the chosen side approx 7–10 cm (3–4 inches) above the puncture site	Increases venous pressure to help vein identification and entry. Careful attention is paid to length of time tourniquet is left on (No more than 1 ½ min or can cause an adverse effect, as below)
4. Apply enough pressure to impede (slow) venous circulation but not arterial blood flow, check for arterial pulse	Prolonged pressure may lead to vein spasm, pain and haematoma (blood in the tissues)
5. To further encourage venous filling consider: • Allow their arm to hang at the patient's side. • Stroke vein lightly. • Ask the patient to wash their hands or place in warm/hot water. • Ask patient to assist by clenching and unclenching their hand.	Aid vein filling and make procedure easier *Take care because this may affect some results, so may not be recommended*
6. Observe and palpate (feel) the selected vein	To identify its course, depth and distinguish structures such as tendons, and to avoid nearby arteries
7. Release the tourniquet. Check that the vein has decompressed (a thrombosed vein will remain firm and palpable)	Reduce the length of time that tourniquet is in situ (see 3) Check for a thrombosed (clotted) vein.
8. Push the tube into the needle adaptor by twisting clockwise	Opens the system
9. Wash hands with liquid soap, and dry hands thoroughly followed by an alcohol hand rub, or wash with an approved antiseptic solution Put on gloves	To minimise the risk of healthcare associated infection. Gloves are worn for the protection of staff against blood spillage. They will not protect against needlestick injuries
10. Ensure the patient's skin is clean. Wash with soap and water and dry thoroughly if visibly dirty	To minimise the risk of infection from the patient's own skin during this invasive procedure
Use alcohol wipe if deemed appropriate, but essential for blood cultures. *Check local policy*	Recommended in hospital patients, but may not be required in a community setting
If using alcohol wipe, cleanse the site in a circular movement from the proposed puncture site for 30 s, then allow to air dry for 30 s	
11. Reapply the tourniquet to the identified site	Encourage venous filling
12. Inspect the needle	To ensure needle is sharp with no barbs (hooks)

Table 12.3 (*continued*)

Action	Reason
13. With the patient's arm in a downward position, line up the needle and collection tube with the vein from which the blood will be drawn. Using the thumb or first finger of free hand anchor the vein by applying manual traction of the skin 2–5 cm below the proposed insertion site. With the bevel of the needle upward insert the needle into the vein. A sensation of resistance will be felt followed by the needle entering the vein	To hold the vein steady and provide countertension, which will facilitate a smooth needle entry
14. Advance the needle a further 1–2 mm into the vein	To stabilise the needle within the vein and prevent it becoming dislodged
15. Secure the needle by holding the guide sheath firmly	To prevent movement of the needle in or out of the vein
16. Using the syringe technique for the initial specimen, fill the blood collection tube by slowly pulling back the plunger, keeping the needle in centre of the vein	To ensure appropriate filling of blood sample tube
17. Remove the tube from the needle by twisting anticlockwise (grip the needle guide sleeve firmly). The needle remains in the vein. Secure next prepared tube onto the needle by twisting clockwise	To minimise the movement of needle and prevent mechanical phlebitis (infection due to friction)
18. The second and subsequent samples may be taken either by the syringe technique or alternatively by the vacuum principle where there is good venous supply Remove the final tube from the needle	To aid blood sampling procedure To ensure the system is 'closed'
19. Release the tourniquet	To release venous congestion Ensure it is not left on
20. Then slip the cotton wool ball down over the puncture site and do not apply pressure until needle has been fully removed Once removed, apply firm finger pressure until bleeding stops (approximately 2 minutes). Do not allow the patient to bend the arm	Prevent bleeding and haematoma formation To prevent pain on removal Prolonged finger (digital) pressure may be required if treatment and/or medical condition interferes with clotting mechanisms Prevent shearing to vein, which causes more bleeding/bruising
21. Once venepuncture site has stopped bleeding, if required, cover site with an Elastoplast dressing, or hypoallergenic dressing if patient has an allergy	To prevent leakage of blood until healing is complete
22. Make no more than two attempts to obtain blood sample/s. If unsuccessful, obtain assistance from more experienced staff	Patient comfort Prevent trauma to vein

(*continued overleaf*)

Table 12.3 (*continued*)

Action	Reason
23. Ensure the patient is comfortable. Advise the patient to inform staff if venepuncture site starts to bleed or is tender or painful, and when to remove any dressing applied Explain to the patient that results may take some time to come back and that they will be informed when they are available	Reduce anxieties
24. Complete the labels on the blood samples you have taken prior to leaving the patient/bedside, checking details with the patient and the blood forms	Ensure that blood samples are correctly labelled

Source: Adapted from NHS Lothian 2007. Reproduced with permission of NHS Lothian.

Table 12.4 Guide to good practice and winged device (butterfly) insertion.

Action	Reason
1. Assess and prepare patient as 1–12 in Table 12.3	
2. Attach adaptor to the tail of the butterfly before attaching the first tube. Fold up wings of butterfly and insert needle into vein as detailed in 13–14 in Table 12.3 (Figure 12.5); bring the device level with skin and then advance along length of the needle, keeping it level and in line with the vein	To prevent blood spillage or leakage
3. Flatten the wings of the butterfly to the skin and secure with Micropore tape	To prevent dislodgement of the butterfly during specimen collection
4. Collect the first specimen using the syringe technique	
5. Complete procedure as 16–24 in Table 12.3	

The ideal volume for an adult is 20 ml evenly distributed between both collection bottles, and not exceeding 12 ml (Ernst 2001). Ernst (2001) also proposed that, if the yield is less than 20 ml, it is better to load (fill) 10 ml into the aerobic bottle (e.g. blue), because 98% of septicaemias are caused by aerobic (need oxygen) organisms, and most of the causative organisms can still be detected, even if the anaerobic (e.g. pink) bottle has less than the optimum volume. Overfilling can lead to false positives, so take care when filling. However, fill the anaerobic (e.g. pink) bottle first, to minimise the risk of air in the syringe getting in and altering the anaerobic (oxygen not needed) environment (Ernst 2001).

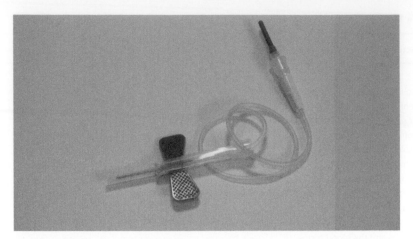

Figure 12.4 Winged device and adaptor.

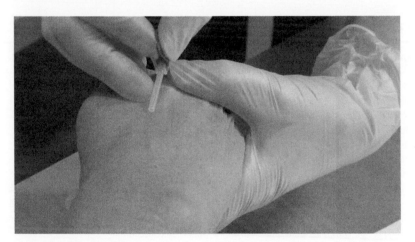

Figure 12.5 Insertion technique.

If a blood culture sample is falsely positive, due to incorrect skin cleansing or contamination from the healthcare assistant's hands, then a patient could have an increased length of hospital stay, which increases costs, with the associated risk of infection. The patient may require transfer if thought to be septicaemic (bacteria in the blood), suffer the unnecessary use of antibiotics and the increased risks associated with this (Figure 12.6). The intravenous (IV) route would be preferred to treat septicaemia, and so would also incur increased costs and pressure on staff time. Thus the longer a patient is in hospital, the more admissions will be restricted, putting more pressure on to limited beds. Therefore extra care is needed when sampling for blood cultures (Table 12.5) (Lavery and Ingram 2005).

Table 12.5 Blood cultures: good practice guide.

Action	Reason
1. Cleanse the proposed venepuncture site as per Table 12.3, Step 10	To prevent contamination of blood sample from microorganisms on the skin
2. Do not re-palpate the vein after the site has been cleansed	As above
3. Remove flip top cap from bottles, wipe the tops with fresh alcohol wipe, allow to dry, then insert clean needle into each	Preventing contamination of the sample
4. Withdraw 20 ml of blood (1–3 ml in neonates) from the adult patient using technique described in Table 12.3	Adequate sample for laboratory testing
5. Fill both bottles and divide blood equally, 10 ml in each	Ensure adequate sample size
6. Dispose of sharps immediately into sharps container	Reducing the possibility of a needlestick injury
7. Decontaminate (cleanse) hands	Preventing infection
8. Minimum data required on samples are surname, forename, date of birth, gender, date and time of sample, type and site of sample, location of patient	Ensuring that laboratory has correct information
9. Minimum data are also required on request form, addressographs can be used including the time and date of sampling, if high risk (e.g. HIV), any antibiotic therapy and relevant clinical details	Ensuring that laboratory has the correct and appropriate information
10. Arrange for transport to the laboratory, if not available immediately, e.g. night-time, leave cultures at room temperature	Appropriate storage of blood cultures

Source: Adapted from NHS Lothian 2007. Reproduced with permission of NHS Lothian.

THINK ABOUT IT

Consider if skin surface bacteria contaminate a sample for blood culture. What might be the outcome for the patient and the service?

Related aspects and terminology

Consent

NHS Choices (2014) reports that, for consent to be valid, it must be voluntary and informed and the person consenting must have the capacity to make the decision. For consent to be voluntary, the decision to either consent or not to consent to treatment must be made by the person themselves, and must not be influenced by pressure from medical staff, friends or family. The person/patient must be given all of the information in terms of what the treatment involves, including

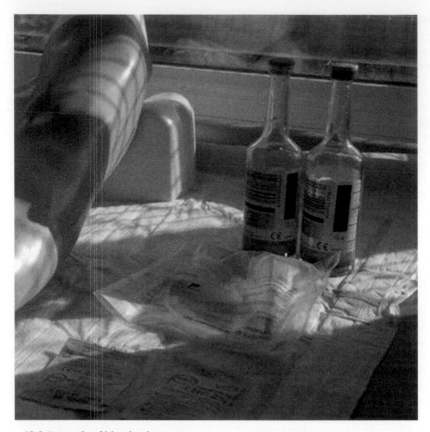

Figure 12.6 Example of blood culture set.

the benefits and risks, whether there are reasonable alternative treatments and what will happen if treatment does not go ahead: this is informed consent. With venepuncture it is sometimes thought that patients have voluntarily consented when their actions support this idea, for example turning up for an appointment or simply rolling up a sleeve and presenting an arm to have the sample of blood taken. For more discussion on consent, refer to Chapters 1 and 4.

Anxiety

In an effort to reduce anxiety, patients should be asked whether they have had venepuncture performed previously. Attention should be paid particularly where there were any adverse (poor) outcomes or experiences, so that reassurance or further action can be taken.

With regard to the actual procedure, anxiety can be caused by a previous bad experience, a degree of 'needle phobia' (fear of a needle) or just a dislike of medical procedures. The RCN (2010) noted the need for skilled practice that minimised pain and anxiety in relation to children or young people, but can be

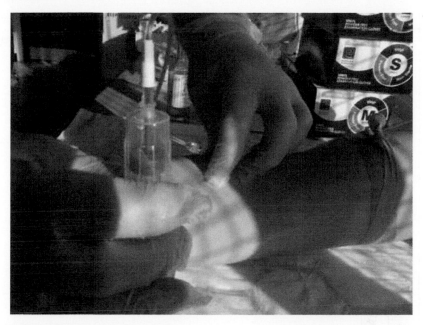

Figure 12.7 Adaptor.

seen as good practice for all. Dougherty (2011) reports a number of approaches have been successful in reducing patient anxiety, including the use of guided imagery (imagining a place where they can feel comfortable and relaxed), music and distraction techniques (RCN 2013b). Distraction therapy is simply a means of taking the mind off a procedure by concentrating on something else, for example there may be a television programme on or a conversation about a subject of interest or even asking the patient to focus on their breathing to relax.

There are a number of local anaesthetic creams that can be applied to the skin to help reduce pain, such as EMLA and Amatop. These are medicines and will need to be prescribed and administered. Dougherty (2011), however, warns us that although less painful, these creams can cause vasoconstriction making venepuncture more difficult. *Please check your local policy to see if this is within the boundaries of your role otherwise you may be breaking vicarious liability* (Boyd 2013).

Common problems

Unsuccessful sampling

This may be due to poor vein assessment, incorrect choice of sampling device or poor technique. Careful review of veins and technique before starting the procedure, as well as consideration of patient comfort and position, is necessary to prevent this. Table 12.6 is a competency framework for venepuncture.

Table 12.6 Competency framework: venepuncture.

Steps	First assessment/reassessment				
	Demonstration/supervised practice				
Venepuncture signature	Date/sign	Date/sign	Date/sign	Date/sign	Date/competent
	1	2	3	4	5
1 Gives explanation of procedure and obtains patient's verbal consent					
2 Selects appropriate equipment and sample tubes					
3 Correctly identifies the patient against the request form					
4 Ensures patient comfort and privacy					
5 Reassures patient, and uses anxiety relieving measures (if appropriate)					
6 Hands washed, gloves and apron worn					
7 Uses appropriate methods to encourage good venous filling					
8 Identifies appropriate vein for venepuncture					
9 Prepares patient's skin as per local policy					
10 Carries out procedure successfully					
11 Removes last sample tube and tourniquet before removing needle					
12 Disposes of sharps immediately					
13 Applies pressure and seals puncture site					
14 Labels and packages samples correctly for transport					
15 Records information in patient's notes					

Supervisor/assessor(s):

Potential complications of venepuncture

Bruising/ecchymosis

Hobson (2008) and Morris (2011) report that bruising is caused by blood seeping into surrounding tissues. Older people, especially if they have fragile skin or are on anticoagulation therapy such as warfarin, are likely to bleed or bruise easily. Good technique is of paramount importance.

Bruising is preventable by the following:

- Accurate identification of a suitable vein.
- The correct insertion technique and angle.
- Ensuring that the tourniquet is not applied with excessive pressure or below previous puncture sites.
- 'Fixing' the vein position by skin traction during the insertion of the needle.
- Ensuring adequate pressure to the puncture site after needle removal, which will prevent further damage (Morris 2011).

Accurate monitoring of the site and documentation of the bruise is also necessary.

Haematoma

A haematoma is described by Hobson (2008) as a complication that results in blood leaking from the vein into surrounding tissue, which is caused by poor technique and failure to select the appropriate vein.

Other causes identified by Morris (2013) are inadequate pressure to the puncture site or failure to remove the tourniquet before removing the needle; poor vein selection; vulnerable patient such as those on anticoagulant therapy; incorrect use of the tourniquet; multiple attempts to access the vein and failure to insert the needle correctly into the vein. In order to manage a haematoma that occurs during the procedure, remove the tube, release the tourniquet and then remove the needle using a sterile swab according to local policy (Dougherty and Lister 2011). The patient should be taken care of and the haematoma monitored and documented (NMC 2015).

Excessive pain

This can be caused by the frequent use of a vein, or poor technique, such as blind plunging manoeuvres (without feeling/assessing for vein); where a nerve or valve is touched; or if the patient is anxious, fearful or has a low pain threshold.

This is prevented by:

- ensuring that the patient is comfortable and the arm supported;
- allowing the alcohol to dry at the skin site;
- carrying out the procedure in a confident unhurried manner.

Consider the use of local anaesthetic cream as previously discussed. *Please check your local practice and policy, because it may not be within the HCA or AP role to apply local anaesthetic cream/gel.*

Arterial puncture

Arterial puncture is characterised by pain and spurting of bright red blood. This is caused by poor technique or inadequate assessment and the healthcare assistant would see bright red blood pulsating into the tube and needle. Prevention is by:

* thorough assessment of the site;
* the use of the correct insertion technique and angle.

Management is to immediately remove the needle and apply prolonged finger pressure for 5 minutes and then a pressure bandage for at least a further 5 minutes. The patient should be under observation, assessment and medical supervision, and the incident should be recorded in the patient's case notes and the local adverse incident reporting mechanisms followed and reported to the nurse in charge (RCN 2013b).

Fibrosis

This is where the vein becomes hard or cord-like and may occur with prolonged use of one site. It is prevented by:

* careful assessment
* rotation of sites.

Phlebitis

This is an infection caused by mechanical irritation (needle rubbing inside the vein) or poor aseptic technique, and is considered a rare complication in venepuncture. The symptoms of phlebitis are pain, oedema, and erythema – often presenting as a red streak along the length of the vein. Prevention is by:

* following sound infection control practice (Morris 2011; RCN 2013b);
* not re-palpating the vein after cleansing the site with alcohol.

Ongoing site monitoring and documentation are critical, as is investigation to identify the cause and plan the steps for future prevention.

THINK ABOUT IT

What action should be taken if an artery is punctured?
  What preventive measures should have been considered?

Summary

Venepuncture is a common procedure and is carried out by many members of the multidisciplinary team both in hospitals and in the community. Thus effective communication and prompt recording are critical for safe patient care. Venepuncture is invasive and is a diagnostic requirement; therefore, it is important practitioners have a theoretical knowledge to underpin the competent performance of this skill.

CASE STUDY 12.1

Mr Robert Walls is an older man aged 90 years and requires samples for full blood count (FBC) and urea and electrolytes (U&Es).

He is frail and dehydrated after a fall, and has an intravenous infusion running into his left median cubital vein. He has a residual weakness in his right arm from a previous stroke (cerebral vascular accident). He is restless and upset at being in hospital, and slightly confused.

Outline the assessment process here and discuss the choice of venepuncture device and describe why you would choose it.

Below is a self-assessment checklist; however, you may also wish to review some of the skills involved in venepuncture, for example infection control is a part of the Skills for Health Care Passport. You might wish to discuss this with your manager.

Self-assessment

Assessment	Aspects	Achieved ✓
Patient	*Have you considered all aspects of this section?* Patient assessment: veins and general condition Infection control and asepsis aspects Consent, communication and education Problem solving	
Procedure	*Have you considered all aspects of this section?* Equipment selection and insertion technique Recording and labelling Reporting concerns Problem solving Disposal of equipment	**Achieved ✓**
Winged device	*Have you considered all aspects of this section?* Selection and insertion of butterfly Recording and labelling Reporting concerns Problem solving Disposal of equipment	**Achieved ✓**
Blood cultures	*Have you considered all aspects of this section?* Infection control and procedure Disposal of equipment	**Achieved ✓**

References

Bishop T (2009) Venepuncture. *Practice Nurse* 37(12): 18–21.
Boyd C (2013) *Student Survival Skills: Clinical Skills for Nurses*. London: John Wiley & Sons.

Dougherty L (2011) Patient's perspective. In: Phillips S, Collins M and Dougherty L (eds) *Venepuncture and Cannulation*. Oxford: Wiley Blackwell, pp. 281–296.

Dougherty L and Lister S (eds) (2011) *The Royal Marsden Manual of Clinical Nursing Procedures*, 8th edn. Oxford: Blackwell Wiley.

Ellson R (2008) Venepuncture and cannulation: In: Richardson R (ed.) *Clinical Skills for Student Nurses: Theory, Practice and Reflection*. Devon: Reflect Press.

Ernst D J (2001) The right way to do blood cultures. *Nursing Journal for Registered Nurses* 64(3): 28–32.

Gilligan P (2012) Blood culture contamination: a clinical and financial burden. *Infection Control and Hospital Epidemiology* 34(10): 22–23.

Hart T (2013) Promoting hand hygiene in clinical practice. *Nursing Times* 109(38): 14–15.

Hobson P (2008) Venepuncture and cannulation: theoretical aspects. *British Journal of Healthcare Assistants* 9(3): 75–78.

Ingram P and Lavery I (2009) *Clinical Skills for Healthcare Assistants*. Oxford: Wiley-Blackwell.

Lavery I and Ingram P (2005) Venepuncture: Best practice. *Nursing Standard* 19(49): 55–65.

Loveday H P, Wilson J A, Pratt R, et al. (2014) epic3: national evidence based guidelines for preventing health care associated infections in NHS hospitals in England. *Journal of Hospital Infection* 86 Suppl 1: S1–S70.

Medicines and Healthcare Products Regulatory Agency (MHPRA) (2013) *Single-Use Medical Devices: Implications and Consequences of Reuse*. London: Medicines and Healthcare Products Regulatory Agency.

Morris W (2011) Complications. In: Phillips S, Collins M and Dougherty L (eds) *Venepuncture and Cannulation*. Oxford: Wiley Blackwell, pp. 281–296.

National Institute for Health Care Excellence (NICE) (2012) Infection Prevention and Control of Healthcare-associated Infections in Primary and Community Care. NICE Clinical Guideline 139 Available at: https://www.nice.org.uk/guidance/cg139/evidence/control-full-guideline-185186701 (accessed December 2015).

NHS Choices (2014) Consent to Treatment. Available at: http://www.nhs.uk/conditions/consent-to-treatment/pages/introduction.aspx (accessed December 2015).

NHS Lothian (2007) *Adult Venepuncture and/or Peripheral IV Cannulation: Clinical Skills Education Package*. Edinburgh: NHS Lothian.

Norris M and Siegfried D (2011) *Anatomy and Physiology for Dummies*, 2nd edn. London: Wiley Publishing Inc.

Nursing and Midwifery Council (NMC) (2015) *The Code: Professional Standards of Practice and Behaviour for Nurses and Nidwives*. London: NMC.

Royal College of Nursing (2010) *Standards for Infusion Therapy*, 3rd edn. London: RCN.

Royal College of Nursing (2012) *Essential Practice for Infection Prevention and Control: Guidance for Nursing Staff*. London: RCN.

Royal College of Nursing (2013a) *Wipe It Out: One Chance to Get it Right. Infection Prevention and Control Information and Learning Resources for Health Care Staff*. London: RCN.

Royal College of Nursing (2013b) *Competencies: An Education and Training Competency Framework for Capillary Blood Sampling and Venepuncture in Children and Young People*. London: RCN.

Royal College of Nursing (2015) *Infection Prevention and Control within Health and Social Care*. London: RCN.

Skills for Health (2015) The Care Certificate Framework (Assessor) Health Education England, Skills for Care and Skills for Health.

Tortora G J and Derrickson B (2014) *Principles of Anatomy and Physiology*, EMEA edn. Hoboken, NJ: John Wiley & Sons Inc.

Witt B (2011) Patient's perspective. In: Phillips S, Collins M and Dougherty L (eds) *Venepuncture and Cannulation*. Oxford: Wiley Blackwell, pp. 108–130.

World Health Organization (2014) Your Five Moments for Hand Hygiene. tinyurl.com/WHO5Moments.

CHAPTER 13

Blood glucose monitoring

LEARNING OBJECTIVES

- Explain what causes diabetes
- Define the different types of diabetes
- List the common symptoms and risk factors
- Describe complications associated with diabetes
- Describe how to measure and record accurate blood sugar levels using appropriate equipment

Aim of this chapter

The aim of this chapter is to understand the fundamental principles of diabetes and apply this to the skill of measuring blood glucose.

What causes diabetes?

The World Health Organisation (2015) describes diabetes as a chronic disease that occurs either when the pancreas does not produce enough insulin or when the body cannot effectively use the insulin it produces. Insulin is a hormone that regulates blood sugar. Hyperglycaemia, or raised blood sugar, is a common effect of uncontrolled diabetes and over time leads to serious damage to many of the body's systems, especially the nerves and blood vessels. The main two types of diabetes are type 1 and type 2, both of which are described later.

Reasons for performing blood glucose measurement

Monitoring and self-monitoring of blood glucose is recognised as an important tool in diabetes management (Wallymahmed 2013). Glucose monitoring is done to obtain information on blood glucose levels at various times to allow

Clinical Skills for Healthcare Assistants and Assistant Practitioners, Second Edition.
Angela Whelan and Elaine Hughes.
© 2016 John Wiley & Sons, Ltd. Published 2016 by John Wiley & Sons, Ltd.

a therapeutic regime to be adjusted, facilitating optimal control avoiding hypoglycaemia and hyerglycaemia (Whitmore 2012).

Blood glucose monitoring is widely undertaken in a number of settings and situations, for example in hospital or at home (Dunning 2014). Point of care testing or near patient testing (where samples are not sent to the laboratory) is a convenient and quick way to obtain blood glucose measurements. Whitmore (2012) identified the need to use equipment correctly and ensuring the readings are accurate. There is a clear link between good blood glucose or glycaemic control and the prevention of long-term complications. It important for staff to work within the boundaries of their role; please check local policy and ensure you have had the required training in order to undertake this procedure. Blood glucose levels are carried out for a variety of reasons, and these are shown in Box 13.1.

Box 13.1 Reasons for taking blood glucose monitoring

- Frequent hypoglycaemic episodes and hypoglycaemic unawareness.
- Unstable or diabetic.
- Managing illnesses at home when recovering from an illness.
- Gestational diabetes mellitus (GDM) pregnancy and in neonates born to women with GDM and diabetes.
- Stabling a new treatment regimen.
- Stabilising Oral Hypoglycaemic Agents (OHA) and/or insulin doses: for example patients with renal failure and/or CVD where signs of hypoglycaemia can be masked; during investigations; during travel and/or to monitor medicine interactions.

There are benefits to patients in keeping their blood glucose levels within acceptable limits, and these include the patient:
- running a smaller risk of developing complications (Wallymahmed 2013) (see later);
- feeling more active and healthy;
- having better clinical outcomes if they have an acute cardiovascular event, for example myocardial infarction (heart attack) or stroke (Ritsinger et al. 2014; Laird 2014).

In order to fully understand diabetes, and the importance of blood glucose monitoring, revision of the anatomy and physiology of the pancreas is necessary.

Relevant anatomy and physiology

The pancreas

The pancreas is situated in the abdominal cavity with the head nesting in the curve of the duodenum (part of the small intestine). It is a pale grey/pink gland that consists of a broad head, body and narrow tail (Tortora and Derrickson

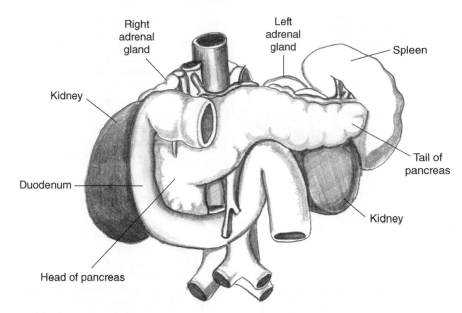

Right
adrenal
gland

Left
adrenal
gland

Spleen

Kidney

Tail of
pancreas

Duodenum

Kidney

Head of pancreas

Figure 13.1 Pancreas shown in relation to the kidneys, duodenum and adrenal glands.

2014). It is the size of an apple and weighs between 70–100 g (Tan 2011). Figure 13.1 shows the position of the pancreas in relation to other organs. The adrenal glands produce steroid hormones, which are essential for well-being and maintenance of life (Tortora and Derrickson 2014).

The pancreas has both an endocrine and an exocrine function: endocrine means excretion of substances directly into the bloodstream – in this case insulin – and exocrine means excretion via ducts and refers to digestive juices.

Only 2% of the pancreas fulfils the endocrine function and this is performed by collections of cells found in clusters irregularly distributed throughout the pancreas, known as the islets of Langerhans. Within the islets of Langerhans there are two types of cells: α (alpha) cells that produce glucagon and β (beta) cells that produce insulin. The body balances these two hormones to maintain a healthy blood glucose level; Figure 13.2 illustrates the variance in their roles.

Related aspects and terminology

Effects of diabetes

Figure 13.2 demonstrates how the body maintains normal blood glucose levels despite periods of fasting or eating. In diabetes, the blood glucose level remains high after the intake of a carbohydrate meal due to defective glucose metabolism by body cells, thus glucose cannot cross the cell membrane and be absorbed by the body. Conversion of glucose to glycogen in the liver and muscles is diminished, leading to protein being broken down instead.

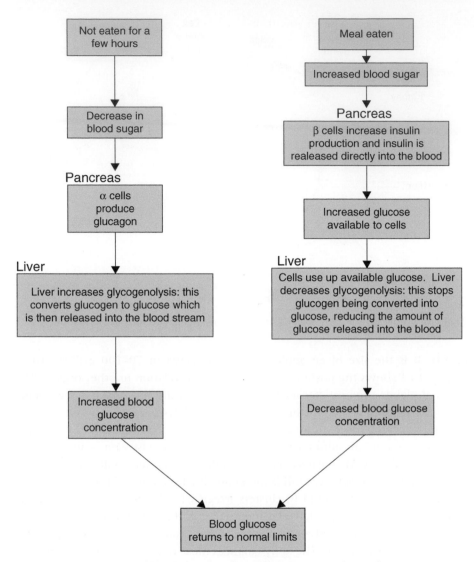

Figure 13.2 Maintenance of blood glucose. Adapted from Tortora and Derrickson (2006), Marieb and Hoehn (2007) and Thibodeau and Patton (2007).

THINK ABOUT IT

List some signs or symptoms of diabetes.

Common terminology

- *Blood glucose*: the amount of glucose (sometimes also called 'sugar') in the circulating blood.

- *Hypoglycaemia*: low blood glucose. This is sometimes referred to as a 'hypo'.
- *Hyperglycaemia*: high blood glucose.
- *DKA (diabetic ketoacidosis)*: dangerously high blood glucose levels. This can result in the patient being in a coma, and may well be the first symptom to be noticed prior to a diagnosis of diabetes.
- *Polydipsia*: increased thirst/appetite (Tortora and Derrickson 2014).
- *Polyphagia*: excess eating (Tortora and Derrickson 2014).
- *Polyuria*: frequently needing to pass urine (micturition) due to excessive urine production and the kidneys being unable to reabsorb excess water (Tortora and Derrickson 2014).
- *Ketonuria*: ketones (a byproduct of red blood cells) present in the patient's urine. This is why people with diabetes often test their urine for both ketones and glucose.
- *HbA1c (glycated haemoglobin)*: percentage of haemoglobin bound to glucose. This is shown in a blood sample that is taken to monitor how well controlled the patient's diabetes is.

Type 1 diabetes

This usually occurs as a result of the progressive destruction of β cells within the islets of Langerhans, which leads to insulin deficiency (Thrower and Bingley 2014). Type 1 diabetes is thought to be triggered by a variety of environmental factors, for example a prolonged period of ill-health, ingestion of certain toxins, dramatic change in life circumstances and perhaps a genetic predisposition (Dunning 2014). The presence of infection can also result in damage to some cells and the subsequent production of antibodies as part of the autoimmune response. Despite these antibodies being detectable before the symptoms of type 1 diabetes become apparent, the antibodies usually disappear within months of the diagnosis (Knipp and Simell 2012). Other symptoms of diabetes usually only appear once 80–85% of all the β cells have been destroyed. The disease is usually of sudden onset in young adults or children, with the cause being generally unknown. The only treatment option for a patient with type 1 diabetes is subcutaneous insulin replacement therapy and the condition cannot be cured, only managed.

Symptoms of type 1 diabetes

- Polydipsia.
- Polyuria.
- Polyphagia.
- Weight loss, due to the body not being able to release insulin, which prevents glucose being released (Tortora and Derrickson 2014).
- Increased incidence of infection.
- Lethargy (extreme tiredness).

- Symptoms of ketoacidosis (see below): collapse, reduced consciousness, rest-lessness, leading to coma and death if undetected.

Ketoacidosis

Diabetic ketoacidosis (DKA) is the result of very low or zero insulin levels, and generally only occurs in type 1 diabetes, because patients with type 2 diabetes have sufficient reserves to prevent this occurring (Noble-Bell and Cox 2014). If it does occur in type 2 diabetes, this is provoked by severe illness and is more likely to develop in people from non-Caucasian ethnic groups (Noble-Bell and Cox 2014). The signs and symptoms Dunning (2014) identifies include polyuria, polydipsia, weakness, fatigue and weight loss and patients tend to present with abdominal pain and vomiting. In severe ketoacidosis there may be tachycardia, hypotension, skin turgour, the smell of acetone (pear drops) on their breath plus deep and/or laboured breathing.

Type 2 diabetes

Type 2 diabetes is related to both reduced insulin sensitivity (insulin resistance) and impaired β cell function (Meier and Bonadonna 2013). It is the most common form of diabetes and occurs in around 90% of cases of diabetes in the developed world and, according to the WHO (2015), is largely the result of excess body weight and physical inactivity. Other causes are thought to include genetic disposition, age and ethnicity. Until recently, this type of diabetes was seen only in adults, but it is now also occurring in children. Whilst the exact cause is unknown, it is thought to relate to lack of physical activity and obesity. The disease is usually late onset and can often be undiagnosed for many years, so in some instances the complications of diabetes will present rather than the disease. Insulin secretion may be below or above normal, but deficiency of glucose inside body cells leads to hyperglycaemia and a high insulin level. This may be due to changes in cell membranes, which block the insulin-assisted movement of glucose into cells.

Symptoms of type 2 diabetes

- Tiredness.
- Blurred vision, this may be due to complications (see below) (Rubin 2008).
- Dry skin.
- Increased appetite and thirst.
- Needing to pass urine more frequently (micturition).

Managing childhood type 2 diabetes (MODY)

This is a form of type 2 diabetes and is due to a β cell defect that reduces the insulin secretion in response to specific blood glucose levels, rather than insulin resistance. Dunning (2014) reports that it requires strict diagnostic criteria, including: diagnosis before the age of 25 years, no requirement for insulin therapy 5 years after diagnosis and a previous familial history spanning several generations.

Gestational diabetes (during pregnancy)

Diabetes can occur for the first time during pregnancy and, after delivery of the baby, glucose tolerance returns to normal. However, it is thought that if gestational diabetes is experienced, the development of type 2 diabetes later in life is more common (Wallymahmed 2007). Treatment involves dietary control and insulin, if required, because the use of oral diabetic medication during pregnancy is not recommended (Dunning 2014).

Blood glucose levels

The two main methods used to monitor blood glucose in people with diabetes are HbA1c and monitoring of blood glucose levels. HbA1c is the gold standard in monitoring and provides information on a person's long-term glycaemic control. To test HbA1c, a venous sample of blood is taken and analysed to determine the amount of glucose attached to red blood cells. This is known as glycated haemoglobin and is recorded as mmol/mol (previously a percentage) with 48 mmol/mol or below being the optimum to achieve (Holt 2014).

Blood glucose level monitoring should be performed to complement HbA1c and provide real time measurement of blood glucose, which is measured in millimoles of glucose per litre of blood and is abbreviated to mmol/l (Dunning 2014). NICE also advises that self-monitoring of blood glucose levels should be used as part of an integrated approach, with pre-meal target levels of 4.0–7.0 mmols/l and post-meal targets of <9 mmol/l for people with type 1 diabetes and <8.5mmol/l for those with type 2 diabetes. The desired range for patients with diabetes is shown in Box 13.2.

Box 13.2 Desired blood glucose levels for patients with diabetes

	Before meals (preprandial)	2 hours after meals (postprandial)
Non-Diabetes	4.0 to 5.9 mmol/l	under 7.8 mmol/l
Type 1 Diabetes	4.0 to 7.0 mmol/l	under 8.5 mmol/l
Type 2 Diabetes	4.0 to 7.0 mmol/l	under 9.0 mmol/l
Children w/ type 1 diabetes	4.0 to 8.0 mmol/l	under 10 mmol/l

NICE recommended target blood glucose level ranges

Sites for blood glucose testing

The most commonly used site to take a blood sample from is the side of the finger using a single-use lancet. It is important to ensure the site of piercing is rotated and overuse of the thumb and index finger is avoided otherwise these areas become very painful (Dougherty and Lister 2011). Alternative site testing is available, which can cause less discomfort but only yields a small quality of blood, and glucose levels vary among sites which may have implications for treatment (Dunning 2014). All readings and sites of piercing should be documented accurately. Diabetes UK advise patients that there are ways to make blood glucose testing easier, such as washing the hand in warm water and shaking them to increase blood flow before you test, and that you should always use the sides of the fingers rather than the more sensitive fleshy pulp at the tips. Many Trusts allow patients to self-test, but patients may need some education if their device is different from that at home. *Check local policies and procedures for further advice on using this site.*

Equipment

There are a variety of blood glucose meters available with varying degrees of technicality and different features (Whitmore 2012; Holt 2014) (Figure 13.3).

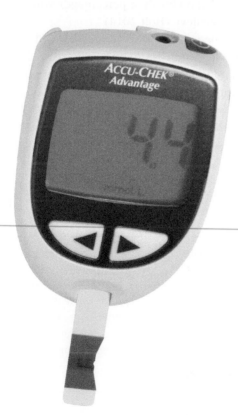

Figure 13.3 Advantage blood glucose meter by Roche. Source: Reproduced with permission of Roche Diagnostics.

Competency based training and comprehensive reading of the manufacturer's instructions regarding both the meter and the associated test strips are essential to ensure safe and accurate measurement. Many meters require daily quality assurance checks to guarantee accuracy of the readings and safety of the patients (Dougherty and Lister 2011) which should be accurately documented. Whitmore (2012), Wallymahmed (2013) and Dunning (2014) emphasise the need for education, training and quality control measures to ensure safe blood glucose monitoring and avoiding errors which can be fatal.

THINK ABOUT IT

Imagine that you are going to take your own blood sugar level. What anxieties would you have? If you can get permission to perform a blood glucose reading on yourself, how did it feel? Consider physical, emotional and psychological aspects.

Taking a blood glucose sample

When considering taking a blood glucose level there are certain contraindications that have been identified and these are listed in Box 13.3.

Box 13.3 Contraindications to blood glucose levels

- Peripheral circulatory failure and severe dehydration, for example, diabetic ketoacidosis, non-ketotic coma, shock and hypotension (low blood pressure). In these situations capillary blood glucose readings can be artificially low due to peripheral shut down (reduced blood to peripheral areas).
- Haematocrit (red blood cells) values: >55% may lead to inaccurate results if the blood glucose level is >11 mmol/l.
- Intravenous infusion of ascorbic acid.
- Some treatments for renal dialysis.
- Hyperlipidaemia (increased fat levels): cholesterol levels >13 mmol/l may lead to artificially raised capillary blood glucose readings.

It would not be expected that a healthcare assistant would identify these contraindications, but it may assist in explaining the treatment plans for some patients. Blood samples for glucose measurement can be capillary, venous or arterial (Dougherty and Lister 2011). Capillary blood is the blood obtained by using a lancing device and is described later. To obtain venous blood the patient would require blood to be taken from their veins (see Chapter 12), which would involve an invasive procedure. An arterial sample would be obtained if the patient has either a central line or similar in place, such as in an intensive care unit (ICU). Table 13.1 describes the procedure for taking a capillary blood sample to measure blood glucose.

Table 13.1 Procedure for taking blood glucose measurements using a capillary blood sample.

Action	Rationale
Before the procedure Collect the required equipment:	
• Blood glucose monitor – check that it is clean, has been calibrated for use with the test strips and has had the quality control test performed and documented (Dougherty and Lister 2011)	A clean meter will prevent cross-infection; follow local policy if it requires cleaning Calibration will ensure the meter is fit for purpose and gives accurate readings
• Test strips, ensure that they are in date and have not been exposed to air (Dougherty and Lister 2011)	To ensure accurate readings
• Single-use disposable finger-pricking device or lancets (MHPRA 2013; Dougherty and Lister 2011)	To prevent cross-infection
• Cotton wool or sterile gauze (Duning 2014)	To stop bleeding at site
• Sharps container	To prevent needlestick injury
The procedure	
1. Describe the procedure to the patient and gain consent Explain that some patients want to look away at the sight of a lancing device (Dougherty and Lister 2011)	To get cooperation from the patient, ensure that they understand the procedure fully Patient comfort and safety; some patients may faint when blood is taken (Dougherty and Lister 2011)
2. Ask the patient to wash and dry their hands with soap and water (Dougherty and Lister 2011)	Prevention of cross-infection (Dougherty and Lister 2011)
3. Position the patient comfortably – either lying down or sitting up	For patient comfort
4. Wash own hands and put on protective gloves and an apron (Wallymahmed 2007)	Prevention of infection
5. Massage the finger from its base to its tip to increase its perfusion (blood flow (Dunning 2014).	
6. Take blood from the side of the finger, using a site that has not been used recently, if possible (Figure 13.4) The finger may bleed without assistance (Figure 13.5) or may need to be milked to form a droplet of blood large enough to cover the test pad (Dougherty and Lister 2011)	As there are comparatively fewer nerve endings in the side rather than the tip of a finger it is less painful (Dunning 2014)
7. Some strips 'suck' blood up automatically, stopping when the correct volume is obtained whilst others may still require blood to be dropped onto the strip (Whitmore 2012)	
8. Read the blood glucose level from the machine, using it as per manufacturer's recommendation.	To provide an accurate reading
9. If there is not enough blood, prick the finger again with a new lancet ensuring the patient is fully informed and offer sympathy to the patient	To ensure accurate results by using disposables as intended by the manufacturer

Table 13.1 (*continued*)

Action	Rationale
After the procedure	
Immediately dispose of the lancet in the sharps box (Dougherty and Lister 2011)	To prevent sharps injury and cross-infection
Apply cotton wool or gauze, with pressure applied	To stop bleeding at the site
When the result is available document into patient's notes/blood glucose chart or patient records, informing the patient	Accurate recording of the results The patient may self-manage their condition and make adjustments themselves to the regimen (Holt 2014)
Inform the nurse in charge of any abnormal or unusual results (Holt 2014)	To allow further intervention if required
Assess the patient clinically, repeating the procedure if they do not appear to correlate (agree) with the results and report to nurse in charge	Incorrect reading, could result in inappropriate management
Dispose of waste as per local policy.	Prevent cross-infection
Observe site for further bleeding, applying further pressure to stop bleeding if necessary	To allow management of any further bleeding
Ensure the patient is comfortable and reassure if necessary	Patient comfort
Wash and dry hands	Prevent cross-infection

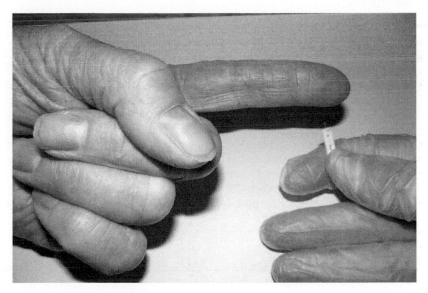

Figure 13.4 Site for blood glucose sampling.

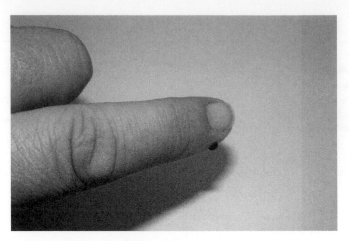

Figure 13.5 Blood specimen for blood glucose testing.

Usually the role of the healthcare assistant and/or AP will be to carry out the procedure following guidance from either nursing or medical staff. This will be based on many factors, some of which are detailed in Box 13.4.

THINK ABOUT IT

A patient with type 1 diabetes is having hip replacement surgery tomorrow. What factors do you think should be considered for this patient with regard to their diabetic control?

Box 13.4 Factors that influence how often blood glucose should be tested

- Patients with type 1 diabetes and people with type 2 diabetes using insulin need to test. Due to financial pressures in the NHS and conflicting research on the usefulness of self-monitoring in non-insulin treated type 2 diabetes, some Trusts have restricted the blood glucose strips to people using insulin (Whitmore 2012).
- The quantity and frequency of the patient's medication.
- The variance of the blood glucose level during the day, increasing if the variance is abnormal.
- If the patient is ill or under stress; this often results in patients who are in hospital requiring more frequent testing (Wallymahmed 2007).
- If dietary intake is altered or eating is prevented, for example fasting before a surgical procedure.
- If more exercise is taken than is normal for the patient.
- If medication has been altered.

Documentation

Results may be recorded in the patient's case notes, care pathway, the patient's own documents or, if an inpatient, on a specific blood glucose chart.

Table 13.2 Symptoms of hypoglycaemia.

Early onset	Severe symptoms
Tremor (Tortora and Derrickson 2011)	Mental disorientation/confusion
Nervousness/shaking (Tortora and Derrickson 2011)	Convulsions
Sweating (Tortora and Derrickson 2011)	Unconsciousness
Increased heart rate (tachycardia) (Tortora and Derrickson 2011)	Shock
Hunger (Tortora and Derrickson 2011)	
Drowsiness	
Abnormal speech (Dunning 2014)	

Hypoglycaemia

This is when the blood glucose level is <4.0 mmol/l, occurring with or without symptoms (Table 13.2). If it is not possible to test the blood glucose, but symptoms are experienced, immediate action (treatment) should be considered. It is sometimes abbreviated to 'hypo'.

Symptoms

The symptoms of hypoglycaemia occur when glucose levels drop, which triggers hormones that result in early onset symptoms. If left untreated it leads to severe symptoms (see Table 13.2).

The causes of hypoglycaemia can be varied and are shown in Box 13.5. These causes should be taught to patients because taking preventive steps could prevent hypoglycaemia occurring.

Box 13.5 Causes of hypoglycaemia

- Too much insulin or oral medication.
- More than the usual amount of exercise or activity.
- Changing the patient's insulin injection site (it is important to rotate sites regularly as overuse of an area may result in the site losing the ability to absorb insulin effectively). Increased uptake of glucose can also occur at a new site.
- Change of insulin schedule.
- Missing or postponing regular meals or eating less than normal.
- Liver failure (Dougherty and Lister 2011).
- Infection (Dougherty and Lister 2011).
- Insulin-secreting tumours (Dougherty and Lister 2011).
- Consuming alcohol.

To ensure patient safety and prevention of late symptoms, where possible treatment should be prompt. Table 13.3 gives the series of actions that should be undertaken, *but check local policy for any variations.*

Table 13.3 Treatment for hypoglycaemia.

Action	Rationale
1. Report to registered staff and/or medical staff	To alert other personnel of patient's condition
2. Assist in giving the patient fast acting glucose, or give on instruction from a registered nurse, without delay. Possible examples include three to six dextrose tables, a sweet soft drink (not diet), or three to five sugar lumps. Glucose gels may also be used	To increase patient's blood glucose
3. Test the patient's blood glucose level both immediately, and after 15 min	To assess if the glucose has entered the patient's bloodstream
If the patient's blood glucose has increased, and it is over an hour and a half until the patient's next meal, a sandwich, some fruit or biscuits, etc. may be given	If the patient eats too soon after the first dose of glucose it will delay the absorption of glucose into the bloodstream
4. If the level has not increased seek further advice	To decide on patient management that may include further glucose
5. Monitor the patient as directed	To ensure that the patient makes a full recovery

---

THINK ABOUT IT

If a patient is hypoglycaemic, explain what action you would take and why.

Hyperglycaemia

Hyperglycaemia is when blood glucose level is too high, usually >10 mmol/l of glucose. The symptoms are shown in Box 13.6.

Box 13.6 Symptoms of hyperglycaemia

- Increased urination.
- Ketones in urine.
- Increased thirst.
- Lethargy.
- Dehydration.
- Weight loss.
- Blurred vision.
- Cramps/weakness caused by excessive urination.
- Increased likelihood of infection.

As with hypoglycaemia the symptoms and causes of hyperglycaemia should be taught to the patient with a view to the patient taking preventive action.

Table 13.4 Treatment for hyperglycaemia.

Action	Rationale
1. Report to registered staff and/or medical staff	To alert other personnel of patient's condition
2. Insulin will be reviewed by medical staff and if prescribed will be administered. The healthcare assistant may assist with this	To reduce blood glucose levels
3. Test the patient's blood glucose level both immediately, and after 15 min	To determine blood glucose level
4. Encourage the patient to drink fluids	Prevent dehydration
5. Monitor the patient as directed	To ensure the patient makes a full recovery

The possible causes of hyperglycaemia are shown in Box 13.7. Hyperglycaemia can affect the patient's well-being and should be treated promptly. Table 13.4 gives the actions required for patients who are hyperglycaemic. *Please check with your local policy.*

THINK ABOUT IT

Go through the possible causes of hypo- and hyperglycaemia and give examples of how they may apply to patients in hospital.

Box 13.7 Possible causes of hyperglycaemia

- Untreated diabetes.
- Decreased mobility/reduction of physical activity.
- Infections/illness.
- Stress.
- Too much food.
- Insufficient medication.
- Overuse of injection sites/poor injection technique.
- Increase in weight.
- Insufficient insulin.
- The wrong type of food.

Common problems

Complications of diabetes

It is of vital importance for the patient with diabetes to have well-controlled blood glucose, because uncontrolled diabetes can lead to either short- or long-term complications. The physical long-term complications of diabetes are generally classified as: macrovascular disease; microvascular disease and neuropathy (Dunning 2014). Table 13.5 summarises some of the common complications.

Table 13.5 Complications of diabetes.

Complication	Type of disease
Macrovascular complications include:	Cardiovascular disease (e.g. heart attack), cerebrovascular disease (e.g. stroke) and peripheral vascular disease (disorders that affect blood vessels outside of the heart and brain known as 'hardening of the arteries') (Dunning 2014)
Microvascular disease includes:	Nephropathy (reduced renal function) damage to the small blood vessels cause damage to the kidneys, one of the main reasons for dialysis Retinopathy (ophthalmic (eye) problems) damage to small vessels that can lead to cataract formation and blindness
Neuropathy (nerve damage)	This can cause sensory deficits, particularly in the feet (Currie 2007b; Sewell 2007) and can increase the incidence of injury, ulcers and infections, resulting in poor circulation Peripheral damage mainly affects the feet and legs and autonomic which can lead to erectile dysfunction, delayed gastric emptying and hypoglycaemic unawareness (Dunning 2014)

Common problems in obtaining a blood glucose measurement

The problems associated with taking a blood glucose measurement can be divided into three areas: the patient, the equipment and technique.

The patient

If the patient has poor circulation, obtaining a sample can be more challenging. Keeping the hand warm can improve circulation and, if the fingers are massaged, this can increase blood flow (perfusion) to the site, allowing the capillaries to bleed more easily (Dougherty and Lister 2011; Dunning 2014). Where the skin has become hardened the patient should be discouraged from using alcohol gel to wash hands (this can also affect the blood glucose reading) (Dougherty and Lister 2011). If the patient is uncooperative with regard to the procedure, despite a full explanation, seek assistance because this may be the first sign of hypoglycaemia.

The equipment

It is essential that the machine be serviced and calibrated as per local policy to ensure that accurate results are obtained. If the machine displays an error code or is malfunctioning another machine should be used. Regular quality control checks are required of both the machine and the strips and these need to be documented (Dougherty and Lister 2011). The strips should be in date, have not been exposed to the air and calibrated for use with the specific machine being used (Dougherty and Lister 2011; Whitmore 2012). The lancets (finger-pricking devices) should be for single-patient use to prevent infection (MHPRA 2013;

Dougherty and Lister 2011). Competency based training with the machine should have been completed as per local policy (Whitmore 2014).

Technique

The site for obtaining a sample (as mentioned earlier) should be the side of the finger and, where possible, a site that has not been used recently to prevent damage. Due to the fact that there are comparatively fewer nerve endings in the side than the tip of the finger, this site is less painful (Dunning 2014). If the finger does not bleed it should be milked but not squeezed because this can give inaccurate results (Dougherty and Lister 2011; Wallymahmed 2007). It is essential that all staff performing this procedure should have had competency based training on the specific machine and accessories being used. When recording the blood glucose level, best practice is also to assess the patient's other observations to ensure that the result appears correct, reporting any concerns immediately. This is highly significant because inaccurate results can lead to mismanagement of patients and can be potentially life threatening.

Summary

Taking blood glucose levels provides important information that affects patient management. It is essential that quality control and good technique be mastered to ensure best practice. Care of the equipment should be followed in line with the manufacturer's guidelines, NICE (2004) and NICE (2009) guidelines, health and safety policy and local glucose monitoring policy and procedure. Where possible, if patients have previously been active in this procedure, they should be encouraged to continue self-care, especially for management of diabetes at home. As with all abnormal or unusual results, the healthcare assistant or assistant practitioner should report these immediately to the nurse in charge or medical staff and act according local policy. An example of competency framework for blood glucose measurement is shown in Table 13.6.

CASE STUDY 13.1

The blood glucose level of an acutely ill patient is taken. Instead of taking the current reading, a value from the previous patient is retrieved from the history function of the machine.
    What do you think are the implications of this error?

CASE STUDY 13.2

Ben is a 17-year-old boy who has taken his own blood glucose level. The level recorded is very high but he appears asymptomatic (he has no symptoms). You notice a bag of sweets on his locker.
    What explanation do you think may be applicable to this patient and what would be your planned actions?

Table 13.6 Competency – blood glucose monitoring.

Steps	First assessment/reassessment					Date/competent/ signature
	Demonstration					
	Date/sign 1	Date/sign 2	Date/sign 3	Date/sign 4	Date/sign 5	
Blood glucose monitoring						
1 Define the types of diabetes						
2 Describe the effect of insulin on the body						
3 Discuss conditions where a patient's blood glucose may require careful monitoring						
4 Identify the contraindications to blood glucose measurement						
5 State the normal range for blood glucose readings						
6 Identify signs and symptoms of hypoglycaemia						
7 Identify signs and symptoms of hyperglycaemia						
8 Discuss the equipment required to undertake this task						
9 Demonstrate an understanding of using appropriate calibration and quality control techniques and what checks should be made on the monitor before use						
10 Demonstrate the proper use of the equipment as laid down by the operating instructions and specifications and discuss the consequences of improper use						
11 Demonstrate that, before taking device to patient, the monitor is checked for the following: That one pack of strips is open and are in date, ensure that the monitor and the test strips have been calibrated together. Discuss the actions that would be taken if there was doubt about the quality of the strips						

12 Check that the quality control test has been carried out that day, when the batteries require changing, when opening new strips and any unusual, unpredicted result

13 Confirm that the quality control check has been recorded in the record book and signed

Blood glucose monitoring procedure	Demonstration					Date/competent/ signature
	1	2	3	4	5	
1 Demonstrate satisfactory explanations of the procedure to the patient						
2 Show awareness of preparation of site before blood sampling						
3 Demonstrate appropriate positioning of patient						
4 Demonstrate safe hand washing according to infection control policy						
5 Demonstrate procedure for safe practice in obtaining a blood sample from the patient to apply to the test pad						
6 Demonstrate safe disposal of lancet						
7 Demonstrate the proper use of the monitor as per individual manual and local policy						
8 Demonstrate the procedure for recording and reporting the result						
9 Show awareness of appropriate disposal of waste						
10 Demonstrate knowledge of care for the patient following the procedure						

Supervisors/Assessors:

Self-assessment		
Assessment	**Aspects**	**Achieved ✓**
Patient/Disease	*Have you considered all aspects of this section?* Types of diabetes and the role of the pancreas Signs and symptoms of diabetes Complications that can occur due to diabetes	
Procedure	*Have you considered all aspects of this section?* Selecting equipment and reasons for blood glucose measurement Technique required Normal values Recording and reporting concerns Safe disposal of sharps	**Achieved ✓**

References

Currie J (2007) Diabetic complications. *Scottish Nurse* 10(11): 28–29.

Dougherty L and Lister S (2011) *The Royal Marsden Hospital Manual of Clinical Nursing Procedures*, 8th edn. Oxford: Blackwell Publishing.

Dunning T (2014) *Care of People with Diabetes. A Manual of Nursing Practice*, 4th edn. Oxford: Wiley Blackwell.

Holt P (2014) Blood glucose monitoring in diabetes. *Nursing Standard* 28(27): 52–57.

Knip M and Simell O (2014) Environmental triggers in Type 1 Diabetes. *Cold Spring Harbour Perspectives in Medicine* 2(7). Available at: http://www.ncbi.nlm.nih.gov/pmc/articles/PMC3385937/ (accessed December 2015).

Laird E (2014) Blood glucose monitoring and management in acute stroke care. *Nursing Standard* 28(19): 52–56.

Marieb E N (2007) *Human Anatomy & Physiology. A Brief Atlas of the Human Body*. San Francisco; Harlow: Benjamin Cummings; Pearson.

Medicines and Healthcare Products Regulatory Agency (2013) *Single-Use Medical Devices: Implications and Consequences of Reuse*. London: Medicines and Healthcare Products Regulatory Agency.

Meier J and Bonadonna R (2013) Role of reduced b-cell mass versus impaired b-cell function in the pathogenesis of type 2 diabetes. *Diabetes Care* 36(2): S113–S116.

National Institute for Health and Clinical Excellence (NICE) (2004) *CG15. Diabetes: Type 1 Diabetes: Diagnosis and Management of Type 1 Diabetes in Children, Young people and Adults*. London: NICE. Available at: http://publications.nice.org.uk/type-1-diabetes-cg15 (accessed 28 February 2015).

National Institute for Health and Clinical Excellence (NICE) (2009) *Type 2 Diabetes: The Management* of Type 2 Diabetes. London: NICE. Available at: http://publications.nice.org.uk/type-1-diabetes-CG66 (accessed 28 February 2015).

Noble-Bell G and Cox A (2014) Management of diabetic ketoacidosis in adults. *Nursing Times* 110(10): 14–17.

Ritsinger V, Malmberg K, Mårtensson A, et al. (2014) Intensified insulin-based glycaemic control after myocardial infarction: mortality during 20 year follow-up of the randomised Diabetes Mellitus Insulin Glucose Infusion in Acute Myocardial Infarction (DIGAMI 1) trial. *The Lancet Diabetes & Endocrinology* 2(8): 627–633.

Rubin A (2008) *Diabetes for Dummies*, 3rd edn. London: Wiley Publishing, Inc.

Sewell J (2007) Diabetes: causes, complications and management. *British Journal of Healthcare Assistants* 1(1): 6–9.

Tan G (2011) The pancreas. *Anaesthesia & Intensive Care Medicine* 12(10): 469–472.

Thibodeau G A and Patton K T (2007) *Anatomy and Physiology*, 6th edn. Elsevier, MO: Mosby.

Thrower S L and Bingley P J (2014) What is type 1 diabetes? Diabetes basic facts. *Medicine* 42(12): 682–686.

Tortora G J and Derrickson B (2014) *Principles of Anatomy and Physiology*, 13th edn. Hoboken, NJ: John Wiley & Sons Inc.

Wallymahmed M (2007) Capillary blood glucose monitoring. *Nursing Standard* 21(38): 35.

Wallymahmed M (2013) Encouraging people with diabetes to get the most from blood glucose monitoring: Observing and acting upon blood glucose patterns. *Journal of Diabetes Nursing* 17: 6–13

Whitmore C (2012) Blood glucose monitoring: an overview. *British Journal of Nursing* 21(10): 58–62.

World Health Organisation (WHO) (2015) Diabetes Fact Sheet No 31 (online). Available at: http://www.who.int/mediacentre/factsheets/fs312/en/ (accessed 14 February 2015)

CHAPTER 14

Fluid balance and intravenous maintenance

LEARNING OBJECTIVES

- Define fluid balance and its importance to nursing practice
- Discuss the body's response to changes in fluid balance
- List the instances when intravenous (IV) fluids are necessary
- Describe how to prime (run through) an IV line
- Describe how to discontinue an IV line
- Identify the common problems with IV administration via gravity infusion sets

Aim of this chapter

This chapter will focus upon the importance of maintaining and monitoring a patient's fluid balance in the clinical environment and the potential need for intravenous (IV) fluids via a peripheral cannula.

To revise the anatomy and physiology of the placement of a cannula, please refer to Chapter 16. Fluids administered by the subcutaneous route are not covered.

Reasons for monitoring fluid balance

Maintaining the balance within the volume and composition of body fluids is essential to health (Tortora and Derrickson 2011). An imbalance in fluid and electrolyte levels can cause changes to a patient's clinical condition and subsequently increase their MEWS score (Shepherd 2011).

Related anatomy and physiology

The total body water for adults is about 60% of the body weight, with a higher percentage in young people and adults of below-average weight (Waugh and

Clinical Skills for Healthcare Assistants and Assistant Practitioners, Second Edition.
Angela Whelan and Elaine Hughes.
© 2016 John Wiley & Sons, Ltd. Published 2016 by John Wiley & Sons, Ltd.

Table 14.1 Regulator of fluid balance.

Organ	Role in fluid balance
Kidneys	If the kidneys reabsorb more water, fluid will remain in the body and prevent loss. This would result in the patient passing concentrated urine
Hypothalamus/Pituitary gland	If there is a reduction in blood volume, e.g. haemorrhage (blood loss) the body will respond by trying to restore normal fluid levels. It does this by releasing the hormone antidiuretic hormone (ADH), which, after being made in the hypothalamus, is released from the posterior pituitary gland. ADH increases the reabsorption of water and therefore increases the circulating blood volume
Adrenal cortex	Reabsorption of sodium is an important part of fluid balance and aldosterone is a hormone secreted to regulate both the reabsorption of sodium and water

Adapted from Dougherty and Coote (2006).

Grant 2010; Tortora and Derrickson 2011). Older people have a reduced amount of water, whereas in infants it is around 75%. Women also tend to have slightly lower water content than men (Thibodeau and Patton 2009). These differences in total body water volume account for the different percentages of lean body tissue. As water isn't stored in fat cells, men and people across the lifespan with greater lean body mass have a higher percentage of total body water compared to women who genetically have more fat cells.

Dougherty and Coote (2006) describe a number of regulators that work together to maintain fluid balance (Table 14.1).

The body's required input can be provided by the patient drinking or eating (as some foods contain fluids) or, after medical intervention and insertion of a cannula, subcutaneous or IV fluids. Excretion is sustained through not only urine output but also insensible losses such as sweating, breathing and faeces, which contribute to small fluid losses (Tortora and Derrickson 2011).

The body is in balance when the required amounts of water and solutes (dissolved substances) are present and are correctly proportioned among the various compartments (Tortora and Derrickson 2011). The body keeps fluid levels constant when water loss equals water gain (Tortora and Derrickson 2011). This is termed homeostasis. Here the body is said to be maintaining its constant internal environment through its own controls, which allows it to return to normal parameters when there has been a change to its balance (Clancy and McVicar 2009). An imbalance in homeostasis can cause problems for some patients and is often associated with diseases, such as renal (kidney) or cardiac (heart) problems. Figure 14.1 shows how the body reacts to a stimulus that caused a decreased volume of fluid in the body. In some very unwell patients a central venous

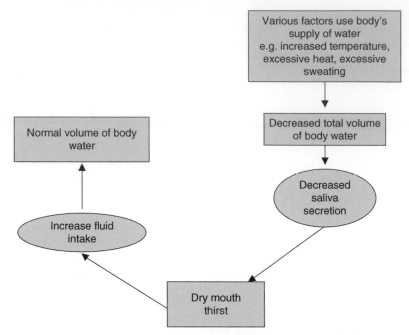

Figure 14.1 Fluid regulation in the body. Source: Thibodeau 2009. Reproduced with permission of Elsevier.

pressure (CVP) line may be inserted into a large vessel where the tip of the cannula sits in the right atrium (top chamber) of the heart to determine the amount of fluid contained within the body. Because of the dangers associated with CVP line insertion, these are always placed by medical staff and the monitoring of this observation is currently the role of a registered nurse (Cole 2007).

Body fluids are distributed within two compartments in the body known as extracellular and intracellular. Extracellular fluid, also called interstitial fluid, can be found outside the cells, consisting of fluids in the blood, lymphatic system (a system that fights infection), spinal fluid (cerebrospinal (CSF)) and fluid that bathes body cells. Intracellular fluid is contained within cells (Waugh and Grant 2010) and both the intracellular and extracellular compartments are separated by a plasma membrane that allows the fluids to move through the compartments (Tortora and Derrickson 2011).

Electrolytes

These are particles that have a positive or negative charge attached to them, and they play an essential role in the body because they control the movement of water between body fluid compartments (Thibodeau and Patton 2009). Patients who have an imbalance in the blood's electrolytes can develop fluid imbalance (Mooney 2007). Examples of some common electrolytes are shown in Box 14.1.

Box 14.1 Common electrolytes in the body

Na$^+$: sodium
Cl$^-$: chloride
K$^+$: potassium
Ca^{2+}: calcium
Mg^{2+}: magnesium

THINK ABOUT IT

Ask to view a patient's blood results and look at the electrolytes contained in the blood. There will be a list of the 'normal' values to which you can compare the results. Identify if they are normal or abnormal. Can you think why this might be? Discuss your thoughts with a registered nurse or a doctor in your clinical area

Related aspects and terminology

- *Hypovolaemia*: loss of fluid (Mooney 2007).
- *Hypervolaemia*: fluid overload (Mooney 2007).
- *Electrolytes*: negatively or positively charged particles within the body.
- *Extracellular*: fluid outside cells.
- *Intracellular*: fluid contained in or around cells.

Hypovolaemia/dehydration

The term 'dehydration' is used to describe the condition that results from excessive loss of body water and electrolytes (Thibodeau and Patton 2009).

Causes of dehydration

- Gastrointestinal problems that cause fluid loss are commonly vomiting and diarrhoea (Tortora and Derrickson 2011). These can be sudden onset and have rapid effects on fluid loss, particularly in vulnerable patient groups such as babies and older people. Some chronic diseases can also cause these symptoms, for example ulcerative colitis (inflammation of the bowel) or irritable bowel syndrome. Patients with a high output ileostomy can also be vulnerable to fluid losses and need to replace lost fluids to prevent dehydration.
- Where there is a reduced oral input, this can be due to altered mental state, for example dementia, depression or where the patient may have a reduced consciousness level or is required to lie flat (Tortora and Derrickson 2011). In such instances the role of the healthcare assistant may be to ensure that the patient is assisted to take regular drinks. Where patients have poor or reduced mobility it is essential to ensure that fluids are within easy reach. Localised problems

in the mouth may also affect the patient's desire to drink because it may cause further discomfort and this should be reported to the nurse in charge.

- Environment can also contribute to a reduced oral input, for example lack of water in a hot climate (Thibodeau and Patton 2009).
- Excessive urination (passing urine) may be due to diuretic medication (encourages increased urine output) with less absorption occurring in the kidneys (Mooney 2007). If fluid balance is being monitored, giving the patient a bed pan or bottle if they are in a care environment to measure urine output can be successful in recording an accurate output. If the patient has mobility problems, ensuring that they are near a toilet after the diuretic medication can reduce any anxiety and prevent incidents of incontinence.
- Any disease or condition that alters fluid loss can cause dehydration, such as haemorrhage, severe burns, diabetes, acute renal failure or gastroenteritis (Marieb and Hoehn 2007).

Signs and symptoms of dehydration

- Changes to cognitive function.
- Muscle weakness, headaches and fatigue.
- Skin that is less elastic, which is sometimes referred to as 'turgor'.
- Poor urine output, which will also be dark in colour.
- Thirst, leading to dry lips and tongue (Campbell 2011; Shepherd 2011).
- Severe dehydration can lead to clinical signs of low blood pressure (hypotension); fast pulse (tachycardia), which can become weak and thready; and cold hands and feet, as the circulating blood is diverted to the major organs (Shepherd 2011).

Treatment

Medical and nursing staff should treat the cause of dehydration; for example, if the patient is vomiting they can be give an anti-emetic (anti-sickness medication) to try to rectify the problem or if the patient is dehydrated following surgery it may be appropriate to supplement their oral intake with IV fluids.

Monitoring and recording the patient's intake and output may be essential to promote recovery for some patients and fluid balance charts can provide vital clues to the patient's level of hydration.

Hypervolaemia (excess fluid)

This is an excess of fluid in the body.

Cause

- Over-infusion of intravenous fluids.
- Congestive cardiac failure, renal (kidney) failure, cirrhosis of the liver due to the kidneys retaining large amounts of sodium and water (Thibodeau and Patton 2009).

Signs and symptoms of excess fluid

- Weight gain.
- Oedema (excess fluid in tissues).
- Breathlessness, which is often made worse when lying flat.
- Increased pulse rate.
- Lung problems – congestion where breathing can sound crackly.
  (Adapted from McMillen and Pitcher 2011.)

Treatment

- Once medical and nursing staff identify the underlying cause, treat it; for example, if the patient has had too much IV fluid, the regimen should be reviewed by medical and nursing staff, and it is essential that any IV infusion is closely monitored.
- If prescribed, assist – if this is in line with your workplace policy – in giving diuretic medication that will promote excretion of fluid from the kidneys, resulting in an increased urine output. Accurate recording of the urine output on fluid balance charts is essential for monitoring the patient's condition

  If a person steadily consumes more water than the kidneys can excrete, water intoxication can occur, which results in the cells within the body swelling dangerously; this can result in death (Tortora and Derrickson 2011).

Fluid balance charts

Fluid balance charts are used to monitor the patient's input and output, and are an important aspect of care, particularly with ill patients. Failure to maintain fluid balance can cause dehydration and can seriously affect the health of patients (Begum and Johnson 2010). Figure 14.2 shows an example of a fluid balance chart. When calculating total losses or gains over a 24-hour period, insensible losses (fluid loss that cannot be directly measured, such as perspiration etc.) should also be considered. For patients with high temperatures or with lung conditions that cause rapid breathing, the increase in insensible losses can lead to dehydration if fluid is not replaced.

The role of the healthcare assistant involves completing the fluid balance chart accurately, therefore training should be undertaken to ensure that the correct information is recorded, given its importance in patient management. Reid et al. (2004) suggest that mandatory education for fluid balance should be incorporated within local training programmes for all staff, to overcome the problems of incomplete charts. Involving patients in completion can be very useful to promote accuracy and can reduce workload for the nursing team (Chung et al. 2002). Box 14.2 shows the potential problems in fluid balance chart completion.

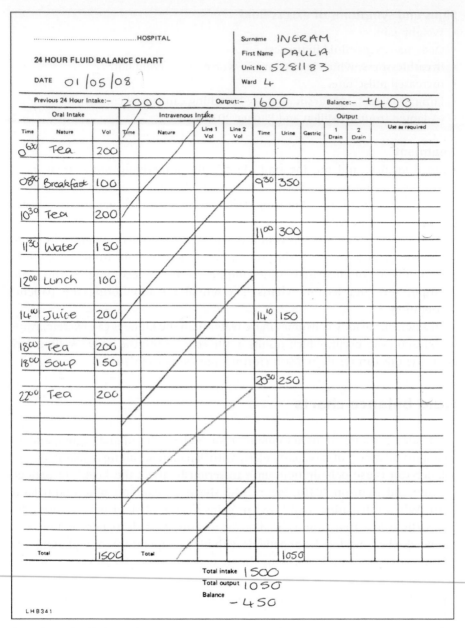

Figure 14.2 Fluid balance chart. Source: NHS Lothian 2008. Reproduced with permission of NHS Lothian.

> **Box 14.2** Potential problems in fluid balance chart completion
>
> - Chart not completed at all.
> - Inaccurate volumes entered, e.g. sips/??? or wet pad/used toilet (Reid et al. 2004).
> - Staff unaware of the volumes in cups/glasses, etc. and estimate wrongly.
> - Patient forgets to measure output.
> - Patient cannot remember input.
> - Patient may be unable to give a history due to previous cerebrovascular accident (stroke) or dementia.
> - Domestic staff remove cups without alerting staff to volume consumed.

In 2007, the NPSA highlighted the importance of hydration in preventing patients from becoming ill (NPSA 2007a). Because of the potential difficulties in monitoring and maintaining fluid balance, some NHS Trusts have implemented hydration care bundles (East of England NHS Trust 2011) to assist both staff and patients in understanding the importance of assessing, planning and monitoring fluid balance. This care bundle allows patients to have input in closely monitoring their hydration and also acts as an educational tool for both staff and patients, thus reducing the risks of dehydration whilst in hospital care. Although this is directed at the hospitalised patient, this has the ability to be adapted for care in other environments helping to reduce the risk of dehydration to all patients.

The intravenous route

When IV fluids would be commenced:
- Patient is nil by mouth, for example before or after surgery.
- Medication is only available in this form.
- Where the patient is feeling nauseous and not taking oral fluids.
- Where the patient is vomiting, so medication cannot be absorbed in the gut.
- To assist in fluid balance maintenance or correct dehydration.
- To correct electrolyte imbalance.

IV fluids are delivered by a cannula inserted into a vein (Figure 14.3; see Chapter 16). Cannulation involves direct entry into the circulatory system and is a route for infection (Lavery and Ingram 2006). Great care must therefore be taken to prevent infection, and this would involve only touching the cannula/IV

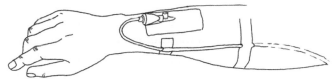

Figure 14.3 Cannula with intravenous line attached.

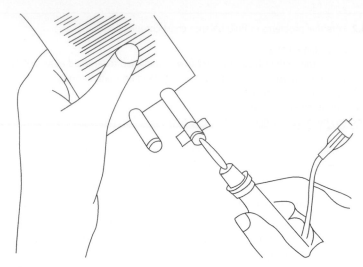

Figure 14.4 Spiking an IV bag.

line when necessary. Preventing equipment coming into contact with potentially harmful organisms can be maximised by using the aseptic or non-touch technique (Rowley 2001). If the healthcare assistant's role involves dealing with IV lines, training and competency in this skill is required.

Priming an IV line

Before administering fluid via the intravenous route the nurse must first fill the line with fluid (primed) to prevent air entering the patient's circulatory system, which could lead to an air embolus (NPSA 2007b; Younger and Kahn 2008). This is important as air emboli, in large volumes, can lead to cardiac arrest. The line, sometimes also referred to as an IV set, comes packed in a sterile pack to prevent infection. Table 14.2 describes the procedure for priming an IV line.

Priming the line should be undertaken only if local policy allows, and when competency training in both aseptic technique and the actual task has been undertaken.

Flushing an IV line

If an IV cannula is in place but is being used only intermittently, often fluid (e.g. sodium chloride or 'saline') will be introduced to keep the line patent (free from blockages). This is known as 'flushing the line'. The administration of IV medication is currently a post-registration role and therefore flushing before, between and after medicine – also seen as good practice – is performed by the registered nurse (National Institute for Health and Clinical Excellence (NICE) 2003; NPSA 2007b). However, it is anticipated that this may change in the future. Where

Table 14.2 The procedure for priming an intravenous (IV) line.

Action	Rationale
1. Ensure that the registered nurse has checked that IV fluid has been prescribed, and not already given. Two practitioners should have checked this, because it is by the IV route Check the IV fluid, ensuring that it is clear, so has no contamination or debris and that in date	Administration of medicines is the role of the registered nurse (Nursing and Midwifery Council (NMC) 2008) IV fluid fit for purpose and within expiry date
2. Collect all other equipment: administration set, gloves/apron, receptacle for any discarded fluid, drip stand, air inlet if the container is glass or rigid, alcohol swab	To ensure that the process can be done timely
3. Wash hands, put on gloves and apron. Where possible undertake procedure in sterile environment, e.g. clinical treatment room in the hospital	Prevent cross-contamination
4. Read the instructions on the IV line packaging, including expiry date if applicable Remove the line from outer packaging and close the roller clamp. Remove the IV fluid from outer bag if applicable	All outward packaging removed
5. Remove the seal on the IV bag where the trocar (spike) will be inserted Insert the trocar into the bag taking care not to spike and puncture the bag (Figure 14.4)	Mis-spiking the bag will allow entry for microorganisms and potentially could cause sharps injury
6. Squeeze the drip chamber at the top to fill around half to two-thirds full (check manufacturer's recommendation) (Figure 14.5)	Some manufacturers' sets may have specific instructions
7. Slowly open the roller clamp allowing the fluid to flow down the IV line	Slow priming of the line will reduce the amount of air in the line
8. Close the roller clamp when the fluid has filled the line completely and come out the end (Figure 14.6)	To expel all air from the line
9. The line is now filled with fluid and ready for connection to the patient. Place a sterile cap over the end ready for connection to the patient	Sterile cap prevents contamination of the line before it is connected to the patient

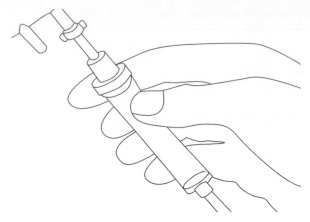

Figure 14.5 Filling the drip chamber.

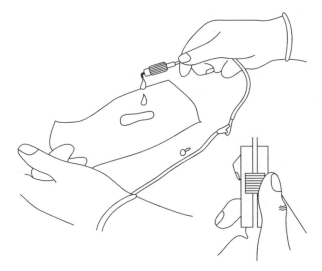

Figure 14.6 Priming the IV line.

this role is permitted in the future it should only be performed by healthcare assistants under local protocols and after competency based training, including aseptic technique.

As mentioned, the medicine used for flushing peripheral lines is usually 0.9% sodium chloride, provided that this does not react with other medications being administered via this route. The volume should be equal to twice the volume of the cannula plus any additional devices, such as needle-free connectors (Royal College of Nursing (RCN) 2010). The recognised technique is a pulsated push–pause (stop–start, stop–start), which creates turbulence with the cannula, removing debris from its internal wall (NHS Grampian 2010).

Care of the cannula

Refer to Chapter 16; however, a summary of care is as follows:
- The cannula site should be inspected regularly to identify potential problems promptly. Phlebitis refers to inflammation of a vein and the use of Visual Infusion Phlebitis (VIP) scales are useful in assessing the need for the removal of the cannula (RCN 2010). Although a healthcare assistant would not necessarily be expected to complete this, having an awareness of its importance in clinical practice is useful in maintaining patient safety. An awareness of this will guide the healthcare assistant in observing the cannula site and reporting its appearance to a registered nurse as appropriate.
- Whenever dealing with an intravenous infusion or a cannula, good handwashing practices and the use of sterile gloves are essential to prevent infection. Always follow your employer's policies over the dressings used for cannulas in your area; and whenever dressings are used it is essential that these do not prevent observation of the cannula or prevent flow of the solution or occlude the vessel in any way (RCN 2010).

Discontinuing an IV infusion

Discontinuing an infusion requires the line to be clamped off (by closing off the roller clamp and then removing it (Figure 14.7)). Disconnection at the cannula

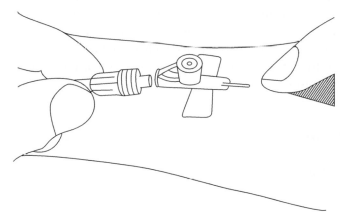

Figure 14.7 Discontinuing an IV line.

Table 14.3 Procedure to discontinue an intravenous infusion.

Action	Rationale
1. Explain the procedure to the patient and obtain verbal consent	To ensure that patient understands and cooperates. Consent for legal purposes
2. Gather all necessary equipment, which includes: gloves, sterile cap, clinical waste bag and sharps bin	To promote safe and efficient removal
3. Close roller clamp on IV line Put on gloves and apron	To prevent spillage of fluid Gloves prevent cross-infection
4. Open sterile cap and place carefully ensuring aseptic technique. Ensure that within easy reach	Prevents contamination
5. Remove IV line carefully (Figure 14.7) asking the patient to elevate the arm upwards if the cannula is in the back of the hand. Application of some light pressure over the cannula (where the cannula enters the vein) can also prevent bleeding (Figure 14.7)	To prevent blood spillage
6. Attach sterile cap	Ensures line is capped off securely
7. Wash hands, dispose of all equipment as per policy	Prevents infection
8. Observe site	To identify any problems with the site
9. Document removal in the patient's notes	Provides a legal record

requires competency in aseptic technique (discussed earlier), and a sterile cap to be applied where the line previously entered the cannula. However, as the role of the healthcare assistant is to monitor fluid balance, it is essential that this is recorded on the fluid balance chart, especially if the infusion is discontinued while there is still fluid in the bag. Understanding the reason for the infusion is important as this can guide the care you provide after removal of the cannula. For example, if the infusion had been in place to keep the patient hydrated whilst nil by mouth, the patient may then need advice and assistance in drinking fluids to ensure hydration. Table 14.3 details the procedure for discontinuing an intravenous infusion (IVI).

Common problems

Despite IV administration being a qualified nursing task, the role of the healthcare assistant may include ensuring that the infusion is running and there are no complications, if competent to do so. As mentioned earlier, patients may well report symptoms of pain, discomfort, swelling or leakage to the healthcare assistant first.

IV infusions can be delivered via infusion devices or by a gravity infusion set (as seen previously). Infusion devices should be used only by individuals who have had competency based training on their use, with local policy dictating which staff are permitted to be involved in this aspect of care. When an infusion device is being used, the role of the healthcare assistant may be to alert staff to infusion problems, which may have resulted from either the patient reporting problems or the alarm on the pump being activated.

A standard gravity set is used for fluid administration, with specialised blood sets for blood and blood products. Table 14.4 details the common problems, presentation and actions that should be taken in relation to gravity infusion sets.

In some instances, the registered nurse may delegate the task to close the roller clamp on the infusion line to a healthcare assistant, but this should only be done when instructed to do so and under local protocol or policy.

Summary

Fluid balance is an important aspect of patient care, which can lead to serious clinical problems where there is an imbalance. The healthcare assistant's role may involve encouraging and recording oral fluids and reporting potential problems where the patient is receiving fluids by the IV route. The healthcare assistant can also assist in monitoring the output either by recording when the patient goes to the toilet or through care of indwelling catheters. The healthcare assistant is often the first person to witness or deal with problems regarding IV infusions, but any interaction must be underpinned by a strong knowledge base and competency based training in accordance with local policies and procedures.

Tables 14.5 and 14.6 are competency frameworks for recording fluid balance and IV maintenance.

CASE STUDY 14.1

Mrs Jones, who is 88 years old, has been admitted to correct dehydration. Her IV infusion has now been discontinued. What is the role of the healthcare assistant in ensuring that a correct fluid balance is both maintained and recorded?

CASE STUDY 14.2

Mr Bob Mills is a 49 year old who has had prostate surgery. He has an intravenous infusion running and is complaining of pain at the site. Describe the actions that you would take.

Table 14.4 Common problems with gravity infusion sets.

Problem	Presentation	Action
The infusion has stopped dripping **Causes:** • Cannula may be blocked • The infusion bag needs to be elevated • The infusion is switched off	No drips evident in the chamber	Inform nurse in charge
The infusion is not running to time **Causes:** • The patient may have interfered with the infusion • The cannula may allow only intermittent flow depending on the position of the patient's arm • The rate has been set incorrectly.	The infusion bag appears to have a volume that is not consistent with the planned infusion duration	Inform nurse in charge
The dressing is not clean, dry and secure **Causes:** • The infusion may have leaked • The patient has caused contamination of the dressing • The patient may have interfered with the infusion	Dressing visually contaminated or dislodged	Change dressing if competent to do so; report
The patient reports pain or wetness at the cannula site (see also Chapter 16) **Causes:** • The IV may have leaked • An acute inflammation of the vein has occurred due to the presence of the cannula, known as phlebitis (Jackson 1998) • Infiltration or extravasation has occurred. This involves leakage of medication into the surrounding tissues. • The classification is linked to the type of medication that has caused the leakage (Ingram and Lavery 2005)	Dressing is wet. Site is painful	Report to nurse in charge. Stop infusion

Table 14.5 Competency framework: record clinical observations (fluid balance).

Steps	First assessment/reassessment					Date/competent/signature
	Demonstration					
	Date/sign 1	Date/sign 2	Date/sign 3	Date/sign 4	Date/sign 5	
Fluid balance						
1 List the two fluid compartments in the body						
2 Describe how the body controls fluid balance						
3 Discuss the symptoms of dehydration/hypervolaemia (excess) fluid						
4 Demonstrate how to complete a fluid balance chart						

Table 14.6 Competency framework: record clinical observations (intravenous (IV) maintenance, including priming and discontinuing an infusion (IVI)).

Steps	First assessment/reassessment					Date/competent/signature
	Demonstration					
	Date/sign 1	Date/sign 2	Date/sign 3	Date/sign 4	Date/sign 5	
IV maintenance						
1 Describe the instances where the IV route is required						
2 Explain why aseptic technique is important when dealing with the IV route						
3 Demonstrate the correct procedure for priming (running through) an IV line						
4 Demonstrate the correct procedure for discontinuing an IV line						
5 Discuss the common problems associated with the IV route, giving the actions expected from a healthcare assistant						

Self-assessment		
Assessment	**Aspects**	**Achieved ✓**
Patient	*Have you considered all aspects of this section?* Describe the regulators that maintain fluid balance in the body The role of electrolytes in the body The symptoms of dehydration/over hydration	
Procedure(s)	*Have you considered all aspects of this section?* Maintaining and recording on fluid balance charts Priming an IV line Common problems with gravity infusion lines Discontinuing an IV line	**Achieved ✓**

References

Begum M and Johnson C S (2010) A review of the literature on dehydration in the institution-alized elderly. *The European e-Journal of Clinical Nutrition and Metabolism* 5(1): e47–e53.

Chung L H, Chong S and French P (2002) The efficiency of fluid balance charting: an evidence based management project. *Journal of Nursing Management* 10(2): 103–113.

Campbell N (2011) Dehydration: Why is it still a problem? *Nursing Times* 107(22): 12–15.

Clancy J and McVicar A (2009) *Physiology and Anatomy for Nurses and Healthcare Practitioners*, 3rd edn. London: Hodder Arnold.

Cole E (2007) Measuring central venous pressure. *Nursing Standard* 22(7): 40–42.

Dougherty B and Coote S (2006) Fluid balance monitoring as part of track and trigger. *Nursing Times* 102(45): 28–29.

East of England NHS Trust (2011) *Adult Intelligent Fluid Management Bundle*. Cambridgeshire: NHS.

Ingram P and Lavery I (2005) Peripheral intravenous therapy: key risks and implications for practice. *Nursing Standard* 19(46): 55–64.

Jackson A (1998) Infection control: a battle in vein; infusion phlebitis. *Nursing Times* 94(4): 68–71.

Lavery I and Ingram, P (2006) Prevention of infection in peripheral intravenous devices. *Nursing Standard* 20(49): 49–58.

Marieb E N and Hoehn K (2007) *Human Anatomy and Physiology*, 7th edn. San Francisco, CA: Pearson Benjamin Cummings.

Mooney G P (2007) Fluid balance. *Nursing Times*. Available at: www.nursingtimes.net/ntclinical/Fluid&uscore;balance.html (accessed 16 October 2008).

National Institute for Health and Clinical Excellence (NICE) (2003) *Infection Control: Prevention of Healthcare-associated Infection in Primary and Community Care. Clinical Guidelines 2*. London: NICE.

NHS Lothian (2008) *Fluid Balance Chart*. Edinburgh: NHS Lothian.

NHS Grampian (2010) *Patient Group Direction for the Administration of Sodium Chloride 0.9% injection for flushing intravenous catheters/cannulae by certified healthcare professionals working within NHS Grampian, Scotland*. Edinburgh: NHS Grampian.

NPSA (2007a) *Water for Health: Hydration Best Practice Toolkit for Hospitals and Healthcare*, London: NPSA.

NPSA (2007b) *Promoting Safer Use of Injectable Medicines*, Alert No. 2007/20, 28th March. NPSA, London.

Nursing and Midwifery Council (NMC) (2008) *Standards for Medicines Management*. London: NMC.

Royal College of Nursing (RCN) (2010) *Standards for Infusion Therapy*, 3rd edn. London: RCN.

Reid J, Robb E, Stone D, et al. (2004) Improving the monitoring and assessment of fluid balance. *Nursing Times* 100(20): 36–39.

Rowley S (2001) Aseptic non-touch technique. *Nursing Times* 97(7): 6.

Sheppherd A (2011) Measuring and managing fluid balance. *Nursing Times* 107(28): 12–16.

Thibodeau G A and Patton K T (2009) *Anatomy and Physiology*, 7th edn. St Louis, MO: Mosby.

Tortora G J and Derrickson B (2011) *Principles of Anatomy and Physiology*, 13th edn. Hoboken, NJ: Wiley & Sons.

Waugh A and Grant A (2010) *Ross and Wilson Anatomy and Physiology in Health and Illness*, 11th edn. Edinburgh: Churchill Livingstone.

Younger G and Khan M (2008) Setting up and priming an intravenous infusion. *Nursing Standard* 22(40): 40–44.

SECTION III
Complex clinical skills

CHAPTER 15

Medicines

LEARNING OBJECTIVES

- Clearly identify the role and accountability of healthcare assistants and assistant practitioners in administration of medicines

- Identify the main components of the Medicine Act that have an impact on the role of the healthcare assistant and assistant practitioner

- Identify the circumstances where nurses can prescribe medication

- Identify the common routes and considerations for administration of medicines with which healthcare assistants and assistant practitioners may assist

- Discuss the circumstances where healthcare assistants and assistant practitioners may check medications

---

Aim of this chapter

A medication is a substance administered for the diagnosis, cure, treatment or therapeutic relief of a symptom or for prevention of disease. In healthcare, the words medication and drug are used interchangeably (Dougherty and Lister 2011).

The role of healthcare assistants and assistant practitioners in relation to medicine administration

The role of healthcare assistants and assistant practitioners in medicine administration is currently under the delegation of a registered nurse who will take accountability for this task (see Chapter 15). This is identified in the Nursing and Midwifery Council (NMC) (2010) Standards for Medicine Management, which set standards for safe practice in the management and administration of medicines by registered nurses, midwives and specialist community public health nurses. The NMC (2010) acknowledge the administration of medicine

---

Clinical Skills for Healthcare Assistants and Assistant Practitioners, Second Edition.
Angela Whelan and Elaine Hughes.
© 2016 John Wiley & Sons, Ltd. Published 2016 by John Wiley & Sons, Ltd.

is not solely a mechanistic task but one that requires thought and the exercise of professional judgement.

The legal limitations and boundaries for medication administration by HCAs and APs is exacerbated by the lack of regulation and registration as well as the incredible diversity of the roles that often include tasks previously considered the domain of the registered professional.

O'Flannaghan (2014) expresses the notion that registration by an independent regulatory body would no doubt give more credibility, especially to the role of the AP, and win confidence from other staff in delegating certain tasks. It would also provide a framework for legal boundaries and possibly give scope for further future development of the role, especially in relation to medication.

This chapter focuses on some of the issues surrounding medicine administration, but local policies will dictate accepted local practice, especially as these roles continue to advance and develop.

Types of medicines

Different classifications of medicines are defined by the Medicines Act 1968, including the following three classification categories provided here.

Prescription-only medicines (POMs)
These are medicinal products that may be supplied, including sold, to a patient on the instruction of a doctor/dentist supplementary prescriber or nurse/pharmacist as an independent prescriber.

Pharmacy-only medicines (Ps)
These are medications that do not require a prescription but can be purchased only from a registered pharmacy, with the sale being supervised by a pharmacist, for example cough medicines.

General sales list medicines (GSLs)
These include all medications that can be bought by the public, for example in supermarkets, and do not require either supervision of a pharmacist or a prescription, for example paracetamol. However, in a hospital setting there is control over these medications and patients cannot take these without prior consultation with medical and nursing staff.

> **THINK ABOUT IT**
>
> Consider the above categories of medicines and give an example of each. If you are unsure, you could take a trip to a supermarket with a pharmacy department and view what is out on the shelves (thus not requiring a pharmacist to be present), and the medications that are behind the counter (requiring a pharmacist to be present). For a prescription-only medication this needs to be prescribed by an approved person either in the community or hospital setting and could be medication for yourself, a family member or a patient.

Medication prescribing and legal aspects

The Medicines Act of 1968 was prompted in part by the consequences of thalidomide in the 1960s. This Act states that only authorised healthcare practitioners can legally prescribe medicines in the UK.

With the evolution of healthcare and the findings of the Crown Reports (1989 and 1992), it was firmly established that there could be significant benefits to nurses having prescribing rights. These rights were extended, initially only to community nurses through the Medicinal Products: Prescription by Nurses Act (1992), then later to nurses and midwives in all aspects of care. More recently, it now includes pharmacists, physiotherapists, chiropodists, podiatrists, optometrists and radiographers; referred to as non-medical prescribers.

In order to enable nurses, midwives and allied health professionals to prescribe legally, this legislation has had to be extended several times. The Amendments to the Prescription Only Medicines (Human Use) Order (2005) is the most recent change enabling the further development of non-medical prescribing.

The Medicines Act (1968) also provides all prescribers with a framework for what medicines require a prescription, and what medicines are available to the public without a prescription and under what circumstances. It outlines the three different categories of medicine.

A brief over view of prescribing legislation in Scotland

Following extensive consultation, nurse and midwifery prescribing was implemented in Scotland in 1996. In 2003 the Health and Social Care Act introduced a new category of prescriber – the supplementary prescriber. Since 2003, legislation has further been amended to extend the powers of supplementary prescribing for nurses, midwifes and pharmacists of all controlled drugs and unlicensed medications. In April 2005, supplementary prescribing was introduced for physiotherapists, chiropodists, podiatrists, radiographers and optometrists.

In May 2006, legislation was amended to extend the independent prescribing powers of nurses and midwives in Scotland to all licensed medication and some controlled drugs.

'Controlled drugs' are, as the name suggests, the most tightly controlled medicines available. The Misuse of Drugs Regulations (2001) set out the requirements for obtaining, storing, prescribing, record keeping and supply (NES 2015).

Any qualified and registered independent prescriber may prescribe all prescription-only medicines for all medical conditions, with some nurse independent prescribers also able to prescribe some controlled drugs (NMC 2010). Supplementary prescribers can prescribe where there is a management plan for the patient, provided that an arrangement with the doctor or dentist and the patient has been formulated (NMC 2010).

Nurses and midwives who have recorded their medication qualification on the NMC register fall into two categories (NMC 2010): practitioner nurse prescribers, where they can prescribe from the community *Practitioner Nurse Prescribers' Formulary*, which includes dressings and some POMs; and independent or supplementary nurse and midwife prescribers, who are trained both to make a diagnosis and to prescribe (independent prescribing) (NMC 2010). These practitioners can also review and change medication as part of a clinical management plan; this is known as supplementary prescribing (NMC 2010).

It is essential to check local policies and procedures about both prescribing and administrating medicines because local policy will dictate current practice.

The law

Legislations relating to medicines are complex and are designed to safeguard patients (Obrey and Caldwell 2013). The administration of medicines has been demonstrated to encompass many areas for potential error. Two pieces of legislation have been identified as important in medicines management: the Medicines Act 1968 and the Misuse of Drugs Act 1971 (Dougherty and Lister 2011).

Medicines Act 1968

This provides a legal framework for manufacture, licensing, prescription, supply and administration of medicines that must be adhered to (NMC 2010). POMs are covered by the Human use order 1997 (SI no. 1830), which gives information and legislation on medicines that require a prescription to be written by specific personnel (NMC 2010).

In the NHS, hospitals adhere to this act by ensuring that a pharmacist supervises the purchasing and supply of medicines, and that supply or administration to a patient is only by personnel authorised to prescribe (Dougherty and Lister 2011).

Within a community setting, doctors, dentists, pharmacists and nurses are exempt from this restriction, allowing them to supply and use medication in the practice of their respective professions without pharmacy supervision (Dougherty and Lister 2011).

Misuse of Drugs Act 1971

This prohibits the possession, supply and manufacture of medicinal and other products unless legal (NMC 2010). It is mostly concerned with 'controlled' drugs, which are medications that are potentially addictive or habit forming, such as morphine substances (Dougherty and Lister 2011).

The role of the healthcare assistant and assistant practitioner in controlled drug administration can exist in the community through local policy, but this is usually advised only where no other registered nurse is available. In this instance, the accountability of the preparation and administration of the medicine still lies with the registered nurse (NMC 2010; NMC 2015) (see the section 'Delegation').

THINK ABOUT IT

You are asked to assist in the preparation and checking of diamorphine for use in an MS26 syringe driver. Do you think this is an appropriate task to be delegated to you? (Think about your knowledge, skills, training and competence.)

In relation to controlled drugs, healthcare assistants and assistant practitioners may be required, through local policy, to witness the preparation and administration of controlled medicines, including in a syringe driver. This is a portable device that is often used for palliative care and delivers medication via a syringe, which is placed in the syringe driver. Where controlled medicines are used, if the unregistered practitioner is assisting with the ingestion or application, the unregistered practitioner must remain under direct supervision at all times (NMC 2010). Competency based training should have been undertaken for all registered nurses undertaking this role to ensure patient safety. Local policies should be in place if a healthcare assistant or assistant practitioner is to assist with this method of administration, and education about palliative care (management of symptoms where there is no cure) and the device should be undertaken.

Related aspects and terminology

Registered nurses' role

The Nursing Midwifery Council's (NMC) (2010a) Standards for Pre-registration Nursing Education: Essential Skills Clusters state: 'People can trust the newly registered nurse to ensure safe and effective practice in medicines management through comprehensive knowledge of medicines, their actions, risks and benefits.'

The nurse's role is clearly defined by the NMC who have set out principles that must be considered by registered nurses before the administration of medicines;

these are detailed in Box 15.1 (NMC 2010). Once the 'direction to supply or administer' principles above have been adhered to, the registered nurse must follow the principles for administration, detailed in Box 15.2. These principles aim to improve and standardise practice, which in turn can reduce errors. Furthermore, Standard 18 of the Code (NMC 2015) clearly states nurses:

18 Advise on, prescribe, supply, dispense or administer medicines within the limits of your training and competence, the law, our (NMC) guidance and other relevant policies, guidance and regulations.

Box 15.1 Methods of supplying and/or administration of medicines (NMC 2010)

Standard 1: Methods

Registrants must only supply and administer medicinal products in accordance with one or more of the following processes:
- Patient specific direction (PSD).
- Patient medicines administration chart (may be called medicines administration record MAR).
- Patient group direction (PGD).
- Medicines Act exemption.
- Standing order.
- Home remedy protocol.
- Prescription forms.

Standard 2: Checking

Registrants must check any direction to administer a medicinal product.

Standard 3: Transcribing

As a registrant you may transcribe medication from one 'direction to supply or administer' to another form of 'direction to supply or administer'.

Box 15.2 Standards for practice of administration of medicines (NMC 2010)

Standard 8

As a registrant, in exercising your professional accountability in the best interests of your patients:
- You must be certain of the identity of the patient to whom the medicine is to be administered.
- You must check that the patient is not allergic to the medicine before administering it.
- You must know the therapeutic uses of the medicine to be administered, its normal dosage, side-effects, precautions and contraindications.
- You must be aware of the patient's plan of care (care plan/pathway).
- You must check that the prescription or the label on the medicine dispensed is clearly written and unambiguous.

- You must check the expiry date (where it exists) of the medicine to be administered.
- You must have considered the dosage, weight where appropriate, method of administration, route and timing.
- You must administer or withhold in the context of the patient's condition, (for example, Digoxin is not usually to be given if pulse below 60) and co-existing therapies, for example, physiotherapy.
- You must contact the prescriber or another authorised prescriber without delay where contraindications to the prescribed medicine are discovered, where the patient develops a reaction to the medicine or where assessment of the patient indicates that the medicine is no longer suitable (see Standard 25).
- You must make a clear, accurate and immediate record of all medicine administered, intentionally withheld or refused by the patient, ensuring the signature is clear and legible; it is also your responsibility to ensure that a record is made when delegating the task of administering medicine.

In addition:

- Where medication is not given the reason for not doing so must be recorded.
- You may administer with a single signature any prescription-only medicine (POM), general sales list (GSL) or pharmacy (P) medication.
  In respect of controlled drugs:
- These should be administered in line with relevant legislation and local standard operating procedures.
- It is recommended that for the administration of controlled drugs a secondary signatory is required within secondary care and similar healthcare settings.
- In a patient's home, where a registrant is administering a controlled drug that has already been prescribed and dispensed to that patient, obtaining a secondary signatory should be based on local risk assessment
- Although normally the second signatory should be another registered healthcare professional (for example doctor, pharmacist, dentist) or student nurse or midwife, in the interest of patient care, where this is not possible, a second suitable person who has been assessed as competent may sign. It is good practice that the second signatory witnesses the whole administration process. For guidance, go to www.dh.gov.uk and search for safer management of controlled drugs: guidance on standard operating procedures.
- In cases of direct patient administration of oral medication from stock in a substance misuse clinic, it must be a registered nurse who administers, signed by a second signatory (assessed as competent), who is then supervised by the registrant as the patient receives and consumes the medication.
- You must clearly countersign the signature of the student when supervising a student in the administration of medicines.

Delegation

The NMC guidelines (2008) state that nurses who delegate the responsibility of administration must ensure that the patient, carer, healthcare assistant or assistant practitioner is competent to carry out the task. This requires education, training and assessment of the patient, carer, healthcare assistant or assistant practitioner, including further support if necessary. This is in the best interests of the registered nurse, the assistant practitioner, the healthcare assistant and patient, with the ultimate responsibility for ensuring the correct patient, dose, drug, time and route lying with the registered nurse who delegated the task (Boyd 2013).

The nurse is also accountable for decisions to delegate tasks and duties to other people (NMC 2015).

Informed consent

All patients have rights, and before administering any medicine it is necessary to obtain informed consent from them (Obrey and Caldwell 2013). A patient who is asked to consent to treatment must be given all the relevant information that they need to make an informed decision. All questions must be answered honestly and fully. If you cannot answer, then find a member of staff who can. Boyd (2013) requires the following points to be worked through:

- Hygiene – do not forget that standard precautions are necessary. Infection control and contamination measures are essential.
- Medicines administration chart – ensure the chart is accurately completed with all the relevant information available.
- Medicine – check the label correctly, including expiry date and measure dose. It should be noted that once some medicines have been opened they have a limited shelf life or are ineffective.
- Patient – check the patient's identity and explain again what you are administering.
- Administer – in an appropriate manner.
- Record – sign record immediately and maintain up-to-date documentation.

There may be times when a patient is unable to take their medication as prescribed. Do not crush or cut tables using tablet cutters if there are swallowing difficulties. Inform the pharmacist that an alternative may need to be prescribed, such as administering the drug in a liquid form. When medication is refused and consent withheld, this must be clearly documented. In the case of children and those whose capacity is lacking, advice must be sought and local policies and procedures followed.

Patient group directions or group protocols

A patient group direction is a specific written instruction for the supply and administration of a named medicine or vaccine in an identified clinical situation (NMC 2010). A pharmacist and a doctor or dentist should have been involved in the development, and then approval must be obtained from the appropriate Health Board, Trust or Division. The role of the healthcare assistant may well be in giving a medicine within specific guidelines, but further training and assessment is essential.

THINK ABOUT IT

Does your clinical area have any patient group directions? If so, identify which medications and patients they cover.

One-stop dispensing

Following the publication of A Spoonful of Sugar in England and Wales (Audit Commission 2002) and The Right Medicine (Scottish Executive 2002) in Scotland, one-stop dispensing has been encouraged within the hospital setting. This is a system of administering and dispensing medicinal products involving the use of patients' own medications while in hospital (NMC 2010). In some instances this may also involve patients administering their own medication via a locked locker at the bedside.

Self-administration

Adult patients who have been screened by the multidisciplinary team may be permitted to self-medicate their medication whilst in hospital (Figure 15.1). The rationale for self-medication is to be proactive in improving compliance and concordance. Boyd (2013) identifies that this is not possible for all patients, for example:

- those patients who are thought of at risk of deliberate overdose;
- those patients being discharged to nursing homes;
- those patients with unstable mental health conditions;
- controlled drugs (patients must not self-administer these);
- those too ill or confused to be ultimately discharged home;
- if patients are identified as having difficulty in opening bottles or reading labels. (This should be brought to the pharmacists' attention so that arrangements can be made for their discharge.)

Record keeping

Accurate records detailing medication given or omitted are essential parts of medicine administration (see Chapter 15 for further information).

Allergies

The need to be vigilant about allergies by asking patients and clearly documenting any allergies cannot be overstated. Please check your local policy and procedure and access anaphylaxis training.

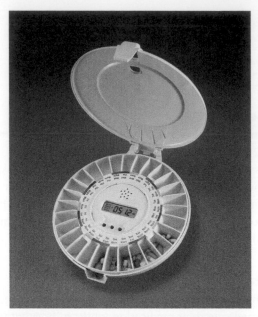

Figure 15.1 Compliance aid for medication delivery. Source: Reproduced with permission of PivoTell® Ltd.

Common medications

The Consumer Protection Act (1987) and Medicines Act (1968) confirm when administering medicines we need to follow what has become known as the 5 Rs:
- **Right** medicine is given.
- To the **right** patient.
- At the **right** time.
- In the **righ**t form.
- At the **right** dose.

There are multiple routes and preparations available, often for the same medication. The choice of route or preparation may be a result of a patient's symptoms; for example, if a patient is vomiting, oral medication may have to be changed to an alternative route, such as rectal administration. Healthcare assistants and assistant practitioners involved in medicine administration will follow local policies and procedure, which will determine the level of knowledge required about the medicine and the side-effects that may present.

Qualified personnel must prescribe all medications and the role of the healthcare assistant and assistant practitioners must be clearly defined. There are many different routes of administration and the most common are discussed below. Before and after all medicine administration, hands should be washed to prevent infection, as discussed previously.

THINK ABOUT IT

Think of some other medication routes and why and when they may be used.

Oral route

This can take the form of either tablets (e.g. paracetamol tablets) or liquids (e.g. amoxicillin preparation for children). Consider if the patient has difficulty swallowing and, if so, report to the nurse in charge where the medicine may need to be changed from tablets to a liquid; for example a patient who has had a cardiovascular accident (CVA or stroke) and who may have dysphagia (problems swallowing), especially if the tablets are large.

When administering tablets, their placement can vary, but this will be clearly indicated on the medicine bottle and the accompanying leaflet. Examples of different oral placement include buccal (which is placement between the gum and the inside of the mouth) or sublingual, which is under the tongue (Dougherty and Lister 2011).

Tablets should not be crushed or opened to release the medication unless the manufacturer states that this is acceptable, because this can alter the chemical properties of the medication (Boyd 2013). The advice on the label or leaflet will show if the medication needs to be administered depending on digestion, such as medication to be taken with/after meals. Tablets can be broken with a file if scored, or a tablet cutter can be used where appropriate, provided that the manufacturer's instructions are consulted.

Accurate measurement of liquid preparations is essential to prevent medication errors, and in some instances this may require a drug calculation to be performed. Local policy dictates whether a healthcare assistant or assistant practitioner can measure liquids. In the case of mixtures, many have a relatively short shelf-life, and some need to be kept in the fridge, for example antibiotics. Tablets and capsules may be susceptible to moisture and need to be kept in a cool dry place (Dougherty and Lister 2011).

Topical creams

This refers to the application of cream, ointments or gels that have been prescribed to relieve symptoms experienced by the patient, for example hydrocortisone (steroid) cream or E45 cream for dermatological (skin) complaints.

As the cream/liquid is the active ingredient and is applied by direct contact, gloves should be worn. This prevents the person applying the cream or ointment receiving a dose of the medication, or a reaction on their skin. Where the application site includes broken skin, an aseptic technique (a technique that involves using sterile gloves and minimal touch to prevent infection) is required.

After application, the site should be observed for a local reaction or worsening of the condition, and reported to the nurse in charge. Patients may require assistance to apply topical creams due to difficulty in the patient reaching the site, for example if the area for application of the medication is on the patient's back.

Storage should be in conjunction with the manufacturer's recommendations, but extremes of temperature should be avoided because deterioration may occur (Dougherty and Lister 2011). Creams and ointments containing a medicine should have a date recorded, preferably on the medication, because many should only be used for a specific time after opening, for example 4 weeks after opening.

Topical creams, such as local anaesthetic creams like emla, can be applied in preparation for a further procedure in either children or anxious patients, for example during venepuncture (taking blood; see Chapters 12 and 16). Please check with your local policies and procedures.

Ear

Administration via the ear canal is to relieve the symptoms of local symptoms, for example eardrops to soften wax. Correct positioning of the patient both before and after administration is essential to ensure that the medication has the desired local effect and does not run out of the ear. This involves the patient tilting the head to the opposite side, which allows access to the ear canal and prevents the medication coming out of the ear. The use of cotton wool can prevent this. Local training and achievement of relevant competencies are required to undertake this task.

Eyes

Administration into the eyes is to relieve local symptoms, for example due to infection, or post-operatively (after surgery), for example after cataract surgery.

Correct positioning of the patient both before and after administration is essential to ensure that the medication has the desired local effect. The patient will need to tilt the head back and look upwards. Care should also be taken to ensure that the medication does not run out of the eye before absorption. Local training and competency are required to undertake this task.

Eyedrops and ointment may become contaminated with microorganisms during use and then pose a danger to the recipient. Therefore, in the hospital environment they are discarded 7 days after they are first opened, but this may be extended to 28 days in the community (Dougherty and Lister 2011). Some products need to be kept in the fridge; ensure that this is checked and guidance followed.

Subcutaneous

This involves a needle administering medication into the subcutaneous tissue (under the skin), for example insulin for a patient with diabetes (see Chapter 13).

It is essential that correct disposal of the needle occurs to prevent needlestick injury.

It may be the patient who usually administers this medicine, but due to illness or lack of dexterity has become unable to do so. Again, training and supervision are essential to ensure competence.

Some injections may need to be kept in the fridge and manufacturer's recommendations should be followed; for example insulin needs to be kept in the fridge.

Suppositories

Suppositories are small, torpedo shaped wax pellets inserted into the rectum. When in the rectum, the suppository melts at body temperature, and dissolves or disperses in the mucous secretion of the rectum. There are a number of different types of suppositories available. Retention suppositories deliver drug therapy, for example, analgesia and antibiotics. Suppositories can often be a useful alternative for the administration of some drugs when the person is unable to take them orally. Those suppositories administered with the intention of stimulating the bowel in order to evacuate it include glycerine and bisacodyl (Peate 2013).

Storage instructions may involve storage in the fridge, check the manufacturer's instructions. Administration by this route should only be undertaken after training and supervision, and in accordance with local policy.

Inhalation

This can include short-term symptomatic relief, for example the use of a Salbutamol inhaler in asthma or a steroidal inhaler for long-term therapy. The actual amount of drug inhaled is small so a good technique is essential. Spacers or a bubble can be used to aid effectiveness (Figure 15.2).

Correct positioning: an upright position may need to be adopted to allow full lung expansion and allow correct medication delivery. A good inhaler technique is essential with this route of administration and, where healthcare assistants are involved in patient education and assessment of inhaler technique, further training and assessment must be undertaken.

Aerosol containers should not be stored in direct sunlight or over radiators, because there is a risk of explosion if they are heated (Dougherty and Lister 2011). Good oral hygiene is also required to avoid patients developing infections due to their medication.

Oxygen

Oxygen is a medication and requires a prescription to allow administration to patients. It is delivered in varying concentrations and is measured in percentages, for example 24, 28, 35 or 40%, depending on the patient's clinical symptoms (Boyd 2013; Dougherty and Lister 2011).

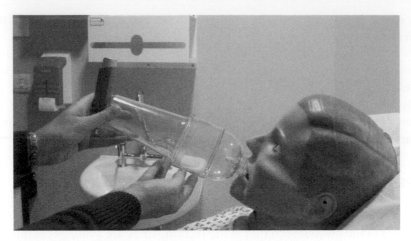

Figure 15.2 A 'spacer' inhaler.

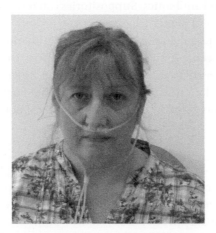

Figure 15.3 Nasal cannula.

Different masks exist that include simple masks with no special features, a non-rebreathing mask, and a Venturi mask, where different coloured fittings dictate the oxygen percentage and flow rate that is required, depending on the prescription (Boyd 2013). Masks are disposable and for single-patient use. They should be changed regularly to prevent infection. Nasal cannulae can be used (Figure 15.3), which make it possible for the patient to eat, drink and talk while receiving oxygen (Dougherty and Lister 2011). In the hospital setting, oxygen is often 'piped', that is available at the bedside with a meter on the wall to apply tubing. In the community or in an ambulance this would involve an oxygen cylinder.

Wound dressings
If the healthcare assistant or assistant practitioner is performing simple dressing, which includes applying a dressing to a wound, a prescription for the dressing

will be required. The district nurse, who has undergone additional training, or the GP may prescribe this.

Best practice would be for the same person to carry out the dressing to monitor improvement or problems at the wound and always report to the nurse in charge. Further training and competence should be undertaken in line with local policy with regard to this skill.

Intravenous (medication administered directly into a vein)

This route should be performed only under strict local policies/procedures and competency based training. It may include administration of fluids or medications. See Chapters 16 and 14 for further information on intravenous flush (administration of 0.9% sodium chloride via a cannula to keep it patent, i.e. prevent blockage).

The NMC (2010) state that, where a registered nurse delegates the task of giving a patient medication, this may be drawn up in advance after a full risk assessment and delegation of the task to a 'named individual' (NMC 2010). Please check your local policies and procedures.

Errors in administration and adverse reactions

The Yellow Card Scheme is vital in helping the Medicines & Healthcare Products Regulatory Agency (MHRA) monitor the safety of all healthcare products in the UK to ensure they are acceptably safe for patients and those that use them. Reports can be made for all medicines including vaccines, blood factors and immunoglobulins, herbal medicines and homeopathic remedies, and all medical devices available on the UK market.

The Scheme collects information on suspected problems or incidents involving:

1 side-effects (also known as adverse drug reactions or ADRs);
2 medical device adverse incidents;
3 defective medicines (those that are not of an acceptable quality);
4 counterfeit or fake medicines or medical devices.

It is important for people to report problems experienced with medicine or medical devices as these are used to identify issues that might not have been previously known about. The MHRA will review the product if necessary, and take action to minimise risk and maximise benefit to the patients. The MHRA is also able to investigate counterfeit or fake medicines or devices and if necessary take action to protect public health (MRHA 2012).

Side-effects to a medicine, vaccine, herbal or complementary remedy

All medicines can cause side-effects (commonly referred to as adverse drug reactions or ADRs by healthcare professionals).

Side-effects reported on Yellow Card are evaluated, together with additional sources of information such as clinical trial data, medical literature or data from international medicines regulators, to identify previously unknown safety issues. These reports are assessed by a team of medicine safety experts made up of doctors, pharmacists and scientists who study the benefits and risks of medicines. If a new side-effect is identified, the safety profile of the medicine in question is carefully looked at, as well as the side-effects of other medicines used to treat the same condition. The MHRA takes action, whenever necessary, to ensure that medicines are used in a way that minimises risk, while maximising patient benefit.

If the healthcare assistant or assistant practitioner is the first person to notice an adverse drug reaction or note that an error has occurred, this must be reported immediately; ensure the patient is safe and follow local policies and procedures. The registered nurse has clear accountability under the NMC Code (2015). Safeguarding the patient is always a priority.

Summary

The evolving role of the healthcare assistant and assistant practitioner would benefit from registration and regulation, but as discussed this has not yet occurred. Whatever and wherever the role, healthcare assistants and assistant practitioners must ensure they have the knowledge, understanding, skills and training before taking on any task involving medication. Drug calculations have not been discussed, but this area remains problematic and can result in catastrophic error. If you are not confident in your numeracy skills, explore options available to you to practice and seek support and training. Many Trusts have already explored the role of healthcare assistants and assistant practitioners in the administration of medication. While medication administration can be fulfilling and rewarding as part of the holistic care of your patient, do not undertake this area of care lightly: be safe, be competent.

References

Audit Commission (2002) *A Spoonful of Sugar*. London: Audit Commission.

Boyd C (2013) *Student Survival Skills: Medicine Management Skills for Nurses*. Oxford: John Wiley & Sons.

Dougherty L and Lister S (eds) (2011) *The Royal Marsden Hospital Manual of Clinical Nursing Procedures*, 8th edn. Oxford: Blackwell Publishing.

Medicines and Healthcare Products Regulatory Agency (MHRA) (2012) *Medicines and Medical Devices: Regulation: What You Need To Know*. London: The Medicines and Healthcare Products Regulatory Agency.

NHS Education for Scotland (NES) (2015) Non-medical prescribing learning resource [online]. Available at: http://www.prescribing.nes.scot.nhs.uk/ (accessed 3 May 2015).

Nursing and Midwifery Council (NMC) (2008) *Standards for Medicines Management*. London: NMC.

Nursing and Midwifery Council (NMC) (2010) *Standards for Pre-registration Nursing Education: Essential Skills Clusters*. London: NMC.

Nursing and Midwifery Council (NMC) (2015) *The NMC Code of Professional Conduct: Standards for conduct, performance and ethics*. London: NMC.

O'Flannagan C (2014) Should assistant practitioners be allowed to administer medicine? *British Journal of Health Care Assistants* 8(12): 594–601.

Obrey A and Caldwell J (2013) Administration of medicines – the nurse role in ensuring patient safety. *British Journal of Nursing* 22(1): 32–35.

Peate I (2013) Clinical skills series/2: enemas and suppositories. *British Journal of Healthcare Assistants* 7(2): 76–80.

Scottish Executive (2002) *The Right Medicine*. Edinburgh: Scottish Executive.

CHAPTER 16

Peripheral intravenous cannulation

LEARNING OBJECTIVES

- Review the anatomy and physiology relating to peripheral intravenous (IV) cannulation (see Chapter 12 for the anatomy and physiology of the arm)

- Review the skills and competence with regard to undertaking peripheral IV cannulation

- Describe possible complications of peripheral IV cannulation and how to manage them

Aim of this chapter

The aim of this chapter is to review the reasons and procedure for undertaking peripheral intravenous (IV) cannulation in the arm, and discuss possible complications and risk prevention. *This may not, however, be a role that is expected of all healthcare assistants; check your local policy and access any approved training via your manager/charge nurse.* Also insertion of a cannula requires a saline flush to confirm patency (that it is working); again many healthcare assistants may not be covered or allowed to administer this because it is classed as a medicine and many clinical areas do not allow healthcare assistants to administer any medicines (see Chapter 15); *again check your local policy for guidance.*

Reasons for cannulation

Peripheral IV cannulation is the introduction of a cannula into a peripheral vein as a means of gaining direct access into the venous circulation. McCallum and Higgins (2012) identify that the quality of care can be significantly influenced by adopting the principles associated with the safe management and care of patients who have these devices in situ (HPS 2012; DH 2011). These procedures may cause trauma and discomfort to the patient, which is even more likely if the person performing them is not competent (Ellson 2008). Demonstrating knowledge and understanding of the effective methods that are used can ensure patient confidence is maintained and their experience of cannulation is positive (McGowan 2014). The Department of Health (DH 2011) developed High Impact Interventions (HIIs), which are evidence-based approaches that relate to key clinical procedures or care processes that can reduce the risk of infection if performed appropriately. They have been developed to provide a practical way of highlighting the critical elements of a particular procedure or care process (a care bundle), the key actions required are a means of demonstrating reliability. The peripheral intravenous cannula HII (DH 2011) highlights the associated risk of infection because of the potential for direct microbial entry to the bloodstream and emphasises the importance of training. *Please ensure that you are given local training and support, to make sure that you are competent in this role before commencing this skill.*

Why perform peripheral IV cannulation

The following list gives some indication of why a patient may require insertion of a cannula; however, many of these are not within the scope of the healthcare assistant to carry out:

• To administer intravenous fluids for the maintenance of fluid and electrolyte balance (elements carried in the blood).
• To administer intravenous medicines (bolus, intermittently or continuously).
• To transfuse blood and blood products.
• Just in case, for example a professional judgement in case the patient collapses.
• Venesection (bleeding a volume of blood from a patient, similar to blood donation).
• To provide access for nutritional support.
• To aid in the monitoring of a patient's condition.

   The decision to insert a cannula will usually be made by a doctor or registered nurse; however, in some practice settings this may also be made based on a care pathway or protocol. *Be aware of your local policy and adhere to local guidance.*

Relevant anatomy and physiology

See Chapter 12 for the anatomy and physiology of the arm. Figures 16.1 and 16.2 are a review of the anatomy and physiology of the arm and hand relating to the veins commonly used in peripheral IV cannulation, and Figure 16.3 shows a cross-section of a vein. It is essential that the healthcare assistant or assistant practitioner undertaking peripheral IV cannulation has a good understanding of the anatomy and physiology of arteries, veins and associated nerves.

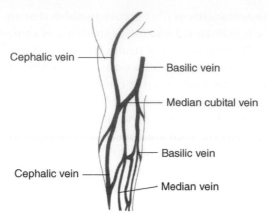

Figure 16.1 Venous anatomy of upper arm.

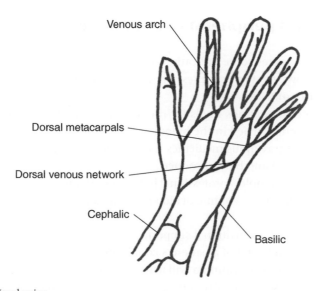

Figure 16.2 Hand veins.

How to insert and remove a peripheral IV cannula

Assessment of the patient and their veins

Patient assessment

A thorough patient assessment is crucial to ensuring the patient receives the most appropriate intervention, the right device in the most appropriate site (Dougherty and Lister 2011). McGowan (2014) highlights the importance of taking into account the patient's age, condition, lifestyle, compliance and preference. Other factors that should be considered include the patient's diagnosis, treatment plan, type of therapy and duration of therapy. It is important to take

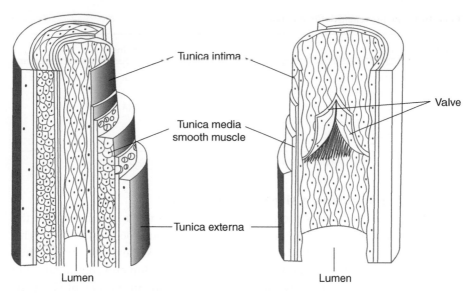

Tunica intima

Valve

Tunica media
smooth muscle

Tunica externa

Lumen

Lumen

Figure 16.3 Cross-section of vein.

time to communicate with the patient to establish their understanding and acceptance and to allay some of their anxieties (Gabriel 2012; McGowan 2014). The patient's experience is important, and yet it is easy to overlook the effect poor IV access and IV device maintenance has on them (Oliver 2015).

Use veins that feel soft and resilient, and refill when depressed, often described by practitioners as 'juicy' or 'bouncy'. Also consider the length of the cannula, so ensure that a straight vein suitable for the length of the cannula is selected, with large veins being preferable over small veins. Patient involvement is essential, so ensure that the procedure is discussed with the patient to gain consent and identify any site preference, for example the patient's non-dominant arm (Dunnnig 2011; Boyd 2013; Dougherty and Lister 2011). Coram (2015) cautions against choosing the site because of a visible vein as it might not necessarily be the best place.

Longmate et al. (2011) describe key interventions to prevent catheter-related blood stream infections that should be considered through the patient's cannulation experience or journey (Table 16.1).

Common sites

See Figure 16.1:
- Dorsal venous arch on hand.
- Forearm vein.
- Cephalic vein on thumb side of wrist.
- Basilic vein.

This might be a useful point to revise your anatomy and physiology. Take care because the most prominent vein is not necessarily the most suitable.

Table 16.1 Key preventative interventions.

Before insertion	During insertion	After insertion
Discuss with the patient	Skin asepsis with	Care of device and area once
Correct vascular access device	chlorhexadine	in situ
(cannula) and site selection	Use of barrier precautions	Prompt removal
Hand hygiene	During insertion	
Competent in skill		

Source: Longmate 2011. Reproduced with permission of BMJ Publishing Group Ltd.

Criteria for selecting a site for cannulation

McGowan (2014) suggests the metacarpal veins found in the hand and the cephalic and basilica veins found in the forearm should be assessed first. This approach is considered best practice as further attempts above the site can then be selected. Gabriel (2012), however, recommends caution and consideration of the ageing process on veins. The ageing process results in the loss of elasticity, with the vein becoming more rigid, plus there is thickening of the vessel walls and the development of arteriosclerosis. Skin is more delicate and haematoma, bruising and damaging the vein more likely. Therefore care and caution is advised when cannulating an older person. Boyd (2013) also cautions about the number of times insertion is attempted and the need to ask a more experienced member of the team.

Witt (2011) sums up veins to avoid as those that are hard, thrombosed, thin, fragile, mobile and/or lying over a bony prominence. She also advises that skin should be intact, free from infection or damage (e.g. a burn) and any existing bruises or swelling. Areas with tattoos should also be avoided as these may also be a potential source of infection.

Choosing the appropriate cannula

As a rule, the smallest cannula should be selected; however, as Boyd (2013) identifies, if the patient is critically ill or this is an emergency situation – for example the patient has hypovolaemic shock – then a larger device is inserted to 'push fluids' into the patient's system quickly for rapid treatment. Please check your local policy

Table 16.2 gives guidance; seek local guidance when necessary.

THINK ABOUT IT

Why is the patient's age a factor that you need to think about when assessing for a site?

Infection

Peripheral IV cannulation breaches the circulatory system, so healthcare assistants and assistant practitioners should consider their role in the prevention of

Table 16.2 Cannula choice guidance.

Cannula size	Care situation
14 gauge	Emergency, e.g. cardiac arrest
16 gauge	Major trauma or surgery, massive fluid replacement
18 gauge	Routine blood transfusions, rapid infusion, surgical or trauma patient
20 gauge	Routine infusions, bolus drug administration, medical, post op patient
22 gauge	Small fragile veins, short-term access
24 gauge	Small or fragile veins, children, older patient

Source: NHS Lothian (2007). Adapted with permission of NHS Lothian.

infection and be aware of predisposing infection risk factors and subsequent management (Box 16.1). Infection control is integral to all care and robust standards of practice are therefore paramount to ensure safe and competent practice both in peripheral IV cannulation and IV care (Lavery 2010). The H.A.N.D.S acronym was created by the IV team at King's College Hospital as an aide memoire to promote safe and evidenced-based practice for the insertion and care of IV devices (Frimpong et al. 2015).

Box 16.1 Predisposing infection risk factors and management

- Skin colonisation (surface bacterial spread) can allow bacteria to enter the circulatory system through the insertion of the needle and cannula, so ensure careful site selection and cleansing.
- Remote infection (e.g. urinary tract infection) can also lead to a risk, the patient should be educated about not tampering with the site, cannula or sterile dressing, and this should reduce the risk of transferring bacteria.
- Multi-use disinfectants can become colonised with bacteria very quickly, so use only single-use sachets when cleansing the site.
- Expired or damaged stock can be a source of infection; ensure stock is in date and has been stored correctly, and is used for its intended purpose; single-use devices must be used (Medicines Devices Agency (MDA) 2000).
- Hands of practitioners are the single most common way in which bacteria are transferred onto devices (equipment), so ensure correct hand cleansing.

(NHS Lothian 2007 with permission.)

H: Hand hygiene

Before, during and after an invasive procedure such as peripheral IV cannulation, for example after contact with a source of microbes (germs): wash hands with liquid soap and warm water for at least 30 seconds; dry thoroughly with paper towels, then use alcogel before accessing the venous access devise (Frimpong et al. 2015).

A: Antisepsis of the skin

The appropriate method of antisepsis to decontaminate the skin site is 2% chlorhexadine in 70% isopropyl alcohol. A single-patient use applicator should be used before insertion for at least 30 seconds using a crosshatch pattern XXX (Frimpong 2015). An area of skin that is equal to the size of the dressing should be cleaned and must be allowed to dry for 30 seconds to achieve maximum bacterial killing effect, which will reduce the risk of infection (Longmate 2011; Loveday et al. 2014).

N: Non-touch technique

Centres for Disease Control and prevention (CDC) (2011) state clearly that the insertion site should not be touched once the skin is cleansed. Aseptic Non-Touch Technique (ANTT) must be performed and observed throughout. If the practitioner cannot cannulate without re-palpating the skin, the use of sterile gloves is strongly advised. Frimpong et al. (2012) also point out that ANTT should be applied when opening giving sets as the bag spike is a key part and must not be touched.

D: Daily inspection; date on the dressing documentation

Daily inspection: is the line still needed?
The removal of IV devices as soon as they are no longer needed is essential and should be part of the daily review for both the nursing and medical staff (MHPRA 3023; Boyd 2013). Loveday et al. (2014) recommend that if the cannula needs to be in situ for longer than the standard duration, the reason should be clearly documented in the patient's medical notes
Date on the dressing
   A sterile, transparent semi-permeable membrane dressing should be used to cover the insertion site. The date, time and initials of the inserting clinician must be written clearly on the dressing without obstructing the insertion site for the cannula. This dressing should be left in place for no longer than seven days and reapplied as required. Please check your local policy.
Documentation: has the line been documented?
   Accurate records must be kept of who inserted the cannula, where on the body it was inserted and the date on which the cannulation was performed. The cannula site should be visually inspected everyday. Local policy should be followed.

S: Scrub the hub; sharps safety

Scrub the hub
Before connecting anything, for example a syringe or a giving set, the hub of the needle-free connector should be scrubbed for at least 15 seconds, cleaning it thoroughly with 2% chlorhexadine 70% isopropyl alcohol, and allowed to completely dry before attaching the giving set or syringe (Frimpong et al. 2015). Loveday et al. (2014) recommend that this procedure is repeated every time the IV device is accessed. It is important that the healthcare assistant or assistant practitioner has been assessed as competent before undertaking any of these procedures.
   Sharps safety
   There is now a greater understanding of the need to be sharp aware and sharp safe. The Health and Safety Executive (HSE) (2013) regulations reinforce the need to dispose of sharps at the point of use. Frimpong et al. (2015) emphasise the importance of the following:
∘ NEVER re-stealth or recap needles.

   ○ ALWAYS dispose sharps at the point of use.
   ○ DO NOT over fill sharps containers.

Protective clothing

Protective clothing should be worn according to local policy; and, as in Chapter 12, care should be taken using latex gloves in case the patient or member of staff has a sensitivity or allergy.

Environment

A safe working environment is important to both the patient and the HCA. Equipment should be at hand, including the sharps bin to avoid any unnecessary hazards to the HCA. To ensure good assessment of the patient and their veins, it is important to have good lighting. The patient should be comfortable and as relaxed as possible through sitting comfortably on a chair or lying on a bed or trolley with their arm supported on a pillow (Dougherty and Lister 2011).

PRACTICE POINT

When using a tourniquet ensure it is either cleaned between patients or use single patient disposable tourniquets.

Performing peripheral IV cannula: requirements and technique

Please refer to Box 16.2 for the equipment required for a cannulation insertion and Table 16.3 for preparation.

Box 16.2 Equipment required for cannulation procedure

- Tourniquet – consider quick release, latex free.
- Non-sterile gloves and apron.
- Alcohol swab (70% isopropyl).
- Appropriate size cannula.
- Closed system (*recommended*), e.g. Smartsite.
- Sterile dressing (e.g. Tegaderm or IV3000).
- Pad to protect from spillage.
- Clean tray/trolley.
- 10 ml syringe.
- 5 ml ampoule sterile 0.9% NaCl flush.
- Sterile green or blue needle or sharps-less needle.
- *Appropriate IV fluid for administration.*[a]
- *Medical device (if required).*[a]
- Sharps bin/container.

[a]As mentioned at the start of the chapter, some healthcare assistants may not be covered to administer either flush or intravenous fluids; check local policy. If this is the case, the healthcare assistant may require a registered nurse or doctor to flush the device once they have inserted the cannula (Figure 16.4).

Table 16.3 Preparation for procedure.

Action	Reason
1. Wash hands with liquid soap, and dry hands thoroughly, followed by an alcohol hand rub, or wash with an approved antiseptic solution	To minimise the risk of healthcare-associated infection (HAI)
2. Assemble all the equipment required for the procedure on a clean trolley or a tray	In order that the procedure is carried out smoothly, efficiently and without interruptions
3. Ensure that all the equipment used is intact and within expiry dates	To maintain asepsis
4. Approach the patient and explain the procedure in a confident manner Allow the patient time to ask questions and express concerns about the procedure, if any	To obtain patient consent and cooperation
5. Help the patient into a comfortable position, e.g. sitting in a chair or lying on bed, and support arm with a pillow Ask patient if they have ever had problems with procedure, e.g. previous fainting episode; if so lay the patient on a bed, to prevent a vasovagal (faint) episode	To maintain the patient's comfort To enable the operator to carry out the procedure with ease
6. Prepare the area, e.g. provide adequate lighting, privacy and heighten the bed, lower cot sides, check positioning	Safe working environment
7. Verbally check the identity of the patient – name, date of birth (DOB) against identification (e.g. patient ID bracelet) and documentation, e.g. care pathway.	Identify the need for the procedure To ensure that the peripheral IV cannula is being inserted into the right patient

Source: NHS Lothian (2007). Adapted with permission of NHS Lothian.

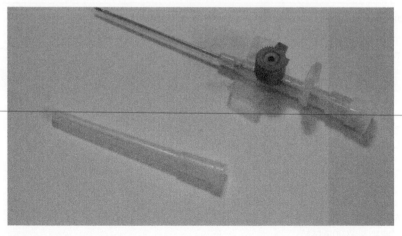

Figure 16.4 Example of cannula.

Table 16.4 outlines the specific actions and observations required throughout the procedure.

Patient education for peripheral IV cannulation

Before and during insertion take care to use language that will not distress the patient. Rosenthal (2005) suggested avoiding the use of words such as 'needle' and 'stick', and use 'plastic tube' and 'insert' instead, and explain to the patient that it is the 'plastic' cannula that is inserted, not the needle.

Table 16.4 Specific actions and observations during the procedure.

Action	Reason
1. Wash hands with liquid soap, and dry hands thoroughly followed by an alcohol hand rub, or wash with an approved antiseptic solution	To minimise the risk of healthcare-associated infection (HAI)
2. Consult with the patient with regard to preferences for cannulation site, based on previous experiences	To actively involve the patient in own treatment. To be aware of the patient's history and factors that may influence choice of vein
3. Apply tourniquet to the arm on the chosen side approximately 7–10 cm (3–4 inches) above selected site for cannulation Apply enough pressure to impede (restrict) venous circulation *Consider the use of a disposable tourniquet, if available*	Increases venous pressure, aiding vein identification and entry Check radial pulse to ensure that arterial flow is not affected Reduce risks of cross-contamination
3. To further encourage venous filling try one of the following; (a) Stroke the vein gently (b) Allow the arm to hang by patient's side (gravity) (c) Immerse limb in warm/hot water for 5–10 mins (d) Ask patient to clench fist and then relax, several times	Helps make vein more prominent and so easier to assess and cannulate
4. Palpate (feel) the selected vein	To identify its course, depth and structures, i.e. tendons, and to avoid nearby arteries or nerves
5. Release the tourniquet and check vein decompresses (returns to normal)	To prevent cell damage due to decreased oxygen (O_2) supply
6. Choose and prepare the smallest practical cannula size (gauge)	Ensure appropriate size
7. Hand antisepsis; use either an alcohol hand rub or wash with an approved antiseptic solution	To minimise the risk of healthcare-associated infection (HAI)
8. Reapply tourniquet to the chosen site	

Table 16.4 (*continued*)

Action	Reason
9. Cleanse the proposed cannulation site with alcohol skin prep, using a firm circular motion from centre to the periphery, for 30 s and at least a 5–7 cm (2–3 inches) area – size of dressing area	To minimise the risk of HAI
Allow the alcohol to air dry, for a minimum of 30 s DO NOT re-palpate the vein after the site has been cleansed; use a mental marker, if necessary, e.g. freckle	Prevent stinging as cannula pierces the skin Increases risk of infection
DO NOT shave the skin at the insertion point	Can cause microscopic damage to skin
10. Put on gloves	Gloves will give some protection from blood spillage
11. Fold down the wings of the cannula	This grip reduces the risk of contaminating the cannula
12. With the patient's arm in a supported downward position, anchor the vein by applying tension to the skin below and to side of the cannulation site	Prevents vein from rolling or moving Prevents risk of injury to nurse inserting
13. Insert the device into the vein at an angle (depending on device used) holding the cannula firmly with a three-point grip and bevel (cut) up *Fragile veins usually require a lower angle of insertion* Watch for the presence of blood in the flashback chamber	Ensures correct positioning between needle and catheter tip, and stabilises cannula within the needle Reduce overshooting This flashback indicates that the needle has successfully entered the vein (Figure 16.5)
14. Lower the angle of the cannula to almost skin level. Advance the cannula a few millimetres into the vein and avoid contamination by holding at the wings or protection cap No resistance should be felt as cannula advances into vein	To prevent puncture of the rear wall of the vessel This ensures that the cannula tip also enters the vein If resistance felt, consider if pierced rear of vein due to angle, or cannula not in vein initially. Remove cannula
15. Withdraw the introducer needle partially (approx. 2–5 mm)	To avoid exit through the rear of vein wall and provide stability to cannula
16. First hold the flashback chamber immobilising the needle. Then advance the cannula forward off the needle into the vein with the other hand; this should be in a smooth single movement	The plastic cannula advances only into the vein Consider point 14 as cannula should advance easily; if not may require removal and new cannula insertion in different vein and site
17. Release the tourniquet	Release venous pressure
18. The needle must never be reinserted while cannula is in the vein (some devices now prevent this, e.g. Vasofix) Apply pressure over the vein distal to the cannula tip (beyond the end of cannula)	To avoid risk of needle severing the cannula and cause plastic embolus To avoid spillage of blood when needle is removed (raising the patient's arm also reduces risk of spillage)

Table 16.4 (*continued*)

Action	Reason
19a. Remove the introducer needle completely, and dispose of immediately into sharps bin, e.g. Vasofix needle cap flips over as it is withdrawn and a slight resistance might occur	Reduces risk of needlestick injury Ensure firm grasp of device while withdrawing needle to prevent accidental removal or dislodging of cannula
19b. Close the cannula with a closed system, e.g. Smartsite, or device cap if closed system not used	Reduce number of times cannula is reconnected to reduce infection rate and mechanical irritation
20. Flush the cannula with 5 ml 0.9% NaCl (physiological saline) or flush volume of twice the length of the cannula, plus any device, e.g. closed system, using push–pause method and positive pressure via the intermittent port or closed system connector[a]	To confirm correct placement of the cannula, the push–pause method helps create turbulence and so maintains flow, and positive pressure means that no blood can backflow into the cannula
21. Secure the cannula in position with sterile dressing, e.g. IV 2000 or Tegaderm IV (Figure 16.6) Skin may be clipped adjacent to, but not at insertion site, to secure the dressing	Good fixation is essential to prevent poor position, rolling or other movements of the cannula, because can cause irritation of the vein Reducing the risk of HAI
22. Make no more than two attempts to insert cannula. If unsuccessful, obtain assistance from more experienced staff	Patient comfort Prevent trauma to vein
23. Ensure that patient is given appropriate education once cannula is in place	Ensure cannula safety and sustain for duration required or 72–96 hours
24. Enter date and time of insertion, site, cannula size and reason for insertion in patient notes, and record signature of operator	Good record keeping and legal requirement Some areas may record date and time on dressing too, to aid monitoring

[a] Push–pause and positive pressure stage 20 – holding plunger with thumb, insert small volume then pause, then repeat, till all the saline is flushed in, then maintain pressure on plunger as syringe is removed.
Source: NHS Lothian (2007). Adapted with permission of NHS Lothian.

Ensure that the patient has also understood the reason for the cannula, and keep them informed about ongoing treatments (Lundgren et al. 1998).

Advise the patient to report any concerns, including if the site becomes painful, swollen, hot or tender, if there is any leakage or the dressing becomes loose. Also advise patients to take care when dressing and undressing because this can dislodge the cannula. Ask them not to tamper with or touch the dressing and to try to minimise movement in the arm, especially if near an area of flexion, such as the wrist or elbow. All these should ensure a safe cannula for the duration and help the patient comply with the procedure (Ingram and Lavery 2007).

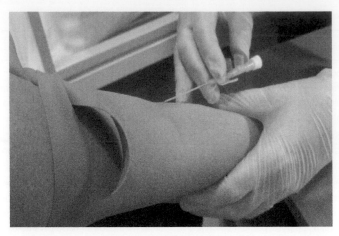

Figure 16.5 Inserting the cannula. Source: Photograph by I Lavery.

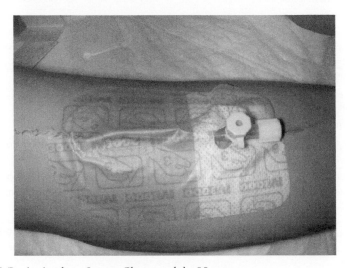

Figure 16.6 Device in place. Source: Photograph by I Lavery.

Refer to Table 16.5 for information on the maintenance and care of a cannula after insertion.

> **THINK ABOUT IT**
>
> While inserting a cannula you encounter resistance. What would you do?

Re-siting of a peripheral IV cannula (*once discussed and agreed locally*)

- Follow the same procedure as for initial insertion.
- After 72–96 hours, if still required, check with senior/charge nurse or notes.
- If inserted in an emergency, re-site after 24 hours (e.g. emergency insertion may not have had time to include appropriate skin cleansing).

Table 16.5 Maintenance and care of the intravenous (IV) cannula after insertion.

Action	Reason
1a. Inspect the cannula each shift or more frequently depending on patient's clinical condition and type of therapy	To ensure cannula is in correct position and observe for potential complications, e.g. phlebitis
1b. Flush cannula with 5 ml 0.9% NaCl or the flush volume is twice the length of the cannula plus any device, e.g. closed system	To maintain patency of cannula and ensure flush volume adequate *Not all healthcare assistants are allowed to administer medicines – check your local policy*
1c. The cannula site should also be monitored each shift or at least daily Recommendations for resiting are after a period of 72–96 h However, cannula may be left in for longer and reason documented, e.g. • when initial cannulation was difficult • when therapy will be completed shortly afterwards	To reduce complications including healthcare-associated infection and to ensure that length of time cannula is in place reflects individual management of each patient and needs To provide reason and justify decisions
2. Use a rigorous aseptic technique when handling the cannula/lines: • reduce manipulations of the system to a minimum • keep number of stopcocks and taps to a minimum • injection sites and bungs cleaned with an alcohol swab and allowed to dry	Any connection in an IV system is a potential point of entry for microorganisms Recommend use of closed system to minimise infection from port
3. Maintain appropriate level of hand hygiene antisepsis before handling the cannula/lines at any time	To minimise risk of infection
4. Document in care plan/notes: • date and time of insertion • gauge (size) of catheter • site of insertion • signature • flush and amount (volume)	Good record keeping and legal requirement

Source: NHS Lothian (2007). Adapted with permission of NHS Lothian.

- If the site becomes infected, the cannula is blocked or leaking or infiltrates the surrounding area (see under Problems).
- Select another vein, alternating between arms if possible, for the new cannula, but proximal (above) to the previously cannulated site.
- Choice of cannulation site will depend on the patient's local anatomy, patient mobility and the required flow rates; however, rotation of sites is essential.
- Continue to use the distal veins of the arms if possible.
- Document reason for removal, including any signs and symptoms of infection or problems and record (see point 4 in Table 16.5).

Use of a tourniquet

Ellson (2008) reminds us that tourniquets are a potential source of infection. Single-tourniquets are available. The tourniquet used should be sufficiently wide that it can be wrapped around the limb and gently tightened so that minimal pressure is used to suppress blood flow and achieve the dilation of the vein (Gabriel 2012). Excess pressure from a narrow tourniquet, for example, can cause trauma to the vein which may result in bleeding and scarring to the vessels, leading to unsuccessful cannulation and distress for the patient.

Related aspects and terminology

Consent

Explain the procedure carefully to the patient so that they understand what the procedure is and why it is being undertaken. Using good interpersonal and communication skills, not only will the patient be able to provide informed consent, but they are less likely to make any sudden movements and are more likely to be relaxed (Hart 2011). Patient education is an important part of patient care and cannot be over-emphasised.

Anxiety

As already discussed in Chapter 12, patients may experience anxiety, so they should be asked if they have had a cannula inserted previously; because, as McGowan (2014) points out, anxiety may be due to a previous bad experience, a degree of 'needle phobia' (fear of a needle) or just a dislike of medical procedures. See Chapter 12 for suggestions on reducing or managing anxiety.

> **THINK ABOUT IT**
> What options might you consider if your patient were very anxious about the procedure?

Terminology

- *Vasovagal episode*: blood pressure drops and patient may feel faint.
- *Erythema*: redness.
- *Cerebrovascular accident (CVA)*: commonly known as a stroke.
- *Phlebitis*: inflammation/infection of the vein.
- *Rigors*: shivering associated with high temperature.
- *Hypotension*: low blood pressure.
- *Malaise*: tiredness, weakness.
- *Venesection*: blood is taken from the patient, for example to reduce the haemoglobin level; commonly this technique is used in patients with chronic bronchitis.

Common problems/potential complications of peripheral IV cannulation

Unsuccessful cannulation

According to Morris (2011), veins might be missed due to: poor skin stabilisation; poor vein choice; or failure to penetrate the vein due to poor insertion angle and physiological changes in the vein due to ageing. A thorough patient assessment, experience and good technique will help the practitioner to avoid or manage these problems. *Ensure that you have followed local policy to achieve competent and safe practice.*

Damaged device

Prior to using the cannula, the packaging needs to be checked to ensure the product is latex free and that it is single use. The packaging will also display the gauge size, lot number and expiry date as well as how many millilitres per minute can be infused (Boyd 2013).

Flushing

In order for the cannula to remain patent it needs to be flushed, usually with sodium chloride 0.9%. Ideally a 10 ml syringe should be used as a smaller syringe creates too much pressure on the vein walls resulting in damage (Boyd 2013). Please check your local policy which should reflect best practice.

Haematoma

Morris (2011) defines this as bleeding (usually uncontrolled) that occurs as a result of infiltration of blood from a punctured vein into the tissue immediately surrounding it. A haematoma can be recognised as a blue/purplish tinged lump at the point of the needle insertion. Once this occurs the procedure should be aborted and the haematoma managed.

Management

If a haematoma occurs during the procedure, release the tourniquet, remove the cannula and apply firm pressure for 2–3 min and elevate the arm. Apply a sterile dressing and ensure that this is documented; also ensure regular monitoring of the site.

Bruising

Bruising is a common risk and can be related to poor technique. Some patients, however, are predisposed to bruising, such as those with delicate skin and/or those taking certain medication (Gabriel 2012). Thorough patient assessment and good technique minimise the possibility of bruising.

Infiltration and extravasation

Infiltration (often referred to as 'tissueing') occurs when the cannula pulls out of the vein and the infusion fluid accumulates in the tissue around the cannula site (Workman 1999; Hadaway 2004). Workman (1999) proposed careful monitoring of the site in an older patient, who may not report discomfort as quickly because loss of skin tone and elasticity mean that tissues around the site have a greater capacity to expand with the leaking fluid.

Extravasation is the infiltration of a vesicant (irritating agent) medicine from an IV line into the surrounding tissue, and can cause severe tissue injury or destruction (Hadaway 2004).

Prevention

- Secure the cannula firmly with a sterile dressing while in place.
- Ensure that appropriate gauge of cannula is selected.
- Replace cannula after 72–96 h (Ingram and Lavery 2007).
- Secure lines and extensions to the limb to prevent accidental pulling (Workman 1999).

Signs

- Swelling.
- Discomfort.
- 'Tightness' at the site.
- Pain.
- Burning sensation – associated with extravasation.
- Blanching and coolness of the skin.

Management

1 Immediately stop the infusion and disconnect the tubing; alert medical staff.
2 If a cannula is needed, re-site in the other arm to allow swelling to subside.
3 Where infiltration has occurred, elevate the arm and apply a warm compress.
4 Intervene rapidly to any suspected extravasation injury; for example, either apply an ice pack or warm compress depending on vesicant (agent), elevate the arm and administer antidote; *this would be the role of registered nurse or doctor only, and would require a local policy.*
5 Reassure the patient that the swelling will subside in a few days.
6 Document and monitor the patient and site to prevent permanent damage (Workman 1999.)

Phlebitis

Mc Callum and Higgins (2012) identify three main types of phlebitis. This is inflammation of the vein and can be caused by mechanical damage, chemical irritation or infection (Ingram and Lavery 2005).

- Mechanical damage is caused by the rubbing of the cannula against the inner (intima) wall of the vein if a cannula is not secured with a sterile dressing.

- Chemical irritation is caused by the infusion of irritant medicines/fluids or a reaction to the cannula material.
- Infection is caused by the contamination of the cannula by microorganisms.

Prevention
- Remove the cannula as soon as it is no longer clinically indicated.
- Change the IV cannula every 72–96 h.
- Regularly inspect the IV site (at least daily).
- Remove the cannula at the first sign of phlebitis.
- Use strict aseptic technique during insertion and manipulation of cannula.
- Secure the device with a sterile dressing.
(Lavery and Ingram 2007.)

Signs
- Erythema.
- Pain at the insertion site.
- Localised skin temperature.
- Swelling.
- Leakage.
- In extreme cases, pus at the insertion site on removal of cannula.

Management
It is recommended to use a phlebitis scale for monitoring (Jackson 1997; Davies 1998; Rosenthal 2004).
- Mechanical and chemical phlebitis: remove cannula and apply warm, moist compress.
- Bacterial phlebitis: remove cannula, take blood cultures, then apply warm compress.
- Post-infusion phlebitis: this can occur 24–96 h after the cannula is removed; apply a warm, moist compress (Macklin 2003).

Thrombophlebitis
Tortora and Derrickson (2006) defined this as inflammation of the vein and clot formation. Thromboembolism occurs when a blood clot on the cannulated vein wall becomes detached, and could pass by venous flow to the heart and pulmonary (lung) circulation.

Prevention
- Use a small gauge cannula, allowing continuous blood flow around it.
- If an infusion stops as a result of clot formation, do *not* flush the cannula because it may dislodge the clot into the circulation; remove the cannula.
- Ensure correct insertion technique.

Air embolism
This is a possible hazard during IV therapy – *however, few healthcare assistants would be involved in administering IV fluids* – and it is caused if lines and connections are

not secure, and any attachment, for example a closed system, is not flushed first before connection.

Prevention
- Air must be removed from all extension lines, stopcocks and administration sets during the priming of the system.
- Ensure that Luer locks are tight fitting.
- Clamp the infusion line before the bag empties completely.

Arterial cannulation
This is identified by bright red blood pulsating into the flashback chamber and is caused by inappropriate assessment and insertion angle.

Prevention
- Plan procedure carefully.
- Apply sound knowledge of venous and arterial structures in the arm.
- Insert cannula at the appropriate angle; consult manufacturer's guide.

Action
- Remove the cannula immediately and apply firm pressure for 5 min, until bleeding stops.
- Apply a pressure bandage for 10–15 min.
- Elevate the arm.
- Check the patient's radial pulse, to ensure that pressure bandage is not too tight.
- Inform medical staff; once they are satisfied that bleeding has stopped the pressure bandage is removed and the site covered with a sterile dressing.
- Do not use that site for a further 24 h.
- Monitor the site over 24 h and document the incident in the patient's notes.

Nerve damage
This is a rare complication caused by poor assessment and inappropriate angle of insertion. The patient may report pain, numbness or tingling in the arm (Dougherty and Lister 2011).

Management
1 Remove the needle/cannula immediately.
2 Apply pressure to stop the bleeding.
3 Inform the doctor.
4 Record the incident in the patient's notes.
5 Observe and advise the patient to report if symptoms worsen.
6 Treatment is symptomatic, so analgesia may be prescribed for pain.
7 Reassure the patient.
8 Physiotherapy may be necessary (Dougherty and Lister 2004).

Delay

In the situation where a patient has collapsed, ensure that help is on the way using the normal emergency procedures. Stay with the patient. It is essential that peripheral IV cannulation be undertaken as soon as possible, as the patient's worsening clinical condition is likely to make cannulation more difficult. *Do not delay* in gaining access (Ingram and Lavery 2007).

THINK ABOUT IT

Consider, if an emergency and a patient had collapsed, whether the insertion of a cannula would be your priority. What is your local policy?

Other complications of peripheral IV cannulation

- Use of inappropriate sites.
- Circulatory overload: too rapid IV rate, wrongly prescribed, wrongly set rate; *this would not be an aspect in which the healthcare assistant would be involved.*
- Kinking of cannula; common if sited in an area of flexion, for example the elbow.
- Plastic embolism: this risk is reduced with safety cannula, for example Vasofix, because it is now not possible to reinsert the needle back into the cannula.
- Tourniquet left in place.
- Septicaemia: result of bacteria entering the bloodstream; patient presents with general malaise, temperature, rigors and hypotension.

  Table 16.7 is a competency framework for peripheral IV cannulation.

THINK ABOUT IT

While removing a cannula, you observe some redness around the site. What might be the cause and what actions will you take?

Removal of peripheral IV cannula

Once a decision has been made to remove the cannula, explain the procedure to the patient, and obtain patient consent and cooperation (see Table 16.6 for the procedure).

  Equipment required: as well as a clinical waste bag and sharps bin:
- Gloves and apron.
- Tray or clean receptacle.
- Cotton ball/gauze swab.
- Pad for spillage.
- Sterile dressing/plaster.
- Tape to secure dressing, if used.

Table 16.6 Specific nursing actions during procedure – removal.

Action	Reason
1. Close the flow clamp to discontinue the infusion of fluid (if necessary and if an accepted part of a healthcare assistant's role)	Prevent fluid leakage
2. Decontaminate (wash) hands, put on gloves	Prevention of infection and of healthcare assistant's hands being contaminated with blood
3. Expose the cannula site and, using aseptic technique, remove the dressing. Do not use scissors	May inadvertently cut the cannula resulting in fragments that can cause embolus (clot)
4. Apply gentle pressure with a swab/cotton ball above the cannulation site while withdrawing the cannula On removal, apply firm pressure for approximately 2–3 min until bleeding stops	Excessive pressure applied to a cannula that is blocked could result in thrombus (fixed clot) being expelled into the blood stream causing an embolus
5. Check patient has no allergy, then cover the site with a plaster/sterile dressing, until the puncture site has healed Continue to observe the site	To prevent bacteria from entering the puncture site Cotton ball may adhere and when removed bleeding restarts
6. Check that cannula removed is undamaged and intact. Discard immediately into a sharps bin However, if there are signs of infection present, report this to a senior nurse and it may be necessary to obtain a swab from the insertion site and the tip of cannula, and send to the laboratory for culture	Ensure no trauma to vein Microbiological investigations
7. Document the date and time of cannula removal and any problems encountered or not	Good record keeping and legal requirement

Source: NHS Lothian (2007). Adapted with permission of NHS Lothian.

Summary

Peripheral IV cannulation is a specialist skill that should not be undertaken lightly, ensuring compliance with local and national policies (Lavery 2010). Care should be taken using the H.A.N.D.S. approach and it should be remembered that this skill is being undertaken on a person. Accurate documentation and good interpersonal skills are important. Perhaps the final words of this chapter that summarise cannulation belong to Lisa Dougherty (2015):

' IV therapy; get it right no matter what.'

Table 16.7 Practical assessment form: competency – peripheral IV cannulation.

Steps	First assessment/reassessment					Date/competent/ signature
	Demonstration	Date/sign 2	Date/sign 3	Date/sign 4	Date/sign 5	
	Date/sign 1					
1 Washed hands and apron worn						
2 Assembled all equipment required on clean tray or trolley and equipment in date and intact						
3 Procedure explained, verbal consent gained						
4 Patient's comfort considered and positioning appropriate for safe practice						
5 Environment prepared – lighting, bed height, privacy if required, and sharps bin ready						
6 Patient's identity confirmed per local policy						
7 Considers with patient; vein of choice by assessing sites and patient comfort						
8 Prepares cannula – depending on patient's condition and reason for cannula						
9 Tourniquet applied 7–10 cm above chosen site, and vein assessed as suitable						
10 Tourniquet released and vein checked decompressed						
11 Hands washed or bactericidal hand rub used						
12 Tourniquet re-applied to chosen site						
13 Site cleansed for at least 30 s and allowed to air dry for minimum of 30 s						
14 Gloves put on						

Table 16.7 (*continued*)

Steps	First assessment/reassessment					Date/competent/ signature
	Demonstration					
	Date/sign 1	Date/sign 2	Date/sign 3	Date/sign 4	Date/sign 5	
15 Vein cannulated successfully following approved local procedure and policy						
16 Tourniquet released						
17 Pressure applied distally to vein, needle is removed, while cannula supported to prevent dislodging						
18 Needle disposed of as per local policy immediately						
19 Considers closed system, e.g. Smartsite, to minimise trauma and infection from port site						
20 Cannula flushed at appropriate rate to confirm patency and position						
21 Secures cannula using appropriate dressing						
22 Patient education given and aware of need for prompt communication if any concerns						
23 Identification of cannula site by recording in appropriate documentation, noting gauge, site, reason for insertion, date, time and signature of operator						

Supervisors/Assessor(s):

CASE STUDY 16.1

Miss Winifred Allsop, aged 72 years, has had a stroke (CVA) affecting her right arm and has rheumatoid arthritis. What assessment factors do you need to consider?

Below, the reader will find a self-assessment checklist; however, the reader may also wish to review Skills for Health (2004) competence HSC72.

Self-assessment

Assessment	Aspects	Achieved ✓
Patient	*Have you considered all aspects of this section?*	
	Patient assessment: veins and general condition	
	Infection control and asepsis aspects	
	Consent, communication and education	
	Problem solving	
Procedure	*Have you considered all aspects of this section?*	**Achieved ✓**
	Selecting equipment and insertion technique	
	Problem solving	
	Recording	
	Monitoring, maintenance and reporting concerns	
	Removal	

References

Boyd C. (2013) Clinical Skills for Nurses. Wiley Blackwell.

Coram J (2015) A collaborative approach: seeking excellence in vascular access. *British Journal of Nursing* 24 Supplement 8: S16.

Davies S (1998) The role of nurses in intravenous cannulation. *Nursing Standard* 12(17): 43–46.

Department of Health (DH) (2011) High Impact Intervention No 2: Peripheral Intravenous Cannula Care Bundle. Available at: http://webarchive.nationalarchives.gov.uk/20120118164404/hcai.dh.gov.uk/files/2011/03/2011-03-14-HII-Peripheral-intravenous-cannula-bundle-FIN%E2%80%A6.pdf (accessed December 2015).

Dougherty L (2015) IV therapy: get it right no matter what. *British Journal of Nursing* 21 Supplement 14: S3.

Dougherty L and Lister S (eds) (2004) *The Royal Marsden Hospital Manual of Clinical Nursing Procedures*, 6th edn. Oxford: Blackwell Publishing.

Dougherty L and Lister S (eds) (2011) *The Royal Marsden Hospital Manual of Clinical Nursing Procedures*, 8th edn. Oxford: Blackwell Publishing.

Dunning T (2011) *A Manual of Nursing Practice*, 4th edn. Oxford: Wiley Blackwell.

Ellson R (2008) Venepuncture and cannulation. In: Richardson R (ed.) *Clinical Skills for Student Nurses Theory*, Practice and Reflection. Reflect Press.co.uk, pp. 115–149.

Frimpong A, Caguioa J and Octavo G (2015) Promoting safe IV management in practice using H.A.N.D.S. *British Journal of Nursing (IV Therapy Supplement)* 24(2): S18–S23.

Gabriel J (2012) Venepuncture and cannulation: considering the ageing vein. *British Journal of Nursing* 21 Supplement 1: S22–S28.

Hadaway L (2004) Preventing and managing peripheral extravasation. *Nursing* 34(5): 66–67.

Health and Safety Executive (HSE) (2013) Health and Safety (Sharp Instruments in Healthcare) Regulations 2013. Guidance for employers and employees. Available at: http://tinyurl.com/cp8sbu5 (accessed 23 February 2015).

Health Protection Scotland (2012) Targeted Literature Review: What are the Key Infection Prevention and Control Recommendations to Inform a Peripheral Vascular Catheter (PVC) Maintenance Care Quality Improvement Tool? tinyurl.com/HPS-PVC-rev.

Ingram P and Lavery I (2005) Peripheral intravenous therapy: key risk and implications for practice. *Nursing Standard* 19(46): 55–64.

Ingram P and Lavery I (2007) Peripheral intravenous cannulation: safe insertion and removal technique. *Nursing Standard* 22(1): 44–48.

Jackson A (1997) Performing peripheral intravenous cannulation. *Professional Nurse* 13(1): 21–25.

Lavery I (2010) Infection control in IV therapy: a review of the chain of infection. *British Journal of Nursing (Intravenous Supplement)* 19(19): S56–S60.

Longmate A G, Ellis K, Boyle L, et al. (2011) Elimination of central-venous-catheter-related bloodstream infections from the intensive care unit. *BMJ Quality and Safety* 20: 174–180.

Loveday H, Wilson P, Pratt R, et al. (2014) epic3: National Evidence-Based Guidelines for Preventing Healthcare-Associated Infections in NHS Hospitals in England . *The Journal of Hospital infection* 86, Supplement 1: S1–S70.

Lundgren A, Ek AC and Wahren L (1998) Handling and control of peripheral intravenous lines. *Journal of Advanced Nursing* 27: 897–904.

Macklin D (2003) Phlebitis: A painful complication of peripheral IV catheterization that may be prevented. *American Journal of Nursing* 103(2): 55–60.

McCallum L and Higgins D (2012) Care of peripheral venous cannula sites. *Nursing Times* 108(34/35): 12–15.

McGowan D (2014) Peripheral intravenous cannulation: managing distress and anxiety. *British Journal of Nursing* 22 Supplement 19: S4–S9.

Medical Devices Agency (MDA) (2000) Single-use Medical Devices: Implications and Consequences of Re-use. MDA DB2000 (04). London: The Stationery Office.

Medicines and Healthcare Products Regulatory Agency (MHPRA) (2013) *Single-Use Medical Devices: Implications and Consequences of Reuse*. London: Medicines and Healthcare Products Regulatory Agency.

Morris W (2011) Complications in venepuncture and cannulation. In: Phillips S, Collins M and Dougherty L (eds) *Venepuncture and Cannulation*. Oxford: Wiley-Blackwell, pp.155–222.

NHS Lothian (2007) *Adult Venepuncture and/or Peripheral IV Cannulation: Clinical Skills Education Package*. Edinburgh: NHS Lothian.

Oliver G (2015) Foreword. Infection prevention in IV therapy. IV3000 dressing meeting the challenge. *British Journal of Nursing* 24 Supplement: S4.

Phillips S, Collins M and Dougherty L (2011) *Venepuncture and Cannulation*. Oxford: Wiley-Blackwell.Rosenthal K (2004) Phlebitis: An irritating complication. *Nursing Made Incredibly Easy* 2(1): 62–63.

Rosenthal K (2005) Tailor your I.V. insertion techniques special populations. *Nursing* 35(5): 36–41.

Skills for Health (2004) *HSC72 Cannulation*. Bristol: Skills for Health. Available at: www.skillsforhealth .org.uk/tools/view_framework.php?id=39 (accessed 2 September 2007).

Tortora G J and Derrickson B (2006) *Principles of Anatomy and Physiology*, 11th edn. Hoboken, NJ: John Wiley & Sons Inc.

Witt B (2011) Patient's perspective. In: Phillips S, Collins M and Dougherty L (eds) *Venepuncture and Cannulation*. Oxford: Wiley Blackwell, pp. 108–130

Workman B (1999) Peripheral intravenous therapy management. *Nursing Standard* 14(4): 53–60.

CHAPTER 17

Recording a 12-lead Electrocardiograph (ECG)

LEARNING OBJECTIVES

- Review anatomy and electrophysiology of the heart as it relates to the ECG
- Review the technique for recording a 12-lead ECG and use of electrocardiograph equipment
- Identify potential problems of the procedure, and discuss actions to prevent or reduce these

---

Aim of this chapter

The aim of this chapter is to provide the healthcare assistant (HCA) and assistant practitioner (AP) with a brief account of the anatomy and electrophysiology of the heart and to provide an overview of how to record an ECG. Emphasis is placed on the holistic care of the patient throughout the chapter, but it does not discuss how to interpret the recording; this is a specialised role and requires specialised training. The Society of Cardiological Science and Technology (SCST) emphasise the need for training and recommend that all personnel who record ECGs should be appropriately trained. They also point out that there are a number of reports and studies that found practitioners' lack of essential knowledge lead to wrongly recorded ECGs, which may result in incorrect diagnoses and inappropriate treatments (SCST 2014).

An ECG is a graphic tracing of electrical patterns produced by the heart (Bayés de Luna 2008). Depending on where they work, the role of the HCA and AP may include recording an ECG (Peate and Wilde 2012). Recording an ECG is an important skill that requires care, competence and confidence: it is not the role of the HCA and AP to make a diagnosis. It is important that the ECG recording is reviewed by a doctor or cardiac practitioner, which Tough (2004) suggests must be within 10 minutes of the initial recording, so you must be aware of to whom results are reported and within what time frame. Check local Trust policy.

Clinical Skills for Healthcare Assistants and Assistant Practitioners, Second Edition.
Angela Whelan and Elaine Hughes.
© 2016 John Wiley & Sons, Ltd. Published 2016 by John Wiley & Sons, Ltd.

Relevant anatomy and physiology

Understanding the anatomy of the heart is essential if skilled, high-quality care is to be provided (Peak and Wild 2012). McChance and Heuther (2014) explain how cardiac activity consists of a number of complex processes including muscular, electrical, neural, emotional and hormonal ones. It might be useful here to review Chapters 5 and 6, which have covered some aspects of how the heart works. Tortora and Derrickson (2011) describe how the heart lies in the thoracic (chest) cavity and consists of four chambers divided by the vertical septum (partition). The upper chambers are known as the left and right atria and the lower chambers as the left and right ventricles. Although the heart consists of four chambers, Hampton (2006) suggests that from the electrical point of view it can be thought of as being two pumps, a right-sided pump and a left-sided pump, because both atria contract together and then both ventricles simultaneously contract. The function of the circulatory system is simple: to circulate oxygenated blood, nutrients and other substances to the tissues via the high-pressure arterial system and to pump deoxygenated blood to the lungs through the low-pressure venous circulation (McChance and Heuther 2014)

The cone-shaped heart, roughly the size of a closed fist (Tortora and Derrickson, 2011), is a muscular organ located in the thoracic cavity, immediately above the diaphragm and between the lungs, that rests in a moistened chamber called the pericardial cavity which is surrounded by the rib cage. The normal adult heart rate is said to be approximately 72 beats per minute, but can fluctuate depending on a variety of factors such as age, fitness and medication (Wild and Peate 2012). Peate and Wild (2012) estimate that since the heart beats tirelessly, it could be calculated that, from the moment it starts to the moment it stops the heart beats approximately 100 000 times per day and about 35 million times in a year. During an average lifetime, that means the human heart will have beat more than 2.5 billion times. Thus the heart pumps more than 6500 litres of blood a day. The volume of blood that reaches the tissues each minute (cardiac output) is the most important index of cardiovascular performance, and in adults with a heart rate of 70 bpm this gives a cardiac output of 4900 ml/minute.

The cardiac conduction system

The heart uses an electrical conduction system to pump blood, as shown in Figure 17.1. An impulse is initiated by the sinoatrial (SA) node that causes the heart muscle to contract or depolarise. Each impulse spreads from the node across both atria, causing them to contract and pump blood through one-way valves into the ventricles. The SA node also controls the pace of the heart (70–80 beats per minute). The electric impulse continues depolarisation (contraction) to the atrioventricular (AV) node, with the electrical discharge passing quickly through

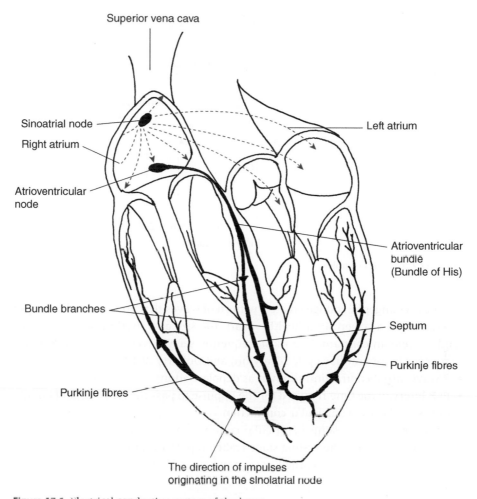

Superior vena cava

Sinoatrial node

Right atrium

Atrioventricular
node

Bundle branches

Purkinje fibres

Left atrium

Atrioventricular
bundle
(Bundle of His)

Septum

Purkinje fibres

The direction of impulses
originating in the sinoatrial node

Figure 17.1 Electrical conducting system of the heart.

the bundle of His – a bundle of specialised fibres within the interventricular septum that divides into right and left Purkinje fibres, which continues to allow
contraction of the ventricles (Stevens 2008).

A 12-lead ECG is a graphical recording of the electrical activity of the heartbeat obtained by placing 10 electrodes on specific positions in the body surface
(four on the limbs and six on the chest) (Stevens 2008). This provides 12 different views of the electrical activity generated by the myocardium as it depolarises
(contracts) and repolarises (relaxes) to produce the heartbeat. An ECG trace is
a series of waves, the size of each wave corresponding to an electrical voltage
(measured in millivolts) generated by the heart as it goes through the cycle of
contraction and relaxation. The currents detected on the skin are weak, hence
the ECG machine contains an amplifier. It will be helpful if you find out about
the type of machine you use.

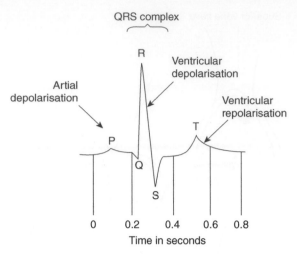

Figure 17.2 The QRS complex.

These changes in voltage create a pattern of waves that are captured on paper or viewed on a screen. In a healthy heart, the size and rhythm of these waves tends to remain constant. The most frequently seen waves are P, Q, R, S and T that occur in one cardiac cycle (Crawford and Doherty 2012).

- P wave: atrial contraction (known as depolarisation).
- P–R interval: the time required for the impulse to pass the AV node and bundle of His, and cause ventricular contraction.
- QRS complex: represents ventricular contraction.
- T wave: represents the resting stage (called repolarisation).

    The QRS complex is recorded as seen in Figure 17.2.

Reasons for recording a 12-lead ECG

Crawford and Doherty (2012) recognise the numerous indications for recording an ECG and point out that it is important to understand that the ECG can only directly measure time and voltage, and so is useful in situations such as detecting the presence of a myocardial infarction but may be of limited use in other areas. Tortora and Derrickson (2011) explain that the standard ECG produces views from different combinations of chest and limb leads. By comparing these tracings with each other and normal records, it is possible to determine three things:

1 If the heart's conduction pathway is abnormal.
2 If the heart is enlarged.
3 If certain regions of the heart have been damaged, for example from a heart attack.

How to perform a 12-lead ECG

The ECG test is inexpensive, uses portable equipment that is easy to operate, and can be undertaken anywhere – including at a patient's bedside, GP surgery or ambulance – giving a prompt result and allowing rapid treatment decisions and actions to be made by relevant healthcare professionals.

Indications for performing an ECG
- The assessment of patients presenting with chest pain.
- Unexplained dizziness and/or syncope.
- The diagnosis·and monitoring of cardiovascular disease.
- The assessment of therapy outcomes, both beneficial and toxic.
- Overdose.
- Presurgical assessment.
- Risk assessment for cardiac disease in individuals with two or more of the following risk factors: diabetes, hypertension, smoking history, obesity, hyper-cholesterolemia, strong family history of cardiac disease.
- A family history of sudden death.
- The assessment of cardiac effects in co-existing systemic disease, for example renal failure.
- Monitoring cardiac transplant success or rejection.
- Adhering to occupational requirements, for example airline pilot, divers.
- Epidemiological studies.

(Crawford and Doherty 2012: 2.)

How to record a 12-lead ECG
This chapter focuses only on a standard 12-lead ECG where electrodes are placed at strategic points of the chest area and limbs as a diagnostic tool, and does not discuss ambulatory and/or continuous ECGs.

Preparation for the procedure

Preparing the patient
A key goal of good practice as identified by SCST (2014) is to ensure the patient has a positive experience and to maintain privacy and dignity, which should also reflect Trust policy. Every effort should be made to ensure the patient has privacy and dignity, and any cultural sensitivities of the patient are addressed and embarrassment minimised. If the patient does not speak English, it may be necessary to provide an interpreter; similarly some patients may use sign language and need the same consideration. Patients should be asked to undress above the waist to allow access to the upper torso for correct placement of the electrodes, removing any jewellery from the patient's neck, arms, and wrists. Assistance should

be offered and given as required. Ensure the patient is comfortable and warm and avoid drafts. The ECG reading can be affected by the position of the patient, where possible, for consistency, the SCST (2014) recommends patients lie in a semi-recumbent position of approximately 45 degrees with limbs supported by the bed to minimise artefact due to muscle tension. Any variation should be noted. Once the electrodes have been attached, the patient maybe covered with a gown to preserve their modesty, avoiding unnecessary exposure. The SCST (2014) also highlights that some patients may want a chaperone present and may also request a relative or carer.

Communication skills have been discussed in Chapter 2 and are emphasised here. The patient having an ECG should be given information about the procedure that they are able to understand. Information should be clear and precise and may take the form of a booklet, information letter or be an oral explanation. The HCA or AP should introduce themselves, explain the procedure and give the patient an opportunity to seek clarification. Reassurance is essential and careful explanations can overcome many fears, especially as many patients feel uncomfortable being touched and having their chest examined (Stevens 2008). A sympathetic, caring, compassionate manner will do much to alleviate some of the patient's apprehension. Peate and Wild (2012) also highlight the importance of explaining to the patient that the ECG is painless, there will be no electrical current entering their body and that small electrodes will be attached to the chest. Leads from the electrodes connected to the ECG machine will produce a printout.

Consent should be gained and the patient positioned comfortably, maintaining dignity at all times. It is important to always remember the person at the centre of this process and treat them with care, compassion and kindness; listen to and talk with them. Check to see if the patient has any allergies, such as electrode adhesive. Confirmation of identity is vital; record the details following local policy, checking the printed recording also has the correct patient details. Only then can consent be gained as discussed in Chapter 1.

THINK ABOUT IT

Mrs Wang, aged 82 years, is to be prepared for a standard 12-lead ECG. What might you need to consider if you were going to carry out this procedure?

Recording a 12-lead ECG

This section looks at the equipment required for the procedure, the patient preparation and the actual procedure. It also reviews the care of the equipment, before moving on to discuss potential problems and means of addressing these.

Equipment

The equipment for a standard 12-lead ECG is an ECG machine (with tracing paper), a patient lead cable (with limb and chest leads labelled accordingly), disposable electrodes and paper towel/tissues (Crawford and Doherty 2012). Stevens (2008) highlights the need to be familiar with local equipment, as showing a lack of familiarity and ability will not result in a calm patient. The equipment should come with a manual to which you can refer. It is also important to know how to change the recording paper; how to charge the machine and where supplies of electrodes and paper are kept; and how to order further supplies. Equipment should be maintained, kept clean and orderly, and all mains leads and cables and connectors be intact with no evidence of damage. Battery operated machines will need to have sufficient charge and mains powered ECG machines should be plugged in and be easily recognisable (SCST 2014).

Electrodes

Peate and Wild (2012) described electrodes as required to detect the electrical energy produced by the heart and transfer the information to the monitoring equipment. External electrodes are used to do this; they consist of adhesive tape and a conductive saline gel, on the other side there is a small metal conductor button that is snap-connected to the monitor via leads.

Manufacturers produce electrodes that are disposable, self-adhesive, latex free and hypoallergenic and prepared with an inner moist conductive gel, that need to be kept stored in the manufacturer's foil packing preventing the conductive gel on each electrode from drying out and protecting the sensor from any damage or contamination (Taylor 2015). The expiry date on the foil pack of electrodes must be checked to ensure they are in date, stored correctly, and that they are all the same product (electrodes not mixed from different packs). When ready, remove the protective electrode backing to expose the gel-covered disc and ensure that gel is still moist and enough covers the disc.

THINK ABOUT IT

You have been asked to carry out a standard 12-lead ECG. What checks of the equipment must you make before proceeding?

Skin preparation and infection control

Skin preparation is important to ensure good skin contact; otherwise the results may be affected or distorted. SCST (2014) identified that care must be taken for patients with sensitive skin. Skin may need cleansing; infection control measures must be taken in accordance with local/Trust policy including handwashing and disposal of clinical waste (SCST 2014). If a patient has body hair this will impair the connection, and so it may be helpful to shave the patient. Exfoliation (removal of hair) may be required and should be undertaken using abrasive tape especially designed for this purpose (SCST 2014). Chest hair may need to be removed to ensure adequate contact with the skin (Peate and Wild 2012).

Caution is advised, as razors may break the skin and pose a potential infection risk. Oral consent should be obtained from the patient and an unused razor should be used and disposed of, as per local policy. After the procedure, remove the electrodes and clean the skin.

Electrode placement

Placement of the four limb electrodes; right arm; right leg; left arm and left leg

The correct positioning of electrodes is essential to obtain a diagnostically accurate recording because each lead records a specific surface of the heart. Misplacing the electrodes may alter the appearance of the ECG (SCST 2014). By attaching electrodes to the right arm, left arm and left leg, just proximal to the wrist and ankle, three major planes for detecting electrical activity can be recorded. These three planes form a hypothetical triangle (Einthoven's Triangle) with the heart in the middle. A fourth electrode is attached to the left leg, but serves only as an earth and is not used for recording purposes (Stevens 2008). The electrodes are usually placed on the outer aspect 3–4 cm above the forearm (wrist) and medial (inner) aspect 3–4 cm above the foreleg (ankle) (Figure 17.3a gives the placement). The electrodes can be placed on another area, such as on the right, if, for example, the patient has a right arm amputation; this should be clearly noted and documented on the recording (SCST 2014) (see Table 17.1 for the procedure).

Placement of the six chest or precordial leads V1, V2, V3, V4, V5, V6

The electrodes are placed on the chest wall at the designated positions (see Figure 17.3 for placement). Clinical Guidelines by Consensus for Recording a standard 12-lead ECG produced by the Society for Cardiological Science and Technology (SCST 2014) clearly identify the correct positioning of the chest leads.

A common error occurs when counting the intercostal spaces from the clavicle: the small space between the clavicle and the first rib is not the first intercostal space. To avoid this error, the manubriosternal joint (also called the Angle of Louis) should be used as the main reference point. To locate the Angle of Louis, a finder should be run down the sternum from the top, until a bony horizontal ridge is met. Sliding the finger down and to the right side will locate the second intercostal space. From here it is possible to count down to the third and fourth intercostal spaces. Slide the finger towards the sternum until the edge is felt and place the electrode for V1 in this position. This procedure should be repeated on the left side to correctly position V2. Note that the left- and right-sided rib spaces may be offset, thus avoiding placing V2 adjacent to V1 without counting the rib spaces.

Next, the V4 electrode should be placed in the fifth intercostal space in line with the mid-point of the clavicle. The V3 electrode should be placed in the fifth intercostal space in line with the mid-point of the clavicle. The V3 electrode should then be placed midway between the V2 and V4 electrodes.

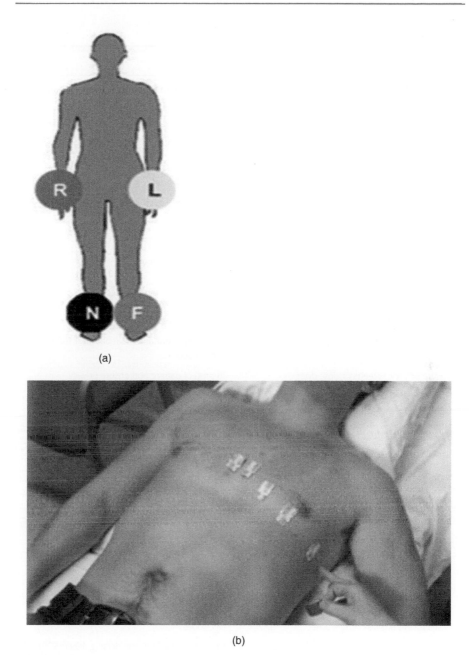

(a)

(b)

Figure 17.3 Electrode and lead placement for standard 12-lead ECG: (a) Limb electrode placement and (b) electrode placement on the chest.

Table 17.1 Procedure for recording a standard 12-lead ECG.

Action	Reason
Position ECG machine close to patient	Minimise risk of leads, cables, etc. becoming disconnected during the procedure
Check that power cable and patient lead fitted correctly to machine, and route power cable away from patient	Working correctly and minimise any electrical interference
Press power on; multi-lead machine will do self-test, then check machine set at:	To ensure that machine set and working correctly
1 mV or 10 small squares (two large squares)	
Paper speed is 25 mm/s	
Filter is on; check local policy	
Introduce self and patient provides name and date of birth (DOB); this is checked against identification, e.g. ID bracelet	Ensure correct patient
Patient explanation given to reassure and inform, to allow questions and gain consent	Understand reason for procedure and how it is done, so relaxed and cooperative
Offer patient chaperone, if appropriate	If female patient and male operator this is good practice
Ensure privacy, screens or close door	To protect patient and ensure privacy
Patient resting comfortably, lying if able (semi-recumbent or supine), with limbs supported, arms at sides	To ensure best recording and patient safety and comfort
Ask or assist the patient to undress exposing forearms, chest and forelegs. Ensure modesty; also the patient may need to remove jewellery	To prepare patient for the procedure and ensure no contact with leads from jewellery, e.g. watch
Wash hands or use alcohol gel	To prevent infection
Check that patient has understood that, once the electrodes are in place and test starts, must keep still and breathe normally	Reduce electrical noise (Henderson 1997)
Clean limbs and chest area as outlined earlier: select flat fleshy areas, avoid bony or muscular areas	To ensure that skin has good contact for electrodes and good placement
Place the 10 electrodes, as per Figure 17.3; first ensure electrodes are in date, in foil pack and gel is still moist, e.g. RA = right arm	To ensure accurate reading, and check the patient has no allergy with the adhesive on the electrodes
Attach leads to electrodes correctly (follow colour coding and labelling), e.g. LA = left arm and yellow (refer to Figure 17.3)	Correct monitoring (Henderson, 1997; SCST 2014). NHS Lothian (2004) noted that manufacturers use different colour schemes so follow UK colour code
Extend patient cable along the side of patient or centre of body from feet to chest	To ensure that all cables fully supported and prevent pulling on the electrodes

Table 17.1 (*continued*)

Action	Reason
Also ensure that the leads are not pulling on the electrodes or lying over each other	To reduce electrical noise from movement and so get good reading
Make sure that patient is ready and relaxed, remind him or her not to talk or cough and allow 10 s for the patient to settle and relax	Procedure proceeds safely
Commence the 12-lead ECG recording by pushing auto-button	Allow machine to automatically run rhythm strip and leads one at a time to obtain ECG recording
Observe that paper strip is moving and recording	Ensure connected and recording correctly
Observe recording; do not alarm the patient; however, if anxious about the recording, seek advice or support, e.g. ask a colleague to get a senior nurse or doctor, and reassure the patient	It is not the role of the healthcare assistant to interpret; however, if any irregularity is observed in the rate or rhythm, it may be prudent to get a doctor or experienced nurse to come and check immediately
During procedure reassure patient and explain what's happening	So patient informed and relaxed
If poor tracing (noise – muscle movement), check electrodes, connections and leads, then redo (repeat) recording	Ensure best recording
Before finishing ECG, check first that the recording is free from artefact (noise) and confirm settings: paper speed 25 mm, standard setting 1 mV, 10 mm	Recording technically accurate, so ready for interpretation by doctor
Let the patient know that procedure is finished, what you will do with recording, and then remove the electrodes. Offer to help wipe off the gel and redress, if necessary	Ensure that patient comfortable and aware of next steps
Document as local policy, suggested that ECG has full patient name, DOB, date and time of recording, relevant clinical details, e.g. chest pain during test, ward/department, operator signs (on the reverse of the ECG recording strip) and before leaving patient	Record maintained and accurate details Avoid errors and risk of ECG being filed in the wrong patient's notes
Turn off machine	Save power
Inform a doctor or senior nurse and ensure that doctor sees recording at earliest or agree time frame, e.g. 10 min (Tough 2004)	To ensure that results acted upon and procedure documented
Remove machine and restock; remember to plug into mains if battery operated	Good practice

Adapted from Dougherty and Lister (2011) and NHS Lothian (2004), with permission from G Brady Education Coordinator Cardiology, NHS Lothian (2004).

The V5 and V6 electrodes should then be positioned in horizontal alignment with the V4 electrode. The V5 electrode should be placed in the anterior axillary line; the V6 electrode should be placed on the mid-axillary line.

It is convention to place the V4, V5 and V6 electrodes beneath the left breast when breast tissue overlies the correct anatomical positions when recording an ECG from female patients. There is some evidence that suggests minimal disruption to the signal may be caused; however, further research is required to confirm or refute this. Using the back of the hand to lift the breast with care and sensitivity to place the electrodes is required.

Times and calibration of ECG

It is of interest to note, as Stevens (2008) identified, that ECG machines are standardised using paper where each large square = 5 mm and this represents 0.2 seconds, so there are five large squares per second and 300 for 1 minute. The standard signal of 1 millivolt (mV) moves the stylus (recording needle) vertically 1 cm (two large squares).

Related aspects and terminology

Even though this chapter does *not cover how to interpret an ECG recording*, it is useful to have an understanding of some terminology relating to the procedure, especially what a normal ECG recording is.

- *Sinus rhythm*: normal rhythm and usually 60–100 bpm; it is regular and complexes (PQRST wave) are identical. The word sinus indicates that the heartbeat originated in the SA node (Hand 2002) (Figure 17.4). Hampton and Adlam (2013) noted that in a child up to 1 year of age, the rate is 140–160 bpm, falling slowly to 80 bpm by puberty (approximately 10 years old).
- *Sinus bradycardia*: regular rate originating from the SA node but less than 60 bpm. Hampton (2003) indicated that this can be due to physical fitness or caused by, for example, hypothermia (low temperature) or some medicines, such as digoxin
- *Sinus tachycardia*: regular rate also from SA node but 100–180 bpm; this can be in response to stressors, for example fever, anxiety, pain, exercise (Hampton 2003). Some stimulants, for example caffeine, alcohol, also can cause tachycardia; check the patient history.
- *Sinus arrhythmia*: a known phenomenon (condition) in younger people; heart rate increases as they breathe in and decreases as they breathe out.
- *Atrial fibrillation (AF)*: rapid chaotic depolarisation (contraction) of impulses through the atrial myocardium, replacing normal rhythmic activity by the SA node; can lead to palpitations as the heart rate is increased (low risk rate below

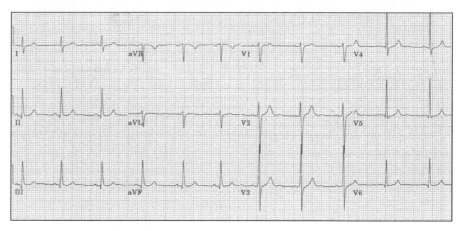

Figure 17.4 Example of sinus rhythm.

100 bpm, medium risk heart rate 100–150 bpm, and high risk if rate over 150 bpm – Hand 2002).

- *Atrial flutter*: less common than AF; in contrast with AF the rate is regular and often the tracing is described as 'saw tooth' and rate is often 150, 100 or 75 bpm (Hand 2002).
- *Ventricular tachycardia*: a serious arrhythmia and requires urgent action
- *Ventricular fibrillation* (VF): the rhythm of cardiac arrest, fast irregular rate as the ventricles contract in a chaotic uncoordinated manner. In VF the heart ceases to pump and after about 10 s, the blood pressure falls and the patient loses consciousness. If left untreated, death follows in 3–5 min (Hand 2002).
- *Artefact*: muscular movement that can affect ECG reading/tracing
- *Electrical noise*: as above, but also occurs if leads or power cables are crossed, or the tracing picks up electrical energy from elsewhere, such as beds or infusion devices (NHS Lothian 2004).

Hampton (2006) also describes the difference in an ECG (with a 12-lead ECG) where the signal is detected by only five electrodes. One electrode is placed on each limb and the fifth is held on by a suction cup and is then manually (by hand) moved to different positions over the patient's chest.

Common problems and actions

Hand (2002) outlines several tracing problems and indicates that they can usually be easily rectified (Table 17.2). Table 17.3 is a competency framework for recording a standard 12-lead ECG.

Table 17.2 ECG recording common problems.

Problem	Action
Poor electrode technique often appears as irregular fluctuations (artefact) on the tracing	Improve skin contact, so remove any body sweat or hair, or change electrodes and ensure good skin preparation
Defective cables or a loss of contact with the electrodes produces sharp waveform fluctuations	Replace cable or insert further into machine
Muscular activity (artefact) appears as fast irregular fuzzy fluctuations	Ensure that patient is comfortable and relaxed or reposition electrodes
AC interference – fuzzy, thickened, regular pattern	Ensure that filter is on, check connections, make sure leads, etc. are not being pulled or crossing over. Do not touch during the procedure, and remind the patient to lie still If possible switch off other electrical source, e.g. bed; discuss with senior nurse first
Wandering baseline – up and down movement of ECG tracing	Ensure good skin contact, re-apply electrodes, make sure that the machine is close to the patient so that there is no pull on the leads or cable, etc.
Incorrect placement of limb leads – commonly right and left arm leads reversed	Check and swap right and left arm leads if incorrect
Misplacement of chest leads/electrodes	Check and confirm placement of electrode, e.g. V1 and V2 fourth rib space

Adapted from Hand (2002) and NHS Lothian (2004). (Reproduced with permission from NHS Lothian 2004.)

Summary

Recording an accurate 12-lead ECG is a crucial skill. This is because the doctor (or registered nurse if a locally accepted role) will use this recording to make a diagnosis and plan appropriate treatment. Preparation and planning for the procedure and appropriate care throughout are therefore essential.

CASE STUDY 17.1

Fred Jones, aged 53 years, has been admitted for cardiac tests. He is anxious and has never been in hospital before. You have been asked to record a standard 12-lead ECG. Describe how you would prepare him for the procedure.

CASE STUDY 17.2

Betty Davis (aged 76 years) has been complaining of chest pain for 5 min and you have been asked to carry out a standard 12-lead ECG recording. Describe how you would position the electrodes and leads and carry out the procedure.

Table 17.3 Competency framework competency: recording a standard 12-lead ECG.

Steps	First assessment/reassessment					Date/competent/ signature
	Demonstration/supervised practice					
Recording a standard 12-lead ECG	Date/sign 1	Date/sign 2	Date/sign 3	Date/sign 4	Date/sign 5	
1 Patient's identity confirmed as per local policy						
2 Procedure explained, verbal consent gained						
3 Assembled all equipment required, checked that ECG machine stocked						
4 Machine checked, cable/leads correctly in place, machine self test done, confirmed all settings set as standard						
5 Patient screened and prepared, undressed and jewellery removed						
6 Patient's comfort considered and positioning appropriate for safe practice						
7 Washed hands or used alcohol gel						
8 Skin sites on limbs and chest area selected correctly						
9 Selected sites correctly cleaned and prepared – sweat or hair removed						
10 Electrodes applied to designated sites, connections pointing in line with direction of cable and lead wires						
11 Confirmed all electrodes/leads connected to power cable correctly and positioned correctly						
12 Explained when procedure starts that patient must not move, talk or cough						

Table 17.3 *(continued)*

First assessment/eeassessment

Steps	Demonstration/supervised practice					Date/competent/ signature
	Date/sign 1	Date/sign 2	Date/sign 3	Date/sign 4	Date/sign 5	
Recording a standard 12-lead ECG						
13 Waited 10 s for patient to settle and tracing to stabilise						
14 Pressed auto button and monitored tracing – ensure working correctly						
15 Confirmed ECG machine working and settings correct during procedure						
16 If problem with recording, checked and corrected problem						
17 Reassured patient during procedure						
18 Acted on concerns, if any, to appropriate person						
19 Checked final recording acceptable quality, then documented required information on paper recording						
20 Switched off machine						
21 Helped patient clean skin and dress, as necessary						
22 Explained next steps to patient						
23 Washed hands						
24 Machine removed and restocked, stored correctly						
25 Procedure reported to designated doctor or senior nurse – check local policy and document as required						

Supervisors/Assessor(s):

Self-assessment		
Assessment	**Aspects**	**Achieved ✓**
Patient	*Have you considered all aspects of this section?*	
	Patient assessment	
	Selection for lead and electrode placements	
	Communication and educational factors	
	Infection control and skin preparation aspects	
	Positioning patient and equipment	
Equipment	*Have you considered all aspects of this section?*	**Achieved ✓**
	Care of the equipment	
	Storage and maintenance of equipment	
Procedure	*Have you considered all aspects of this section?*	**Achieved ✓**
	Equipment and technique	
	Consent, communication and education	
	Problem solving	
	Recording	
	Reporting concerns and procedure completion	

References

Bayés de Luna A (2008) *Basic Electrocardiography: Normal and Abnormal ECG Patterns.* Oxford. John Wiley & Sons.

Crawford J and Doherty L (2012) *Practical Aspects of ECG Recording.* Keswick: M&K Update Ltd.

Dougherty L and Lister S (eds) (2011) *The Royal Marsden Hospital Manual of Clinical Nursing Procedures,* 8th edn. Oxford: Wiley-Blackwell.

Hampton J R (2006) *The ECG in Practice,* 4th edn. Edinburgh: Churchill Livingstone.

Hampton J R and Adlam D (2013) *The ECG in Practice,* 6th edn. Edinburgh: Churchill Livingstone.

Hand H (2002) Common cardiac arrhythmias. *Nursing Standard* 16(28): 43–53.

Henderson H (1997) Electrocardiography. *Nursing Standard* 11(44): 45–56.

McChance K and Heuther S (2014) *The Pathophysiology: The Biologic Basis for Disease in Adults and Children,* 7th edn. London: Elsevier.

NHS Lothian (2004) *Recording a Standard 12-lead ECG NHS Lothian – University Hospitals Division.* Edinburgh: NHS Lothian.

Peate I and Wild K (2012) Taking ECGs: being skilled, competent and confident. *British Journal of Healthcare Assistants* 6(7): 328.

Society for Cardiological Science and Technology (SCST) (2014) Clinical Guidelines by Consensus. *Recording a 12-lead Standard ECG. An Approved Methodology by the Society for Cardiological Science and Technology Guidance.* London: Society for Cardiological Science and Technology.

Stevens N (2008) 12-lead ECG recording. *Practice Nurse* 36(9): 1.

Taylor Industries Inc. (2015) Electrode Reference Guide Taylor Industries. http://www.taylor-ind.com/.

Tortora G J and Derrickson B (2011) *Principles of Anatomy and Physiology,* 13th edn. Hoboken, NJ: Wiley & Sons.

Tough J (2004) Assessment and treatment of chest pain. *Nursing Standard* 18(37): 45.

Wild K and Peate I (2012) Clinical observations 2/6: assessing the pulse rate. *British Journal of Healthcare Assistants* 6(6): 274–278.

Index

Page numbers in *italic* type indicate figures; those in **bold** indicate tables or boxes.

Clinical Skills for Healthcare Assistants and Assistant Practitioners, Second Edition.
Angela Whelan and Elaine Hughes.
© 2016 John Wiley & Sons, Ltd. Published 2016 by John Wiley & Sons, Ltd.